ANXIETY DISORDERS IN
CHILDREN AND ADOLESCENTS

Anxiety Disorders in Children and Adolescents

Second Edition

Edited by

TRACY L. MORRIS
JOHN S. MARCH

THE GUILFORD PRESS
New York   London

© 2004 The Guilford Press
A Division of Guilford Publications, Inc.
72 Spring Street, New York, NY 10012
www.guilford.com

Printed in the United States of America

This book is printed on acid-free paper.

Last digit is print number: 9   8   7   6   5   4   3   2   1

Library of Congress Cataloging-in-Publication Data

Anxiety disorders in children and adolescents / edited by Tracy L.
Morris, John S. March.—2nd ed.
      p. cm.
Includes bibliographical references and index.
  ISBN 1-57230-981-4 (hbk. : alk. paper)
  1. Anxiety in children. 2. Anxiety in adolescence. I. Morris, Tracy
L. II. March, John S., MD.
  RJ506.A58A58 2004
  618.92′8522—dc22

                                              2003017062

To Boris M. Kieslowski, teacher extraordinaire.
—T. L. M.

To my Dad, Ralph March,
who first introduced me to the joys of science.
—J. S. M.

About the Editors

Tracy L. Morris, PhD, is Associate Professor of Psychology at West Virginia University (WVU). She received BS and MS degrees in psychology from Pittsburg State University (Kansas) and a PhD in clinical psychology from the University of Mississippi. Dr. Morris completed a clinical internship and postdoctoral fellowship at the Medical University of South Carolina specializing in child clinical psychology prior to joining the faculty at WVU. Currently she serves as Associate Chair of the department, as well as coordinator of the doctoral program in child clinical psychology. Dr. Morris's primary research focus is on the developmental psychopathology of anxiety disorders, with a special interest in the etiology, assessment, and treatment of shyness and social anxiety.

John S. March, MD, MPH, is Professor of Psychiatry and Chief of Child and Adolescent Psychiatry at Duke University Medical Center. He received a BA from the University of California at Riverside and an MS in molecular biology from the University of California at Berkeley. He obtained an MD-MPH (epidemiology) from the UCLA School of Medicine, and later completed a residency in family practice at that institution. Following several years as a family practitioner in rural Montana, Dr. March trained in general and child and adolescent psychiatry in the Department of Psychiatry, University of Wisconsin–Madison. He has extensive experience developing and testing the efficacy and effectiveness of cognitive-behavioral and pharmacological treatments for pediatric mental disorders and is widely published in the areas of obsessive–compulsive disorder, posttraumatic stress disorder, anxiety, depression, attention-deficit/hyperactivity disorder, and pediatric psychopharmacology.

Contributors

Paula M. Barrett, PhD, School of Applied Psychology, Griffith University, Mount Gravatt, Australia

Deborah C. Beidel, PhD, ABPP, Maryland Center for Anxiety Disorders, University of Maryland, College Park, Maryland

Joseph Biederman, MD, Pediatric Psychopharmacology Research Program, Massachusetts General Hospital, Cambridge, Massachusetts

Boris Birmaher, MD, Department of Psychiatry, University of Pittsburgh School of Medicine, Pittsburgh, Pennsylvania

Scott N. Compton, PhD, Department of Psychiatry and Program in Child and Adolescent Anxiety Disorders, Duke University Medical Center, Durham, North Carolina

Kristen Schoff D'Eramo, PhD, The Bradley School, East Providence, Rhode Island

Andreas Dick-Niederhauser, PhD, Child Anxiety and Phobia Program, Florida International University, Miami, Florida

Sara P. Dow, MD, private practice, Seattle, Washington

Thalia C. Eley, PhD, Social, Genetics, and Developmental Research Center, Institute of Psychiatry, King's College London, London, United Kingdom

Ellen C. Flannery-Schroeder, PhD, Department of Social Sciences, University of the Sciences in Philadelphia, Philadelphia, Pennsylvania

Edna B. Foa, PhD, Center for the Treatment and Study of Anxiety, University of Pennsylvania, Philadelphia, Pennsylvania

Greta Francis, PhD, The Bradley School, East Providence, Rhode Island

Martin E. Franklin, PhD, Center for the Treatment and Study of Anxiety, University of Pennsylvania, Philadelphia, Pennsylvania

Jennifer B. Freeman, PhD, Department of Child and Family Psychology, Rhode Island Hospital, Providence, Rhode Island

Abbe M. Garcia, PhD, Department of Child and Family Psychology, Rhode Island Hospital, Providence, Rhode Island

Laurie A. Greco, PhD, Division of Adolescent Medicine and Behavioral Science, Vanderbilt University Medical Center, Nashville, Tennessee

Alice M. Gregory, BA, Social, Genetics, and Developmental Research Center, Institute of Psychiatry, King's College London, London, United Kingdom

Dina R. Hirshfeld-Becker, PhD, Pediatric Psychopharmacology Research Program, Massachusetts General Hospital, Cambridge, Massachusetts

Neville J. King, PhD, Faculty of Education, Monash University, Victoria, Australia

Henrietta L. Leonard, PhD, Department of Child and Family Psychology, Rhode Island Hospital, Providence, Rhode Island

John S. March, PhD, Department of Psychology, Duke University Medical Center, Durham, North Carolina

Sara G. Mattis, PhD, Department of Psychology, Boston University, Boston, Massachusetts

Catherine D. McKnight, BS, Department of Psychology–Social and Health Sciences and Program in Child and Adolescent Anxiety Disorders, Duke University Medical Center, Durham, North Carolina

Lauren M. Miller, BA, Department of Psychology, Virginia Commonwealth University, Richmond, Virginia

Tracy L. Morris, PhD, Department of Psychology, West Virginia University, Morgantown, West Virginia

Peter Muris, PhD, Department of Medical, Clinical, and Experimental Psychology, Maastricht University, Maastricht, The Netherlands

Thomas H. Ollendick, PhD, Department of Psychology, Virginia Polytechnic Institute, Blacksburg, Virginia

Daniel S. Pine, MD, Mood and Anxiety Disorder Program, National Institute of Mental Health, Bethesda, Maryland

Jerrold F. Rosenbaum, MD, Department of Clinical Psychopharmacology, Massachusetts General Hospital, Cambridge, Massachusetts

Soraya Seedat, MB, ChB, FCPsych, Medical Research Council Unit on Anxiety and Stress Disorders, Department of Psychiatry, University of Stellenbosch, Cape Town, South Africa

Wendy K. Silverman, PhD, Department of Psychology, Florida International University, Miami, Florida

Murray B. Stein, MD, Department of Psychiatry, University of California at San Diego, La Jolla, California

Cynthia M. Turner, PhD, School of Applied Psychology, Griffith University, Mount Gravatt, Australia

Marquette W. Turner, PhD, Counseling Center, Morgan State University, Baltimore, Maryland

Roma A. Vasa, MD, Neurobehavior Unit, Kennedy Krieger Institute, Johns Hopkins School of Medicine, Baltimore, Maryland

Preface

Anxiety disorders in children and adolescents are common and, left untreated, cause considerable suffering. Fortunately, the past decade has seen considerable progress in the diagnosis and treatment of anxious youth. Now in its second edition, this book is designed to help clinicians from a variety of disciplines learn about the etiology, assessment, and treatment of children and adolescents with anxiety disorders.

The book is organized in three parts. In Part I, *Foundations*, we set out a framework for the later chapters on specific phobic and anxiety disorders by providing a broad and integrative view of issues that affect the psychopathology, assessment, and treatment of the various childhood anxiety disorders. Specific chapters cover neurobiology, behavioral inhibition, social development, behavioral genetics, and assessment.

In Part II, *Disorders*, we focus on the DSM-IV anxiety disorders themselves. Each chapter includes sections on clinical manifestation or phenomenology of the disorder, diagnosis and classification (including differential diagnosis and comorbidity), and developmental course of the disorder, before turning to evidence-based treatments for the disorder(s) in question.

In Part III, *Treatment*, we take a broader view of the treatment landscape, with the aim of blending treatments that cross disorders and comorbidities. Specific topics covered in this section include cognitive-behavioral psychotherapy, pharmacotherapy, and, importantly, combining treatment in an evidence-based fashion. The final chapter, on prevention, is a new addition to this volume and encompasses the considerable strides that have been made in this regard and our general philosophy concerning the merits of early intervention in enhancing the quality of life for children at risk for disorder.

In editing this book, we were fortunate to have as collaborators an outstanding group of psychologists and psychiatrists who are expert in their respective areas. Much if not most of what is known arises from work conducted by these pioneering scientists and their students. We are grateful to them for conveying their accumulated wisdom, which highlights the extraordinary progress made in pediatric anxiety disorders over the past 10–15 years.

Most of all, we owe a special debt of gratitude to the many patients and their families who have taught us so much about anxiety disorders in young people. With so much of mental health care still driven by poorly standardized assessments and ineffectual and unproven treatments, it seems to us that our patients and their parents frequently are ahead of the practitioner community in their understanding of mental illness and its treatment. Their resolve in the face of anxiety and their willingness to work with us to find the answers they need have been and remain professionally rewarding and personally inspiring.

We of course could not do this work without support of family and friends. I (TLM) want to thank my friend Joe for his unwavering support and patient ear through trials large and small. His depth of understanding and creativity of mind have enriched my life in more ways than can be expressed. I (JSM) want to thank my wife, Kathleen, and my children, Matthew and Maggie, for their indulgence as we put this volume together. Their love and support make possible the varied tasks of academic life. Because research is a collaborative endeavor, we also thank the members of our research groups, without whom our own small scientific contributions would soon founder.

Finally, as in most areas of psychiatry and psychology, controversy thrives. This book, while bursting with new information, may not do justice to the edge of the field nor will the reader agree with everything we say. The errors of fact are ours; the controversies will eventually yield to good science. Our goal in producing this text is to help children and adolescents with anxiety disorders lead more normal, happy, and productive lives. We hope we have achieved this goal.

Contents

I. FOUNDATIONS

II. DISORDERS

III. TREATMENT

ANXIETY DISORDERS IN
CHILDREN AND ADOLESCENTS

Part I

FOUNDATIONS

Chapter 1

Neurobiology

ROMA A. VASA
DANIEL S. PINE

Pediatric anxiety disorders are among the most prevalent forms of childhood psychopathology, affecting approximately 20% of children and adolescents at some point in their lives (Shaffer et al., 1995; Verhulst, van der Ende, Ferdinand, & Kasius, 1997). Although prior research indicates that these anxiety disorders are often transient (Last, Perrin, Hersen, & Kazdin, 1996; Pine, Cohen, Gurley, Brook, & Ma, 1998), recent studies suggest that some children may have anxiety disorders that persist into adulthood (Alpert, Maddocks, Rosenbaum, & Fava, 1994; Costello & Angold, 1995; Ferdinand & Verhulst, 1995; Manfro et al., 1996; Newman et al., 1996; Pine et al., 1998; Pollack et al., 1996; Schneier, Johnson, Hornig, Liebowitz, & Weissman, 1992). Because adult anxiety disorders are often associated with serious and debilitating comorbid conditions such as substance abuse disorders, depression, and suicidality (Achenbach, Howell, McConaughy, & Stangor, 1995; Ferdinand & Verhulst, 1995; Klein, 1995; Pine et al., 1998), there is an imperative to identify risk characteristics that predispose certain children to chronic anxiety. Investigating the neural underpinnings of anxiety disorders may identify this subset of children who face a particularly high risk for long-term morbidity.

Prior reviews on the neurobiology of pediatric anxiety disorders have focused on results from a wide spectrum of studies comparing behavioral, physiological, cognitive, and neuroimaging variables between anxious and control participants (for reviews of these studies, see Pine et al., 1999, 2000; Sallee & Greenawald, 1995). This chapter

3

explores the pathophysiology of these conditions through the lens of a relatively new research perspective, the field of affective neuroscience. Affective neuroscience research integrates information from clinical psychiatry, cognitive psychology, and neuroscience to elucidate the neural circuitry involved in the experience and expression of emotion (Pine & Grun, 1999). With regard to anxiety, some of this research considers the relevance of animal models to normal anxiety states in humans. Understanding the neural mechanisms that mediate normal fear and anxiety subsequently may allow researchers to postulate etiological models regarding pathological anxiety, as dysregulation of emotion represents a basic aspect of many psychiatric disorders (Davidson, Putnam, & Larson, 2000).

This chapter describes the central principles of affective neuroscience research and considers the relationship between two areas of research: fear conditioning and information processing, and the development of normal and pathological anxiety. Neurobiological data from adult and child studies are reported based on the underlying premise that there may be continuity in the neural pathways that mediate child and adult anxiety syndromes.

A HIERARCHY OF PATHOPHYSIOLOGICAL FACTORS

Although the past decade has witnessed an explosion of adult studies that investigate the neuroanatomy of anxiety and other emotional disorders, few studies examine the neurobiological underpinnings of these conditions in children. One major obstacle to such research, in both children and adults, is phenotypic heterogeneity, a phenomenon that exists both within and across specific diagnostic categories (Merikangas, Avenevoli, Dierker, & Grillon, 1999). Perhaps the strongest data on phenotypic heterogeneity derive from studies demonstrating high rates of comorbidity and strong diagnostic overlap among anxiety disorders (Gurley, Cohen, Pine, & Brook, 1996). From a nosological perspective, these data illustrate the problems confronting efforts to establish diagnostic specificity and demonstrate the need for research that identifies more precise phenotypes. Defining homogeneous phenotypes can facilitate the development of neurobiological models regarding the etiology of these disorders.

One approach to understanding the origins of phenotypic heterogeneity involves a focus on specific biological profiles such as physiological, cognitive, neurohormonal, neuroanatomical, or neurophysiological measures. These measures, collectively termed "biomarkers," may be more readily linked to the underlying pathophysiology and genetic etiology of anxiety (Pearlson, 2000). Enhanced understanding of the relationships between biomarkers and anxiety disorders could clarify the degree to which phenomenologically distinct DSM-IV anxiety disorders are related on the basis of underlying neurocircuitry. These markers may ultimately serve as an invaluable tool to identify at-risk children.

Consistent with this approach, factors contributing to the pathophysiology of anxiety disorders can be conceptualized along a hierarchy, which extends from overt clinical symptoms to the underlying neural substrata (Figure 1.1). Symptoms of DSM-IV anxiety disorders are hypothesized to represent clinical expressions of broad behavioral tendencies, such as temperament types (e.g., behavioral inhibition), or abnormal reactions to motivational stimuli and stress. These behavioral tendencies may reflect functions in more elementary behavioral, physiological, or cognitive operations, which are subserved by functional activity in various neural systems. Research on the neural contributions to various cognitive and physiological operations suggests that these functions are subserved by networks of neural structures distributed throughout the brain rather than in one or more particular brain regions. As an example of this hierarchical approach, Kagan, Reznick, and Snidman (1987) demonstrated associations between physiological variables (e.g., increased heart rate and increased blood pressure) that are regulated by select neural networks and behavioral inhibition, which is viewed as a broad behavioral disposition or temperament type. Biederman and colleagues (2001), in turn, demonstrated a link between behavioral inhibition and social anxiety disorder.

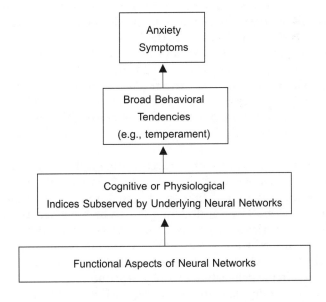

FIGURE 1.1. Heirarchy of pathophysiological factors underlying anxiety disorders.

Efforts to understand the neural mechanisms mediating anxiety can therefore be divided into two parts: identification of the cognitive or physiological operations that distinguish anxious from nonanxious children and delineation of the neural circuits underlying each of these operations (Reiman, 1988). The development of functional magnetic resonance imaging (fMRI) has provided an ideal opportunity to examine associations between brain activity and a broad range of cognitive and physiological parameters. The majority of fMRI studies have examined the neural correlates of anxiety in adults; research that identifies these same correlates in children may provide evidence linking childhood and adult anxiety syndromes.

AFFECTIVE NEUROSCIENCE PERSPECTIVE

The field of affective neuroscience shares similar aims with prior neurobiological research in its search for cognitive and physiological correlates of anxiety. Theoretically, however, this perspective uniquely differs because it uses information from animal models of emotion to generate hypotheses regarding the neuroanatomy of emotions in humans. This approach is based on the premise that humans and lower animals share a common set of neural circuits involved in emotion regulation (Panksepp, 1998). With regard to the specific emotion of fear, this premise implies that the neural systems involved in detecting danger and producing defensive responses are similarly organized across all species (LeDoux, 1995, 1998); that is, considerable behavioral, physiological, and anatomical data note cross-species parallels in the regulation of fear-related behavior. As a result, laboratory-based behavioral observations provide an excellent forum in which the precise relationships between changes in neuronal activity and corresponding changes in complex behaviors can be observed. These models can ultimately be extrapolated to the realm of normal and pathological anxiety in humans.

Although an abundance of research exists on the neural basis of fear and other emotions, much of this work has been fraught with significant controversy regarding the definition of emotion (see reviews in LeDoux, 1993, 1995, 2000b). Historically, emotion has been defined as a subjective psychological experience originally thought to be mediated by the "primitive" architecture that forms the limbic system. In recent years, however, this model has been challenged both anatomically and theoretically because of imprecision in the delineation of limbic structures and in the mechanisms responsible for producing emotions (LeDoux, 1993, 1998, 2000a, 2000b). More recent theorists define emotion empirically (LeDoux, 1993, 2000b). For example, Rolls (1999) conceptualizes emotions as a family of brain states elicited by stimuli with reinforcing properties, either rewards or punishments; the terms "reward" and "punishment" refer respectively to positive or negative stimuli that an organism will expend effort to obtain or avoid. Specifying goals rather than particular behavioral patterns of responses broadens the definition of emotion to include a variety of behavioral strategies that can manifest in response to a given stimulus (Rolls, 2000). According to this definition, fear and anxiety are defined as brain states associated with punishment.

As noted, fear represents an ideal emotion for affective neuroscience research because of cross-species similarities in the physiology of this emotion. This facilitates comparability of experimental procedures for eliciting and measuring fear in humans and experimental animals (LeDoux, 1995). The next two sections review human and animal research on the relationships between the presentation of threatening stimuli and two psychological processes: fear conditioning and information processing. As the ultimate goal of affective neuroscience research is to link behavior to brain function, both sections emphasize the potential utility of fMRI to correlate these psychological processes with brain function.

FEAR CONDITIONING MODELS

Fear Conditioning

Fear conditioning is a form of classical or associative learning that involves linkage between a neutral stimulus and an aversive stimulus. In a fear-conditioning experiment, a neutral stimulus, such as a light or a tone, serves as the conditioned stimulus (CS). This stimulus is paired with an unconditioned stimulus (UCS), such as a shock or a loud noise. After one or more pairings, the CS acquires the capacity to elicit a repertoire of behavioral, autonomic, and endocrine responses that typically appear in response to the UCS (LeDoux, 2000a). Although the pairing of CS and UCS is learned, the responses are not learned but rather species-typical responses to threat that are automatically activated when confronting dangerous stimuli (LeDoux, 2000a). The brain state associated with the response to the CS is labeled "cue-specific" fear (LeDoux, 1995). In addition, when a CS is paired with a UCS, the organism also develops a fear-related response to the background or contextual stimuli in which the CS was presented, a process known as contextual conditioning (LeDoux, 1995).

Enthusiasm for efforts to extend fear conditioning research to clinical anxiety disorders results from at least two sets of findings (Gorman, Kent, Sullivan, & Coplan, 2000). First, fear conditioning in animals and clinical fear states in humans are both characterized by similar response patterns, that is, avoidance behavior, changes in vigilance and autonomic regulation, and a decrease in hedonic activity. Second, lesions of the amygdala, a paramount structure in the fear conditioning process, produces deficits in fear conditioning and related processes in both animals and humans (Bechara et al., 1995; Davis, 1998; LaBar, LeDoux, Spencer, & Phelps, 1995; LeDoux, 1995, 1998).

Some efforts to apply fear conditioning models in animals to human anxiety disorders treat threatening stimuli or situations as representative of the UCS; for example, considerable research, reviewed later, uses emotional facial expressions as stimuli to compare responses between healthy and anxious subjects. Support for this approach is derived from neuroscience perspectives that demonstrate that the presentation of emotionally valent stimuli results in activation of motivational networks in the brain, which leads to the organization of visceral and behavioral responses (Lang, Bradley, & Cuthbert, 1998). Data from adult and child studies demonstrate that patients with select anxiety disorders exhibit enhanced subjective, as well as physiological, responses to a standard set of mildly threatening stimuli or situations (UCS; Barlow, 2002; Birbaumer et al., 1998; Lang et al., 1998; Pine et al., 2000). Because fear conditioning is influenced by the magnitude of the response to the UCS, it is unclear whether heightened responses to the UCS are related to particular aspects of the anxiety disorder that follow from conditioning associated with UCS presentation or to factors associated with the differential response to the UCS independent of the CS. These considerations may account for possible similarities and differences across anxiety disorders.

At least three additional factors also need to be considered when examining the association between anxiety disorders and heightened susceptibility to provocation by a UCS. First, specificity of the response to the UCS needs to be empirically established. For example, although data from adult studies demonstrate that social anxiety disorder is associated with heightened response to both complex evaluative social situations and relatively simple stereotyped facial displays of emotion (Birbaumer et al. 1998; Davidson, Marchall, Tomarken, & Henriques, 2000; Lundh & Ost, 1996), more detailed studies are needed to determine the precise aspects of face processing that may be unique to this disorder. Second, state versus trait factors may play an important role in the abnormal response to anxiety-provoking situations, as prior studies demonstrate that acute emotional states can exert robust effects on various psychological processes (Barlow, 2002; Cahill, 1999; Daleiden & Vasey, 1997; Lang et al., 1998). Third, responses to the UCS may be complex, consisting of a combination of autonomic, cognitive, and neurophysiological measures that are all mediated by distinct brain circuits (Davis, 1998). For example, patients with social anxiety disorder demonstrate increased heart rate and increased right-sided cortical activation in the anterior temporal and prefrontal regions during states of high social anxiety (Davidson, Marchall, et al., 2000).

Despite interest in fear conditioning research, the precise role played by fear conditioning in certain types of human anxiety disorders remains unclear. For example, although fear conditioning models may be applicable to the neural mechanisms that underlie some anxiety disorders, such as simple phobia (Pine & Grun, 1999), other types of anxiety, such as fear of failure or fear of authority, are difficult to simulate in the laboratory setting. In addition, although amygdalar lesions impair fear conditioning in animals and humans, these lesions typically do not produce marked changes in clinical components of anxiety (Davis, 1998). Cue-specific fear conditioning also appears normal in many individuals with anxiety disorders (Merikangas et al., 1999). Similarly, inconsistencies emerge in the effects of pharmacological agents on fear conditioning in rodents as opposed to anxiety disorders in humans (Cassella & Davis, 1985). Two possible underlying processes may account for these inconsistencies. First, fear conditioning may confer risk for anxiety or broad dispositional tendencies, as opposed to clinical disorders, as suggested by some data that report enhanced fear conditioning processes in children at risk for anxiety disorders (Merikangas et al., 1999). Second, other processes associated with fear conditioning, such as contextual conditioning, may relate more closely to anxiety disorders than to fear conditioning per se. For example, the ability to proficiently distinguish dangerous stimuli or situations from similar but harmless situations (a bear in the woods vs. in the zoo) may be impaired in anxious individuals (Crestani et al., 1999; LeDoux, 1995).

Neural Substrates Involved in Fear Conditioning

Brain circuits that mediate fear conditioning in animals have been delineated at both the anatomical and molecular levels (Crestani et al., 1999; Squire & Kandel, 1999). Fear conditioning involves changes in neural pathways that correspond to changes in an organism's response (CR) to a previously innocuous stimulus (CS). Lesion-deficit studies in animals and humans provide converging evidence demonstrating that the amygdala plays a critical role in the fear conditioning process (Bechara et al., 1995; Davis, 1998; LaBar et al., 1995; LeDoux, 1998).

The amygdala is a complex structure that is composed of multiple nuclei that subserve various functions, one of which includes evaluating and responding to potentially threatening stimuli (LeDoux, 1992, 1998). Situated within the temporal lobe, the amygdala is anatomically well placed to integrate sensory inputs from the cortex, the thalamus, and the hippocampus and to project efferent connections to the hypothalamus, the brain stem, and the cortex; these different brain regions are involved in the behavioral and cognitive aspects of the fear response (Davis, 2000; LeDoux, 1995, 2000a, 2000b). In fear conditioning, it is hypothesized that amygdalar activation results in changes in connecting brain structures, which leads to expression of a complex behavioral response (Davis, 2000; LeDoux 1995, 2000a, 2000b). At the molecular level, conditioning may be mediated by an N-methyl-D-aspartate (NMDA)-dependent long-term potentiation (LTP)-like phenomenon within the amygdala (LeDoux, 1992, 1993, 1995, 2000a; Rogan & LeDoux, 1995).

During the past decade, the development of functional neuroimaging techniques, particularly fMRI, has allowed researchers to directly visualize activity in the intact human amygdala during fear conditioning or presentation of a UCS. With regard to fear conditioning in adults, many fMRI studies in normal and clinically anxious participants examine brain regions engaged during fear conditioning experiments using a variety of conditioned and unconditioned stimuli; the effects of fear conditioning are measured by comparing the neuronal and physiological responses to presentation of conditioned and unconditioned stimuli (Buchel & Dolan, 2000). Most of these studies document activation of similar brain regions implicated in animal models of fear conditioning, that is, the amygdala, the hippocampus, and associated cortical regions, such as the ventral prefrontal cortex (Buchel & Dolan, 2000; Buchel, Dolan, Armony, & Friston, 1999; LaBar, Gatenby, Gore, LeDoux, & Phelps, 1998; Schneider et al., 1999).

In addition to fear conditioning, the amygdala is involved in the processing of innately evocative stimuli, particularly fearful facial expressions. As a result, facial stimuli are often used as examples of UCS in fear conditioning research. Amygdala engagement during facial recognition of emotion was originally documented through animal electrophysiological studies that showed that the amygdala contains neurons that respond selectively to faces (Leonard, Rolls, Wilson, & Baylis, 1985; Rolls, 1984) and through human lesion-deficit studies (Adolphs, Tranel, Damasio, & Damasio, 1994; Young, Hellawell, Van De Wal, & Johnson, 1996) that demonstrated relationships between amygdalar damage and impaired fear recognition. More recently, fMRI studies investigated the role of the amygdala in face processing using paradigms that compare neural activity in response to neutral, happy, or fearful facial expressions. Consistent with data from lesion-deficit studies, these studies demonstrate preferential activation of the amygdala and related structures in response to fearful versus neutral or happy faces in normal participants (Breiter et al., 1996; Morris et al., 1996; Whalen et al., 1998). Some of these studies also report neuroanatomical specificity across various emotional facial displays, that is, the amygdala appears particularly sensitive to fearful expressions, whereas the striatum and insula appear sensitive to disgust and the ventral prefrontal regions appear sensitive to anger (Breiter et al., 1996; Phillips et al., 1999; Whalen et al., 1998).

Although extensive fMRI data in adults implicate the amgydala in fear conditioning and face-emotion processing, minimal research examines the role of this structure in normal and anxious children. With regard to fear conditioning research, Merikangas and colleagues (1999) report some evidence of abnormal fear-conditioning processes in children at risk for anxiety disorders, though some consistencies emerge across studies, genders, and age groups. With regard to research on face-emotion processing, Thomas, Drevets, Dahl, and colleagues (2001) found a relationship between amygdalar engagement and anxiety ratings in children with anxiety disorders.

In healthy children, four studies report on the relationship between amygdalar activation and face-emotion viewing. Baird and colleagues (1999) demonstrated amygdalar activation during recognition of fearful faces, suggesting that the amygdala may play a role in affect recognition prior to adulthood. Killgore, Oki, and Yurgelun-Todd (2001) similarly note engagement of the amygdala to fearful faces, as well as developmental changes in the amygdala and prefrontal cortex during face viewing. In contrast, Thomas, Drevets, Whalen, and colleagues (2001) document differences in amygdalar activity between healthy children and adults, with children exhibiting greater responses to neutral as opposed to fearful faces. Similarly, Pine and colleagues (2001) failed to engage the amygdala in either healthy adolescents or adults using a masked-face task, but they did report enhanced activation in the association cortex among adolescents, suggesting that emotional faces may provide more salient stimuli for adolescents than for adults. Taken together, these data, although conflicting, provide a prelude to future research investigating the neurobiological and developmental aspects of fear conditioning and face processing in children, specifically as it relates to the pathophysiology of anxiety disorders.

Summary

A continuum may exist between fear conditioning in animals and humans based on two broad conclusions that can be gleaned from the literature. First, adults and children with anxiety disorders exhibit enhanced subjective and physiological reactivity in response to presentation of threatening stimuli. Second, considerable fMRI data in adults and, to some extent, in children demonstrate a relationship between fear elicitation and amygdalar activation. Although much work remains in terms of understanding how fear conditioning models can be correlated with anxiety disorders, mounting evidence supports a role for this construct in understanding the patho-physiology of these conditions.

INFORMATION-PROCESSING MODELS

According to cognitive-behavioral conceptualizations, anxiety disorders originate from distorted beliefs about the dangerousness of certain stimuli or situations (Clark, 1999; Mogg & Bradley, 1998). These beliefs are thought to stem from biases that occur when information is manipulated and modified as it progresses through the cognitive system (Daleiden & Vasey, 1997). The majority of information-processing studies consider the effect that potentially dangerous stimuli exert on two cognitive functions, attention and memory (Mogg & Bradley, 1998). In adults, most of these studies report a relationship between clinical anxiety and attentional and mnemonic biases that favors the processing of threatening information. Although the relationship between anxiety and these cognitive processes is considered bidirectional, direct evidence of an etiological role remains sparse.

Extrapolation of information-processing theories to childhood anxiety has only begun to emerge. Applying an information-processing perspective to the pathophysiology of childhood anxiety carries significant implications for assessment and treatment. For example, identifying the source of deficient and distorted cognitive processes that characterize anxious children may lead to the development of performance-based measures of anxiety that would complement the existing self-report measures (Daleiden & Vasey, 1997). This, in turn, may lead to more focused treatments that promote cognitive changes in anxious children.

Attention

The ability to rapidly allocate attention to threatening stimuli represents a critical component of fear states (McNally, 1996). Considerable research with adults and children demonstrates an attentional bias favoring the selective processing of threat cues in clinical anxiety. In adults, numerous studies reveal such biases using two sets of attention paradigms, the "emotional Stroop" and the "dot probe" tasks (Bradley, Mogg, Millar, & White, 1995; Bradley, Mogg, White, Groom, & deBono, 1999; Bradley, Mogg, & Williams, 1995; McNally, 1996; Mogg & Bradley, 1998, 1999; Williams, Mathews, & MacLeod, 1996). The results of these studies show that attention is selectively shifted toward threat in patients and away from threat stimuli in healthy participants. Interestingly, depression is also associated with an attentional bias, though the temporal characteristics of this bias differ from those in anxious participants (Bradley, Mogg, Millar, & White, 1995; Williams et al., 1996).

In the emotional Stroop test, anxious participants are shown emotionally valent words printed in different colors. Participants are asked to name the color of the word while ignoring the word meaning (Mathews & MacLeod, 1985; McNally, 1996). Color-naming delay occurs when the word's meaning interferes with the person's ability to attend to the word's color (McNally, 1996). Attentional biases are measured when anxious participants show increased color-naming delay in response to threatening words in comparison with neutral words (Mathews & MacLeod, 1985; Mogg & Bradley, 1998). Using the emotional Stroop test, attentional biases can be revealed for every type of anxiety disorder (McNally, 1996)—for example, simple animal phobia (Watts, McKenna, Sharrock, & Trezise, 1986), social phobia (Hope, Rapee, Heimberg, & Dombeck, 1990; Mattia, Heimberg, & Hope, 1993), obsessive–compulsive disorder (Foa, Ilai, McCarthy, Shoyer, & Murdock, 1993), panic disorder (Ehlers, Margraf, Davies, & Roth, 1988; McNally, Reimann, & Kim, 1990), posttraumatic stress disorder (McNally, Kaspi, Reimann, & Zeitlin, 1990) and generalized anxiety disorder (Mathews & MacLeod, 1985). To a degree, these studies also report some degree of content specificity in underlying effects; that is, the closer a word relates to the patient's focus of anxiety, the greater the likelihood is that it will result in color-naming latency (e.g., social phobics are more likely to demonstrate latency for social threat words such as "stupid" than for physical threat words such as "fatal"; McNally, 1996).

The dot-probe task provides a more direct measure of visual attention allocation than the Stroop paradigm. In this paradigm, a pair of words, one threatening and one neutral, are briefly (500 ms) presented on a computer screen, after which one of the words immediately disappears and is replaced by a dot; participants are required to respond as quickly as possible to the dot probe by pressing a computer button. The effects of threatening stimuli on attention are inferred from measuring reaction times to various stimuli. Participants with generalized anxiety disorder respond more quickly to dot probes that replace threat words than neutral words, relative to depressed and normal controls (MacLeod, Mathews, & Tata; Mogg & Bradley, 1998; Mogg, Mathews, & Eysenck, 1992). In contrast to these findings, some data indicate that participants with high social anxiety demonstrate an attentional bias away from threat cues (Clark, 1999). From a clinical perspective, these findings conform to a model of social phobia that proposes that avoiding eye contact and looking away from other's faces may provide a psychological escape by reducing threat associated with these stimuli (Clark & Wells, 1995).

Accumulating evidence demonstrates attentional biases in anxious children using both the dot-probe and Stroop paradigms (Table 1.1). Consistent with adult data, the majority of these studies report enhanced attentional bias for threat cues in anxious children, suggesting that there may be some link between information-processing abnormalities in anxious children and adults. These data, however, must be interpreted in the context of several limitations, such as the failure of some studies to include the presentation of positively valenced stimuli and interference effects associated with both attentional paradigms. Furthermore, data from several animal studies show that pharmacological and behavioral treatments abolish attentional biases, suggesting that cognitive biases are sensitive indicators of clinical state (McNally, 1996). These limitations underscore the need for further research using more specific attentional probes in clinically anxious children.

Memory

Anxiety disorders are characterized by recurrent intrusive and illogical thoughts related to personal harm. Although the process by which these anxious thoughts are acquired and stored remains unclear, considerable enthusiasm has emerged for the process known as emotional learning or emotional memory (LeDoux, 1993). Emotional memory involves the acquisition, storage, and retrieval of information about the emotional significance of experiences (LeDoux, 1993). Fear conditioning provides one particularly salient example of emotional learning whereby an environmental event (pairing of aversive and neutral stimulus) is transformed into an emotional response (conditioned response). The phenomenology of some anxiety disorders suggests that threatening information may be selectively encoded or more easily recalled. This implies that pathological anxiety states may be associated with a memory bias for threatening information (McNally, 1997).

Emotional memory systems can be probed implicitly or explicitly, with fear conditioning providing one possible example of an implicit memory process. Explicit or declarative memory refers to the ability to consciously recall past experiences, either via free recall, cued recall, or recognition (McNally, 1996). Implicit memory refers to memory that is based on facilitated performance on a behavioral measure or changes in physiology without conscious recollection (McNally, 1996). Besides the considerable work on fear conditioning, most memory research examines explicit rather than implicit memory in adults with a variety of anxiety disorder diagnoses. In general, the majority of these studies document a memory bias for threat in panic disorder (Becker, Rinck, & Margraf, 1994; Cloitre & Liebowitz 1991; Cloitre, Shear, Cancienne, & Zeitlin, 1994). Studies of adult partici-

TABLE 1.1. Attentional Biases Associated with Childhood Anxiety

Study	Task	Age (yr)	Diagnosis	Results
Martin, Horder, & Jones (1992)	Stroop	6–13	Spider fear versus no spider fear	Bias toward spider-relevant words in spider-fear group
Vasey, El-Hag, & Daleiden (1996)	Dot probe	11–14	High versus low test anxiety	Bias toward threat words in high-test-anxious group; bias away from threat material in low-test-anxious group
Vasey, Daleiden, Williams, & Brown (1995)	Dot probe	9–14	Clinically anxious versus healthy controls	Bias toward threat words in clinically anxious group
Kindt, Brosschot, & Everaerd (1997)	Stroop	8–9	High anxious versus low anxious	Bias toward threat in high- and low-anxious groups
Kindt, Bierman, & Brosschot (1997)	Stroop	8–12	Spider fear versus no spider fear	Bias toward spider words in spider-fear and control groups
Moradi, Taghavi, Neshat-Doost, Yule, & Dalgleish (1999)	Stroop	9–17	Posttraumatic stress disorder versus healthy controls	Bias toward trauma-related material in PTSD group
Taghavi, Neshat-Doost, Moradi, Yule, & Dalgleish (1999)	Dot probe	9–18	Clinically anxious versus anxious/depressed versus healthy controls	Bias toward threatening words in clinically anxious group only
Dalgleish, Moradi, Taghavi, Neshat-Doost, & Yule (2001)	Dot probe	9–17	PTSD versus healthy controls	Bias toward socially threatening words in PTSD group

pants with other anxiety disorders (generalized anxiety disorder, social anxiety disorder, specific phobia) find inconsistent associations between clinical anxiety and an enhanced memory for threatening stimuli (Mathews, Mogg, May, & Eysenck, 1989; Mogg & Mathews, 1990; Mogg, Mathews, & Weinman, 1987; Otto, McNally, Pollack, Chen, & Rosenbaum, 1994; Rapee, McCallum, Melville, Ravenscroft, & Rodney, 1994; Watts & Coyle, 1993). Some contend that these conflicting results may be influenced by the type of encoding task, the type of cognitive processing, the particular nature or emotional valence of the stimulus, or state versus trait factors (Becker, Roth, Andrich, & Margraf, 1999; Daleiden, 1998). Interestingly, considerable data supports a robust association between memory biases for negative information in depression (Becker et al., 1999; Bradley, Mogg, Millar, & White, 1995). In fact, more evidence implicates memory biases in depression than in anxiety.

Research on the relationship between anxiety and implicit memory has yielded mixed results. These studies use a word-stem completion paradigm (Mathews et al., 1989) that involves studying words of varying valence (e.g., *coffin*, *charm*) and subsequently asking participants to complete word stems (e.g., *cof*) with the first word that comes to mind; implicit memory is demonstrated when participants complete a greater proportion of stems with previously presented words (e.g., *coffin*) compared to words that were not previously studied (e.g., *coffee*; McNally, 1996). An implicit memory bias occurs if more threat than nonthreat stems are completed (McNally, 1996). Although two studies report implicit memory biases in generalized anxiety disorder (Mathews et al., 1989) and social anxiety disorder (Lundh & Ost, 1996), other studies have failed to replicate these findings (Mathews, Mogg, Kentish, & Eysenck, 1995; Otto et al., 1994; Rapee et al., 1994). These inconsistencies indicate that further research is needed in order to clarify the discrepant memory biases across diagnostic categories, as well as to explain why some disorders are associated with attentional but not memory biases.

At least four studies demonstrate an association between memory deficit and anxiety in children (Table 1.2). Although these studies differ in the neuropsychological paradigms used and in the clinical and demographic characteristics of the samples studied, the data collectively illustrate that a common theme may be emerging to implicate memory abnormalities among children with anxiety. The results of two particular studies are of noteworthy significance. First, Pine, Wasserman, and Workman (1999) demonstrated that mnemonic abnormalities predicted increases in anxiety over time, suggesting a temporal relationship between mnemonic abnormalities and risk for future anxiety. Second, Merikangas and colleagues (1999) reported that a family history of an anxiety disorder predicted mnemonic abnormalities in children, suggesting that cognitive dysfunction may confer risk for anxiety.

Neural Substrates Involved in Attention and Memory

The relationship between cognitive processes and fear is based on the hypothesis that enhanced interactions may exist between the amygdala and

TABLE 1.2. Relationship between Memory and Childhood Anxiety

Study	Memory	Age (yr)	Diagnosis	Results
Daleiden (1998)	Semantic and procedural memory	11–13	High versus low trait anxiety	Memory bias toward threat material in high-trait-anxious group
Merikangas (1999)	Visual and spatial memory	7–17	Family history of anxiety versus no family history	Family history of anxiety predicted mnemonic abnormalities
Pine et al. (1999)	Visual and spatial memory	7–11	Boys at risk for disruptive behavior disorders	Memory abnormalities predicted anxiety at 1 year
Moradi, Doost, Taghavi, Yule, & Dalgleish (1999)	Verbal, visual, visuospatial memory	11–17	PTSD versus no PTSD	Poorer overall memory performance in PTSD group
Toren et al. (2000)	Verbal memory	6–18	Anxiety disorder versus no anxiety disorder	Lower verbal memory scores in anxiety disorder group
Moradi, Taghavi, Neshat-Doost, Yule, & Dalgleish (2000)	Verbal memory	9–17	PTSD versus no PTSD	Poorer overall memory performance and memory bias for negative material in PTSD group

brain networks devoted to cognitive processes. Two neural hypotheses have been proposed to describe the interactions between fear and cognition (LeDoux, 1995). The first hypothesis postulates that amygdalar activation by dangerous stimuli may exert a neuromodulatory effect on cortical and other sensory processing areas, which may subsequently affect a variety of cognitive processes, notably attention or memory (Mogg & Bradley, 1998). For example, amygdalar projections to the nucleus basilis may result in widespread cholinergic modulation of cortical arousal and, hence, regulation of attentional processes (Gallagher, 2000). The second hypothesis postulates that cortical afferents to the amygdala can influence the evaluation of dangerous stimuli, thereby triggering fear reactions (LeDoux, 1995).

Activation of these reciprocal pathways may be enhanced in anxious participants but may of course not be mutually exclusive.

In support of the first hypothesis, brain circuits implicated in attentional conflict or allocation are thought to involve activity in a variety of cortical regions, particularly components of the cingulate gyrus, a region implicated in coordinating and integrating activity in multiple attentional systems (Carter et al., 2000; Peterson et al., 1999). In situations in which there are competing demands on attentional systems, the cingulate may be involved in the weighing of alternative choices for further processing. During such weighing of alternative choices, individuals at risk for anxiety disorders are hypothesized to display a bias for potentially dangerous stimuli. Such bias may manifest as abnormal reaction times during conflict tasks, such as the Stroop, in which existing fMRI studies document the engagement of the anterior cingulate gyrus (Isenberg et al., 1999; Peterson et al., 1999). However, the degree to which engagement of this region varies as a function of performance remains unclear. Given performance differences among patient groups, fMRI studies of such attentional processes may provide an avenue for mapping neural circuits involved in risk for anxiety disorders. Nevertheless, interpretation of between-group differences in brain activation patterns becomes complicated for fMRI tasks in which performance differences exist between groups (Callicott et al., 1998).

As with research on attention, fMRI studies also document involvement of distinct brain circuits in various aspects of memory, that is, encoding, storage, and retrieval. The neural networks mediating emotional memory are stored through both the amygdala and the hippocampus, in contrast to the systems that mediate storage of experiences devoid of emotion, which draw less consistently on the amygdala. With regard to mood and anxiety disorders, considerable research examines the manner in which the emotional content of to-be-remembered material influences recall and brain activation patterns (Blaney, 1986). These data indicate that the brain region that is most clearly implicated in emotional memory is the amygdala. Functional neuroimaging data demonstrate that the emotional content or arousing nature of a stimulus influences the degree to which it is encoded (Cahill et al., 1996) and may be later recalled, with arousing material being more readily recalled than unarousing stimuli (Lang et al., 1998). Prior studies with positron emission tomography (PET) and fMRI suggest that this modulatory effect of arousal may derive from amygdalar influences on hippocampal activity (Cahill, 1999; Cahill et al., 1996). During encoding, both amygdala activity and correlations between amygdala and hippocampal activity may predict the degree to which emotional material will be recalled. Threatening information may also be easily recalled due to chronic partial activation of fear structures, which may decrease the activation threshold at which ongoing processing is influenced (Daleiden, 1998; Foa & Kozak, 1986).

Summary

Information-processing models of anxiety provide another perspective by which researchers can conceptualize the pathophysiology of anxiety disorders. The most compelling data in this field demonstrate associations between anxiety and selective attentional biases toward threatening stimuli. Evidence of memory biases in anxiety is also emerging, especially in children and adolescents. These findings highlight the need to consider cognitive influences in the regulation of anxiety.

CONCLUSIONS

Affective neuroscience research has created new possibilities for investigating the physiology of normal and pathological anxiety. Preliminary evidence demonstrates that some of the behavioral and neural abnormalities in fear conditioning and information processing that have been identified in adults may also be present in children. FMRI may be a useful tool with which to study the developmental neurobiology of anxiety disorders in children because it allows researchers to integrate information from cognitive, behavioral, and biological perspectives.

REFERENCES

Achenbach, T. M., Howell, C. T., McConaughy, S. H., & Stangor, C. (1995). Six-year predictors of problems in a national sample of children and youth: I. Cross-informant syndromes. *Journal of the American Academy of Child and Adolescent Psychiatry, 34,* 336–337.

Adolphs, R., Tranel, D., Damasio, H., & Damasio, A. (1994). Impaired recognition of emotion in facial expressions following bilateral amygdala damage to the human amygdala. *Nature, 372,* 669–672.

Alpert, J. E., Maddocks, A., Rosenbaum, J. F., & Fava, M. (1994). Childhood psychopathology retrospectively assessed among adults with early onset major depression. *Journal of Affective Disorders, 31,* 165–171.

Baird, A. A., Gruber, S. A., Fein, D. A., Maas, L. C., Steingard, R. J., Renshaw, P. F., Cohen, B. M., & Yurgelun-Todd, D. A. (1999). Functional magnetic resonance imaging of facial affect recognition in children and adolescents. *Journal of the American Academy of Child and Adolescent Psychiatry, 38,* 195–199.

Barlow, D. H. (2002). *Anxiety and its disorders: The nature and treatment of anxiety and panic* (2nd ed.). New York: Guilford Press.

Bechara, A., Tranel, D., Damasio, H., Adolphs, R., Rockland, C., & Damasio, A. R. (1995). Double dissociation of conditioning and declarative knowledge relative to the amygdala and hippocampus in humans. *Science, 269,* 1115–1118.

Becker, E., Rinck, M., & Margraf, J. (1994). Memory bias in panic disorder. *Journal of Abnormal Psychology, 103,* 396–399.

Becker, E. S., Roth, W. T., Andrich, M., & Margraf, J. (1999). Explicit memory in anxiety disorders. *Journal of Abnormal Psychology, 108,* 153–163.

Biederman, J., Hirshfeld-Becker, D. R., Rosenbaum, J. F., Herot, C., Friedman, D., Snidman, N., Kagan, J., & Faraone, S. V. (2001). Further evidence of an association between behavioral inhibition and social anxiety in children. *American Journal of Psychiatry, 10,* 1673–1679.

Birbaumer, N., Grodd, W., Diedrich, O., Kose, U., Erb, M., Lotze, M., Scheider, F., Weiss, U., & Flor, H. (1998). fMRI reveals amygdala activation to human faces in social phobia. *NeuroReport, 9,* 1223–1226.

Blaney, P. H. (1986). Affect and memory: A review. *Psychological Bulletin, 99,* 229–246.

Bradley, B. P., Mogg, K., Millar, N., & White, J. (1995). Selective processing of negative information: Effects of clinical anxiety, concurrent depression, and awareness. *Journal of Abnormal Psychology, 104,* 532–536.

Bradley, B. P., Mogg, K., White, J., Groom, C., & deBono, J. (1999). Attentional bias for emotional faces in generalized anxiety disorder. *British Journal of Clinical Psychology, 38,* 267–278.

Bradley, B. P., Mogg, K., & Williams, R. (1995). Implicit and explicit memory for emotion-congruent information in clinical depression and anxiety. *Behaviour Research and Therapy, 33,* 755–770.

Breiter, H. C., Etcoff, N. L., Whalen, P. J., Kennedy, W. A., Rauch, S. L., Buckner, R. L., Strauss, M. M., Hyman, S. E., & Rosen, B. R. (1996). Response and habituation of the human amygdala during visual processing of facial expression. *Neuron, 17,* 875–887.

Buchel, C., & Dolan, R. J. (2000). Classical fear conditioning in functional neuroimaging. *Current Opinions in Neurobiology, 10,* 219–223.

Buchel, C., Dolan, R. J., Armony, J., & Friston, K. J. (1999). Amygdala–hippocampal involvement in human aversive trace conditioning revealed through event related fMRI. *Journal of Neuroscience, 19,* 10869–10876.

Cahill, L. (1999). A neurobiological perspective on emotionally influenced, long-term memory. *Seminars in Clinical Neuropsychiatry, 4,* 266–273.

Cahill, L., Haier, R. J., Fallon, J., Alkire, M. T., Tang, C., Keator, D., Wu, J., & McGaugh, J. L. (1996). Amygdala activity at encoding correlated with long-term, free recall of emotional information. *Proceedings of the National Academy of Sciences of the USA, 93,* 8016–8021.

Callicott, J. H., Ramsey, N. F., Tallent, K., Bertolino, A., Knable, M. B., Coppola, R., Goldberg, T., van Gelderen, P., Mattay, V. S., Frank, J. A., Moonen, C. T., & Weinberger, D. R. (1998). Functional magnetic resonance imaging brain mapping in psychiatry: Methodological issues illustrated in a study of working memory in schizophrenia. *Neuropsychopharmacology, 18,* 186–196.

Carter, C. S., MacDonald, A. M., Botvinick, M., Ross, L. L., Stenger, V. A., Noll, D., & Cohen, J. D. (2000). Parsing executive processes: Strategic vs. evaluative functions of the anterior cingulate cortex. *Proceedings of the National Academy of Sciences, 15,* 1944–1949.

Cassella, J. V., & Davis, M. (1985). Fear-enhanced acoustic startle is not attenuated by acute or chronic imipramine in rats. *Psychopharmacology, 87,* 278–282.

Clark, D. (1999). Anxiety disorders: Ehy they persist and how to treat them. *Behaviour Research and Therapy, 37,* S5–S27

Clark, D. M., & Wells, A. (1995). A cognitive model of social phobia. In R. G. Heimberg, M. R. Liebowitz, D. A. Hope, & F. R. Schneier (Eds), *Social phobia: Diagnosis, assessment, and treatment* (pp. 69–93). New York: Guilford Press.

Cloitre, M., & Liebowitz, M. R. (1991). Memory bias in panic disorder: An investigation of the cognitive avoidance hypothesis. *Cognitive Therapy and Research, 15,* 371–386.

Cloitre, M., Shear, M. K., Cancienne, J., & Zeitlin, S. B. (1994). Implicit and explicit memory for catastrophic associations to bodily sensation words in panic disorder. *Cognitive Therapy and Research, 18,* 225–240.

Costello, E. J., & Angold, A. (1995). Epidemiology. In J. S. March (Ed.), *Anxiety disorders in children and adolescents* (pp. 109–124). New York: Guilford Press.

Crestani, F., Lorez, M., Baer, K., Essrich, C., Benke, D., Laurent, J. P., Belzung, C., Fritschy, J. M., Luscher, B., & Mohler, H. (1999). Decreased GABA-receptor clustering results in enhanced anxiety and a bias for threat cues. *Nature Neuroscience, 2,* 833–839.

Daleiden, E. L. (1998). Childhood anxiety and memory functioning: A comparison of systemic and processing accounts. *Journal of Experimental Child Psychology, 68,* 216–235.

Daleiden, E. L., & Vasey, M. W. (1997). An information-processing perspective on childhood anxiety. *Clinical Psychology Review, 17,* 407–429.

Dalgleish, T., Moradi, A. R., Taghavi, M. R., Neshat-Doost, H. T., & Yule, W. (2001). An experimental investigation of hypervigilance for threat in children and adolescents with post-traumatic stress disorder. *Psychological Medicine, 31,* 541–547.

Davidson, R. J., Marchall, J. R., Tomarken, A. J., & Henriques, J. B. (2000). While a phobic waits: Regional brain electrical and autonomic activity in social phobics during anticipation of public speaking. *Biological Psychiatry, 47,* 85–95.

Davidson, R. J., Putnam, K. M., & Larson, C. L. (2000). Dysfunction in the neural circuitry of emotion regulation: A possible prelude to violence. *Science, 289,* 591–594.

Davis, M (1998). Are different parts of the amygdala involved in fear versus anxiety? *Biological Psychiatry, 48,* 51–57.

Davis, M. (2000). The role of the amygdala in conditioned and unconditioned anxiety. In J. P. Aggleton (Ed.), *The amygdala* (2nd ed., pp. 213–288). New York: Oxford University Press.

Ehlers, A., Margraf, J., Davies, S. O., & Roth, W. T. (1988). Selective processing of threat cues in subjects with panic disorder. *Journal of Abnormal Psychology, 101,* 371–382.

Ferdinand, R. F., & Verhulst, F. (1995). Psychopathology from adolescence into young adulthood: An eight-year follow-up study. *American Journal of Psychiatry, 152,* 586–594.

Foa, E. B., Ilai, D., McCarthy, P. R., Shoyer, B., & Murdock, T. B. (1993). Information-processing in obsessive–compulsive disorder. *Cognitive Therapy and Research, 17,* 173–189.

Foa, E. B., & Kozak, M. J. (1986). Emotional memory of fear: Exposure to corrective information. *Psychological Bulletin, 99,* 20–35.

Gallagher, M. (2000). The amygdala and associative learning. In J. P. Aggleton (Ed.), *The amygdala* (2nd ed., pp. 311–330). New York: Oxford University Press.

Gorman, J. M., Kent, J. M., Sullivan, G. M., & Coplan, J. D. (2000). Neuroanatomical hypothesis of panic disorder, revised. *American Journal of Psychiatry, 157,* 493–505.

Gurley, D., Cohen, P. Pine, D. S., & Brook, J. (1996). Discriminating depression and anxiety in youth: A goal for diagnostic criteria. *Journal of Affective Disorders, 39,* 191–200.

Hope, D. A., Rapee, R. M., Heimberg, R. G., & Dombeck, M. J. (1990). Representations of the self in social phobia: Vulnerability to social threat. *Cognitive Therapy and Research, 14,* 177–189.

Isenberg, N., Silbersweig, D., Engelien, A., Emmerich, S.,Malavade, K., Beattie, B., Leon, A. C., & Stern, E. (1999). Linguistic threat activates the human amygdala. *Proceedings of the National Academy of the Sciences of the USA, 96,* 10456–10459.

Kagan, J., Reznick, J. S., & Snidman, N. (1987). The physiology and psychology of behavioral inhibition in children. *Child Development, 58,* 1459–1473.

Killgore, W. D. S., Oki, M., & Yurgelun-Todd, D. A. (2001). Sex-specific developmental changes in amygdala response to affective faces. *NeuroReport, 12,* 427–433.

Kindt, M., Bierman, D., & Brosschot, J. F. (1997). Cognitive bias in spider fear and control children: Assessment of emotional interference by a card format and a single-trial format of the Stroop task. *Journal of Experimental Child Psychology, 66,* 163–179.

Kindt, M., Brosschot, J. F., & Everaerd, W. (1997). Cognitive processing of children in a real-life stress situation and a neutral situation. *Journal of Experimental Child Psychology, 64,* 79–97.

Klein, R. G. (1995). Anxiety disorders. In M. Rutter, E. Taylor, & L. Hersov (Eds.), *Child and adolescent psychiatry: Modern approaches* (3rd ed., pp. 351–374). London: Blackwell Scientific.

LaBar, K. S., Gatenby, J. C., Gore, J. C., LeDoux, J. E., & Phelps, E. A. (1998). Human amygdala activation during conditioned fear acquisition and extinction: A mixed-trial fMRI study. *Neuron, 20,* 937–945.

LaBar, K. S., LeDoux, J. E., Spencer, D. D., & Phelps, E. A. (1995). Impaired fear conditioning following unilateral temporal lobectomy in humans. *Journal of Neuroscience, 15,* 6846–6855.

Lang, P. J., Bradley, M. M., & Cuthbert, B. N. (1998). Emotion, motivation, and anxiety: Brain mechanisms and psychophysiology. *Biological Psychiatry, 44,* 1248–1263.

Last, C. G., Perrin, S., Hersen, M., & Kazdin, A. E. (1996). A prospective study of childhood anxiety disorders. *Journal of the American Academy of Child and Adolescent Psychiatry, 35,* 1502–1510.

LeDoux, J. E. (1992). Brain mechanisms of emotion and emotional learning. *Current Opinions in Neurobiology, 2,* 191–197.

LeDoux, J. E. (1993). Emotional memory systems in the brain. *Behavioural Brain Research, 58,* 69–79.

LeDoux, J. E. (1995). Emotion: Clues from the brain. *Review of Psychology, 46,* 209–235.

LeDoux, J. E. (1998). Fear and the brain: Where have we been, where are we going? *Biological Psychiatry, 44,* 1229–1238.

LeDoux, J. E. (2000a). The amygdala and emotion: A view through fear. In J. P. Aggleton (Ed.), *The amygdala* (2nd ed., pp. 289–310). New York: Oxford University Press.

LeDoux, J. E. (2000b). Emotional circuits in the brain. *Annual Review of Neuroscience, 23,* 155–184.

Leonard, C. M., Rolls, E. T., Wilson, F. A., & Baylis, G. C. (1985). Neurons in the amygdala of the monkey with responses selective for faces. *Behavioural Brain Research, 15,* 159–176.

Lundh, L. G., & Ost, L. G. (1996). Recognition for critical faces in social phobics. *Behaviour Research and Therapy, 34,* 787–794.

MacLeod, C., Mathews, A., & Tata, P. (1986). Attentional bias in emotional disorders. *Journal of Abnormal Psychology, 95,* 15–20.

Manfro, C. G., Otto, M. W., McArdle, E. T., Worthington, J. J., III, Rosenbaum, J. F., & Pollack, M. H. (1996). Relationship between stressful life events to childhood and family history of anxiety and the course of panic disorder. *Journal of Affective Disorders, 41,* 135–139.

Martin, M., Horder, P., & Jones, G. V. (1992). Integral bias in naming of phobic related words. *Cognition and Emotion, 6,* 479–486.

Mathews, A., & MacLeod, C. (1985). Selective processing of threat cues in anxiety states. *Behaviour Research and Therapy, 31,* 57–62.

Mathews, A., Mogg, K., Kentish, J., & Eysenck, M. W. (1995). Effect of psychological treatment on cognitive bias in generalized anxiety disorder. *Behaviour Research and Therapy, 33,* 293–303.

Mathews, A., Mogg, K., May, J., & Eysenck, M. W. (1989). Implicit and explicit memory bias in anxiety. *Journal of Abnormal Psychology, 98,* 31–34.

Mattia, J. I., Heimberg, R. G., & Hope, D. A. (1993). The revised Stroop color-naming task in social phobics. *Behaviour Research and Therapy, 31,* 305–314.

McNally, R. J. (1996). Cognitive bias in the anxiety disorders. In D. Hope (Ed.), *Nebraska Symposium on Motivation: Vol. 43. Perspectives on anxiety, panic, and fear* (pp. 211–250). Lincoln: University of Nebraska Press.

McNally, R. J. (1997). Memory and anxiety disorders. *Philosophical Transactions of the Royal Society of London, Series B: Biological Sciences, 352,* 1755–1759.

McNally, R. J., Kaspi, S. P., Riemann, B. C., & Zeitlin, S. B. (1990). Selective processing of threat cues in posttraumatic stress disorder. *Journal of Abnormal Psychology, 99,* 398–402.

McNally, R. J., Riemann, B. C., & Kim, E. (1990). Selective processing of threat cues in panic disorder. *Behaviour Research and Therapy, 28,* 407–412.

Merikangas, K. R., Avenevoli, S., Dierker, L., & Grillon, C. (1999). Vulnerability factors among children at risk for anxiety disorders. *Biological Psychiatry, 46,* 1523–1535.

Mogg, K., & Bradley, B. P. (1998). A cognitive-motivational analysis of anxiety. *Behaviour Research and Therapy, 36,* 809–848.

Mogg, K., & Bradley, B. P. (1999). Some methodological issues in assessing attentional biases for threatening faces in anxiety: A replication study using a modified version of the probe detection task. *Behaviour Research and Therapy, 37,* 595–604.

Mogg, K., & Mathews, A. (1990). Is there a self-referent mood-congruent recall bias in anxiety? *Behaviour Research and Therapy, 28,* 91–92.

Mogg, K., Mathews, A., & Eysenck, M. W. (1992). Attentional bias to threat in clinical anxiety states. *Cognition and Emotion, 6,* 149–159.

Mogg, K., Mathews, A., & Weinman, J. (1987). Memory bias in clinical anxiety. *Journal of Abnormal Psychology, 96,* 94–98.

Moradi, A. R., Doost, H. T., Taghavi, M. R., Yule, W., & Dalgleish, T. (1999). Everyday memory deficits in children and adolescents with PTSD: Perfomance on the Rivermead Behavioural Memory Test. *Journal of Child Psychology and Psychiatry, 40,* 357–361.

Moradi, A. R., Taghavi, M. R., Neshat-Doost, H. T., Yule, W., & Dalgleish, T. (1999). Performance of children and adolescents with PTSD on the Stroop color-naming task. *Psychological Medicine, 29,* 415–419.

Moradi, A. R., Taghavi, R., Neshat-Doost, H. T., Yule, W., & Dalgleish, T. (2000). Memory bias for emotional information in children and adolescents with posttraumatic stress disorder: A preliminary study. *Journal of Anxiety Disorders, 14,* 521–534.

Morris, J. S., Frith, C. D., Perrett, D. I., Rowland, D., Young, A. W., Calder, A. J., & Dolan, R. J. (1996). A differential neural response in the human amygdala to fearful and happy facial expressions. *Nature, 83,* 812–815.

Newman, D. L., Moffit, T. E., Caspi, A., Magdol, L., Silva, P. A., & Stanton, W. R. (1996). Psychiatric disorder in a birth cohort of young adults: Prevalence, comorbidity, clinical significance, and new case incidence from ages 11 to 21. *Journal of Consulting and Clinical Psychology, 64,* 552–562.

Otto, M. W., McNally, R. J., Pollack, M. H., Chen, E., & Rosenbaum, J. F. (1994). Hemispheric laterality and memory bias for threat in anxiety disorders. *Journal of Abnormal Psychology, 103,* 828–831.

Panksepp, J. (1998). *Affective neuroscience: The foundation of human and animal emotions.* New York: Oxford University Press.

Pearlson, G. D. (2000). Neurobiology of schizophrenia. *Annals of Neurology, 48,* 556–566.

Peterson, B. S., Skudlarski, P., Gatenby, J. C., Zhang, H., Anderson, A. W., & Gore, J. C. (1999). An fMRI study of Stroop word-color interference: Evidence of cingulate subregions subserving multiple distributed attentional systems. *Biological Psychiatry, 45,* 1237–1258.

Phillips, M. L., Williams, L., Senior, C., Bullmore, E. T., Brammer, M. J., Andrew, C., Williams, S. C., & David, A. S. (1999). A differential neural response to threatening and non-threatening negative facial expressions in paranoid and non-paranoid schizophrenics. *Psychiatry Research: Neuroimaging, 92,* 11–31.

Pine, D. S. (1999). Pathophysiology of childhood anxiety disorders. *Biological Psychiatry, 46*, 1555–1566.

Pine, D. S., Cohen, P., Gurley, D., Brook, J., & Ma, Y. (1998). The risk for early-adulthood anxiety and depressive disorders in adolescents with anxiety and depressive disorders. *Archives of General Psychiatry, 55*, 56–64.

Pine, D. S., & Grun, J. (1999). Childhood anxiety: Integrating developmental psychopathology and affective neuroscience. *Journal of Child and Adolescent Psychopharmacology, 9*, 1–12.

Pine, D. S., Grun, J., Zarahn, E., Fyer, A., Koda, V., Li, W., Szeszko, P. R., Ardekani, B., & Bilder, R. M. (2001). Cortical brain regions engaged by masked emotional faces in adolescents and adults: An fRMI study. *Emotion, 1*, 137–147.

Pine, D. S., Klein, R. G., Coplan, J. D., Papp, L. A., Hoven, C. W., Martinez, J., Kovalenko, P., Mandell, D. J., Moreau, D., Klein, D. F., & Gorman, J. M. (2000). Differential carbon dioxide sensitivity in childhood anxiety disorders and a nonill group. *Archives of General Psychiatry, 57*, 960–967.

Pine, D. S., Wasserman, G. A., & Workman, S. B. (1999). Memory and anxiety in prepubertal boys at risk for delinquency. *Journal of the American Academy of Child and Adolescent Psychiatry, 38*, 1024–1031.

Pollack, M. H., Otto, M. W., Sabatino, S., Majeher, D., Worthington, J. J., McArdle, E. T., & Rosenbaum, J. F. (1996). Relationship of childhood anxiety to adult panic disorder: Correlates and influence on course. *American Journal of Psychiatry, 153*, 376–381.

Rapee, R. M., McCallum, S. L., Melville, L. F., Ravescroft, H., & Rodney, J. M. (1994). Memory bias in social phobia. *Behaviour Research and Therapy, 32*, 89–99.

Reiman, E. M. (1988). The quest to establish the neural substrates of anxiety. *Psychiatric Clinics of North America, 2*, 295–307.

Rogan, M. T., & LeDoux, J. E. (1995). LTP is accompanied by commensurate enhancement of auditory-evoked responses in a fear conditioning circuit. *Neuron, 15*, 127–136.

Rolls, E. T. (1984). Neurons in the cortex of the temporal lobe and the amygdala in the monkey with responses selective for faces. *Human Neurobiology, 3*, 209–222.

Rolls, E. T. (1999). *The brain and emotion.* New York: Oxford University Press.

Rolls, E. T. (2000). Precis of the brain and emotion. *Science, 2*, 177–191.

Sallee, R., & Greenawald, J. T. (1995). Neurobiology. In J. S. March (Ed.), *Anxiety disorders in children and adolescents* (pp. 3–34). New York: Guilford Press.

Schneider, F., Weiss, U., Kessler, C., Muller-Gartner, H. W., Salloum, J. B., Grodd, W., Himmelmann, F., Gaebel, W., & Birbaumer, N. (1999). Subcortical correlates of differential classical conditioning of aversive emotional reactions in social phobia. *Biological Psychiatry, 45*, 873–871.

Schneier, F. R., Johnson, J., Hornig, C. D., Liebowitz, M. R., & Weissman, M. M. (1992). Social phobia: Comorbidity and morbidity in an epidemiological sample. *Archives of General Psychiatry, 49*, 282–288.

Shaffer, D., Fisher, P., Dulcan, M. K., Davies, M., Piacentini, J., Schwab-Stone, M. E., Lahey, B. B., Bourdon, K., Jensen, P. S., Bird, H. R., Canino, G., & Regier, D. A. (1995). The NIMH Diagnostic Interview Schedule for Children Version 2. 3 (DISC): Description, acceptability, prevalence rates, and performance in the

MECA study. *Journal of the American Academy of Child and Adolescent Psychiatry, 35,* 865–877.

Squire, L. R., & Kandel, E. R. (1999). *Memory: From mind to molecules.* New York: Scientific American Library.

Taghavi, M. R., Neshat-Doost, H. T., Moradi, A. R., Yule, W., & Dalgleish, T. (1999). Biases in visual attention in children and adolescents with clinical anxiety and mixed anxiety-depression. *Journal of Abnormal Child Psychology, 27,* 215–223.

Thomas, K. M., Drevets, W. C., Dahl, R. E., Ryan, N. D., Birmaher, B., Eccard, C. H., Axelson, D., Whalen P. J., & Casey, B. J. (2001). Amygdala response to fearful faces in anxious and depressed children. *Archives of General Psychiatry, 58,* 1065–1071.

Thomas, K. M., Drevets, W. C., Whalen, P. J., Eccard, C. H., Dahl, R. E., Ryan, N. D., & Casey, B. J. (2001). Amygdala response to facial expression in children and adults. *Biological Psychiatry, 49,* 309–316.

Toren, P., Sadeh, M., Wolmer, L., Eldar, S., Koren, S., Weizman, R., & Laor, N. (2000). Neurocognitive correlates of anxiety disorders in children: A preliminary report. *Journal of Anxiety Disorders, 14,* 239–247.

Vasey, M. W., Daleiden, E. L., Williams, L. L., & Brown, L. M. (1995). Biased attention in childhood anxiety disorders: A preliminary study. *Journal of Abnormal Child Psychology, 23,* 267–279.

Vasey, M. W., El-Hag, N., & Daleiden, E. L. (1996). Anxiety and the processing of emotional stimuli: Distinctive patterns of selective attention among high- and low-test-anxious children. *Child Development, 67,* 1173–1185.

Verhulst, F. C., van der Ende, J., Ferdinand, R. F., & Kasius, M. C. (1997). The prevalence of DSM-III-R diagnoses in a national sample of Dutch adolescents. *Archives of General Psychiatry, 54,* 329–336.

Watts, F., McKenna, F. P., Sharrock, R., & Trezise, L. (1986). Color naming of phobia-related words. *British Journal of Psychology, 77,* 97–108.

Watts, F. N., & Coyle, K. (1993). Phobics show poor recall of anxiety words. *British Journal of Medical Psychology, 66,* 373–382.

Whalen, P. J., Rauch, S. L., Etcoff, N. L., McImerney, S. C., Lee, M. B., & Jenike, M. A. (1998). Masked presentation of emotional facial expressions modulate amygdala activity without explicit knowledge. *Journal of Neuroscience, 18,* 411–418.

Williams, J. M., Mathews, A., & MacLeod, C. (1996). The emotional Stroop task and psychopathology. *Psychological Bulletin, 120,* 3–24.

Young, A. W., Hellawell, D. J., Van De Wal, C., & Johnson, M. (1996). Facial expression processing after amygdalaotomy. *Neuropsychologia, 34,* 31–39.

Chapter 2

Behavioral Inhibition

DINA R. HIRSHFELD-BECKER
JOSEPH BIEDERMAN
JERROLD F. ROSENBAUM

Identifying early precursors to anxiety disorders can inform both our understanding of the etiology of these disorders and our selection of candidates for early intervention. Research on such precursors has focused over the past 10–15 years on the temperamental construct "behavioral inhibition to the unfamiliar," or BI (Kagan, Reznick, & Snidman, 1988). BI represents the tendency to exhibit fearfulness, restraint, reticence, and withdrawal in the face of novel events or situations, including unfamiliar rooms, toys, peers, and adults. First studied in depth by Kagan and colleagues, the stability and correlates of BI have since been examined by a growing number of researchers, with converging evidence suggesting that BI represents a diathesis for anxiety disorder, and in particular for social anxiety disorder. Despite this promising evidence, the construct itself is subject to methodological limitations in the way it is defined, operationalized, and measured, in its inconsistent associations with physiological variables, and in the uncertainty about the specificity of the risk it confers. In this chapter, we review the evidence on BI and its associations with anxiety disorder, discuss the strengths and limitations of the studies conducted to date, and suggest directions for further research.

COURSE AND HERITABILITY
OF BEHAVIORAL INHIBITION

Because of developmental changes, BI manifests differently at different ages. Inhibited toddlers react to unfamiliar settings with distress, fear, and avoidance and by clinging to parents. They may shrink away from unfamiliar adults, refuse to approach new toys or enter new rooms, and withdraw from unknown peers. Inhibited preschool-age children may not show overt fear or distress but tend to exhibit quiet restraint and hesitancy to smile, approach, or initiate spontaneous conversations with new peers or adults. In older children, the restraint and reticence may be especially evident with groups of unfamiliar peers. Inhibited children may be more likely to remain solitary in group settings (e.g., birthday parties, classrooms). In addition, older children may show anticipatory anxiety with regard to transitions to new settings or activities.

Stability of Behavioral Inhibition

Kagan and colleagues followed two cohorts of white, mainly middle-class, Boston-area children selected in toddlerhood (at age 21 or 31 months) as either extremely inhibited or extremely uninhibited (Kagan, 1994). The laboratory situations observed at the initial assessment included a series of interactions with unfamiliar adults and toys, and the indices of BI included counts of the child's distress vocalizations, withdrawals, and absence of spontaneous interactions with the examiner, as well as measures of latencies to interact with the toys or adults (Garcia-Coll, Kagan, & Reznick, 1984). They observed the children again at ages 4, 5½, and 7½ years and found that the inhibited children preserved their inhibition to a moderate degree through middle childhood. Over three-fourths (77%) of children originally classified as inhibited at age 21 months remained above the sample median on the overall aggregate of inhibition at 7½ years (Kagan, Reznick, Snidman, Gibbons, & Johnson, 1988).

To examine early precursors of BI, Kagan and Snidman and colleagues studied two cohorts of infants originally assessed at age 4 months (total N of 462) and found that high reactivity, the tendency to respond to novel or surprising events with high motor activity and distress, was moderately correlated with inhibited behavior in toddlerhood. In both samples, over one-third (36% and 35%) of high-reactive infants showed high fear in laboratory episodes involving interaction with an unfamiliar woman and objects at both 14 and 21 months, compared with 3–4% who showed low fear (Kagan, 1994, p. 183). At age 7, children from the first cohort who had been high reactive were significantly less likely than low-reactive and other children to speak spontaneously with or smile at an unfamiliar female examiner and significantly more likely to be above the sample median on anxious symptoms reported by mothers and teachers on an author-constructed questionnaire (45% vs. 15% and 21%; Kagan, Snidman, Zetner, & Peterson, 1999). Using similar methods, Calkins, Fox, and Marshall (1996) found, among 81 children from the Washington, DC, area, that high motor activity and distress at 4 months predicted BI at age 14 months, based on laboratory observations of behavior with an unfamiliar examiner and unfamiliar toys. At age 4, these children were more likely to be rated by their mothers as high in shyness on the Colorado Child Temperament Inventory (Schmidt et al., 1997).

Kagan and colleagues regard inhibited children as a distinct subset of children, rather than seeing BI as a dimensional measure. This distinction is based on the observation that BI is more stable over time among children who start out extreme in this tendency (Kagan, Reznick, & Snidman, 1988; see Table 2.1).

The stability of BI across childhood has been largely supported by other longitudinal observational studies, which varied in the ways they operationalized BI, as summarized in Table 2.1. Studies in the table are categorized according to whether they include unselected samples or samples selected as extreme in inhibition or uninhibition. Although the two studies that directly compare selected and unselected groups found higher stability for children extreme in inhibition or uninhibition (Kagan, Reznick, & Snidman, 1988; Kerr, Lambert, Stattin, & Klackenberg-Larsson, 1994), results of the other studies are not as conclusive. For example, although stabilities in two of the three studies using selected samples were reasonably high (r's ranging from .54 to .67), the study by Scarpa, Raine, Venables, and Mednick (1995) of a large sample of children on the island of Mauritius did not fit this pattern. However, this study used a broader definition of "extreme," used multimethod comparisons (initial laboratory observations and later teacher reports), and used less exact follow-up definitions of BI (including measures of distress, school refusal, and emotionality), all of which may have reduced the stability of the construct measured.

In contrast, with the exception of Asendorpf's (1990, 1994) study, the unselected samples typically had slightly lower stabilities of BI (ranging from .18–.42). It is possible that Asendorpf's observational assessments may have captured initial shyness with strangers rather than sustained inhibition, as the interactions he observed ranged from 2–15 minutes, as opposed to the 30- to 60-minute assessment periods in Kagan's studies. Considering the evidence summarized in Table 2.1, BI appears to have moderate stability during early and middle childhood, with the suggestion that stability is higher among children who are initially extreme in inhibition.

Less is known about the stability of BI during adolescence and adulthood. The study of this question is limited by uncertainty as to how to measure BI among adults, because observed behavior reflects influences other than temperament (e.g., learning, psychopathology). Several long-term longitudinal studies have, however, suggested that inhibited children maintain their cautiousness and restraint into adulthood. Caspi and Silva (1995) followed 800 unselected children from a birth cohort recruited in the early 1970s in Dunedin, New Zealand, from age 3 to early adulthood. Assessments of inhibition at age 3 were based on ratings of behaviors during cognitive and motor testing that reflected inhibition in novel settings, shyness, fearfulness, minimal vocalization, and tendency to be upset by the examiner. At age 18, those who had been inhibited reported an increased tendency toward caution, restraint, avoidance of thrills, and endorsement of social norms. These young adults also reported a decreased propensity for taking leadership roles, influencing others, and desiring to be the center of attention. Gest (1997) found that BI (conceptualized as stranger wariness) in 203 individuals recruited from elementary schools in Minneapolis was preserved from ages 8 to 12 years to 17 to 24 years. Inhibited young adults were more likely to be ill at ease, hesitant, and inexpressive in conversations with strangers, as well as less likely to initiate contact through talking, smiling, or joking. In addition, inhibition in young adulthood was associated with greater negative emotionality and emotional distress in men and with a less positive, less active social life in both genders. In a birth cohort from the late 1920s, Caspi, Bem, and Elder (1989) found that shyness in middle childhood, based on mother's descriptions of social ease and reserve, predicted older age at marriage, fatherhood, and establishment of career for men and a greater likelihood of not working outside of the home for women.

Gender and Cultural Differences in Behavioral Inhibition

Among toddlers and young children, some investigators have found slightly higher rates of BI among girls (Robinson, Kagan, Reznick, & Corley, 1992), whereas others have reported no differences (Broberg, Lamb, & Hwang, 1990; Chen et al., 1998). Several studies have found BI to be more persistent among girls (Hirshfeld et al., 1992; Kerr et al., 1994; Schwartz, Snidman, & Kagan, 1999). With regard to cultural differences, Chen and colleagues (1998) found that BI was significantly more common among 2-year-olds in a sample from the People's Republic of China than in a Canadian sample. In contrast, however, another study found that rates of high reactivity (motor activity and fretting) were higher among groups of 4-month-old infants in the United States (Boston), intermediate among a sam-

TABLE 2.1. Stability of Behavioral Inhibition in Childhood

Investigators	Sample characteristics	Ages	Means of assessing behavioral inhibition (situation observed, and types of behaviors rated)	Stability
			Studies of selected samples (children selected as extreme in inhibition and uninhibition)	
Kagan, Reznick & Snidman (1988)	46–58 Caucasian middle-class children from the Boston area (the most extreme on inhibition or uninhibition—upper and lower quartiles—from a larger sample selected at 21 mo)	21 mo 4 yr 5.5 yr 7.5 yr	21 mo: Interaction with unfamiliar female adult (20 min); distress, withdrawals, and latencies to interact with toys or adult	2–7.5 yr: .67 4–7.5 yr: .54 5.5–7.5 yr: .57
			4 yr: Two dyadic play interactions with unfamiliar peers (40 min); latencies to interact, time proximal to mother	
			5.5 yr: Risk room with unfamiliar toys, interaction with an unfamiliar adult, dyadic play with an unfamiliar peer; latencies to interact, latencies and frequencies of comments and smiles	
			7.5 yr: Free play and games with 8–10 unfamiliar peers (80 min); time spent alone, frequencies of interaction, smiling, cheering	
			Interaction with unfamiliar adult (90 min); latencies to spontaneous comments, frequency of comments and smiles, time looking away	
			Aggregate indices at each age	
Fordham & Stevenson-Hinde (1999)	50 children from Cambridge, England, who had been selected from a pool of children nominated by preschool teachers as "shy" or "confident"	4.5 yr 7.5 yr 8.4–10.6 yr	4.5 yr: Questionnaire ratings of shyness by mother and meeting in the home with an unfamiliar examiner; global ratings of verbal and nonverbal interaction; child had to be either "high shy" or "not high shy" on both to be included	4.5–latest: .66 7–latest: .60 The investigators note that the correlations in this study represented consistent linear trends and were not due to extreme ratings only.
			4.5 and 7.5 yr: Laboratory interaction with an unfamiliar examiner who invited child to approach a toy and began administering a vocabulary test; global 9-point ordinal rating of inhibition based on verbal responsiveness and nonverbal interactions	
			8.4–10.6 yr: Interview with an unfamiliar adult examiner conducted in the child's home; examiner global ratings of nonverbal anxiety and low verbal responsiveness (same scale as above)	

(continued)

TABLE 2.1. *(continued)*

31

Investigators	Sample characteristics	Ages	Means of assessing behavioral inhibition (situation observed, and types of behaviors rated)	Stability
Scarpa et al. (1995)	All 3-year-old children in two towns on the island of Mauritius (N = 683–1,795)	3 yr 8 yr 11 yr	3 yr: Psychophysiological and cognitive testing with an unfamiliar examiner; averaged standard global ratings made of crying, sociability, approach–avoidance, degree of verbalization, ease of relationship with tester, and social involvement with other children 8 yr: Teacher ratings (on the Rutter Scale) of a child's solitariness, distress, fear of new situations, and tears on arrival or school refusal 11 yr: Teacher ratings of sociability, emotionality, and talkativeness; correlations are between inhibition indices with sample limited to children in the upper or lower 40th percentile	3–8 yr: .11 3–11 yr: .21
			Studies of unselected samples	
Broberg et al. (1990)	144 Swedish toddlers	16 mo 28 mo 40 mo	Initial interaction with unfamiliar examiner in the child's home (5 min); ratings of the child's sociability Dyadic peer play with a familiar peer at home (30 min); rating of child's noninvolvement Parent ratings on the fearfulness scale of the Rothbart Infant Behavior Questionnaire (initial assessment only)	16–40 mo: .38 28–40 mo: .42
Robinson et al. (1992)	324–356 Colorado twins from the MacArthur Longitudinal Twin Study	14 mo 20 mo 24 mo	Interactions with novel toys and a stranger (20–25 min); latencies to leave mother and approach toys and/or stranger (aggregate indices at each age)	14–20 mo: .33 20–24 mo: .30 14–24 mo: .18
Asendorpf (1990, 1994)	99 German preschoolers	3.9 yr (mean) 4.9 yr (mean) 5.9 yr (mean) 6.9 yr (mean) 8 yr, 10 yr	Laboratory interaction with an unfamiliar adult (5 min in yr 1 and 3) or play interaction with 1–3 peers (10–15 min in yr 2 and 4); latency to first spontaneous comment Conversation with an unfamiliar adult (2 min); percentage of silence (ages 8 and 10) (measures of "stranger inhibition")	3.9–6.9 yr: .64 4–8 yr: .59 4–10 yr: .44

32

Study	Sample	Age	Measures	Results
Asendorpf (1990, 1994)	Same as above	Same as above	Parent ratings on eight questions tapping inhibition with unfamiliar adults and peers (ages 3.9–6.9); teacher ratings of classroom behavior (ages 8, 10)	3.9–6.9 yr: .73[a] 4–8 yr: .52 4–10 yr: .32
Stevenson-Hinde & Shouldice (1995)	70 second-born children from Cambridge, England	4.5 yr 7.5 yr	4.5 and 7.5 yr: Laboratory interaction with an unfamiliar examiner who invited child to approach a toy and began administering a vocabulary test; global 9-point rating of inhibition based on verbal responsiveness and nonverbal interactions	4.5–7 yr: .24

Studies comparing selected and unselected samples

Study	Sample	Age	Measures	Results
Kerr et al. (1994)	170–210 Swedish children	3 mo 6 mo 9 mo 12 mo 18 mo 24 mo Yearly thru age 6	Through age 6 yr: Behaviors during clinic interviews and testing over the first 6 yr of life; averaged 5-point global ratings by psychologists of initial ease of adjustment, tendency to cling to mother, nervousness (including timidity, restriction of play, and silence), positive social behaviors (including smiling and vocalization), and social confidence	Betas from regressions predicting BI at 3–6 yr from scores at 21 mo: Whole sample: Boys: .18 Girls: .22 Extremes (10–15%): Boys: .54 Girls: .39
Kagan, Reznick, & Snidman (1988)	100 European American middle-class children from the Boston area	14 mo 20 mo 4 yr	14 and 20 mo: Interaction with unfamiliar female adult; distress, withdrawals, and latencies to interact with toys or adult 4 yr: Interaction with an unfamiliar female adult, dyadic free play with an unfamiliar peer, behavior in a risk room with unfamiliar toys (similar measures to other Kagan studies cited above) Aggregate indices at each age	Whole sample: 14–48 mo: NS 20–48 mo: NS Extremes (upper and lower 20% at 14 and 20 mo): Inhibited and uninhibited groups differed significantly at 4 yr

Note. Only significant correlations (*p* < .05) are reported.
[a] Corrected for attenuation.

ple from Ireland (Dublin), and lowest among those from China (Beijing; Kagan et al., 1994).

Physiological Underpinnings

Kagan, Reznick, and Snidman (1988) hypothesize that the physiological underpinnings of BI include a lower threshold to limbic and sympathetic nervous system arousal in response to novelty; specifically, higher reactivity of the basolateral and central nuclei of the amygdala and their projections to the striatum, hypothalamus, sympathetic chain, and cardiovascular system. They have examined physiological markers associated with BI, and in their first longitudinal cohort they found correlations between BI and increased urinary MHPG (at age 5½ years), increased baseline morning salivary cortisol levels (at age 5½ and 7½ years), and high and stable heart rates (at ages 21 months, 4 years, and 5½ years) with a tendency for heart rate to accelerate across laboratory batteries. The children who remained consistently inhibited in visits at 21 months and at 4, 5½, and 7½ years had the highest heart rates. However, these findings have not been consistently replicated in other cohorts or by other groups.

With regard to cardiac findings, several groups have noted increased heart rate or reduced variability among inhibited children (Marshall & Stevenson-Hinde, 1998; Schmidt, Fox, Schulkin, & Gold, 1999). Findings on cortisol levels have been less consistent. For example, Schmidt and colleagues (1997) found that 4-year-olds who displayed high social wariness during play with peers had significantly higher average morning cortisol levels compared with others. However, Schmidt, Fox, and colleagues (1999) found no differences in cortisol levels between shy and nonshy 7-year-olds before or after a stressful period anticipating a self-presentation task. Other studies have suggested that contextual factors influence associations with cortisol. For example, Nachmias, Gunnar, Mangelsdorf, Hornik Parritz, and Buss (1996) found that postsession levels of cortisol among seventy-seven 18-month-old BI children were elevated only among those classified as having insecure attachments to their mothers. However, in this correlational study, BI was coded solely on inhibition of approach and not on displays of distress to novel stimuli, whereas distress displays were correlated with insecure attachment quality; therefore, it may be that the children classified as both inhibited and insecurely attached were the ones most comparable to those in Kagan's cohort (i.e., those with most extreme inhibition). Similarly, two studies found that associations between rises in cortisol from morning to afternoon in preschool-age children in child care were associated with teacher-reported shyness or anxiety in boys (Dettling, Gunnar, & Donzella, 1999; Tout, de Haan, Campbell, & Gunnar, 1998). It may be that shyness renders boys more vulnerable to the stress of full-day child care. Elevated cortisol secretion in this study was not specific to shyness but was associated, in addition, with impulsivity (in boys), poor inhibitory control (in girls), and verbal aggression (in both genders; Dettling et al., 1999).

Others explain the neuroanatomical underpinnings of BI with reference to Gray's recently revised theory, which describes different affective–motivational brain systems, including a behavioral activation system that mediates approach behaviors in response to signals of reward and nonpunishment, and an opposing behavioral inhibition system that inhibits ongoing behaviors in responses to signals of novelty, punishment, and nonreward and that mediates anxiety (Gray, 1982, 1991; Gray & McNaughton, 1996). The latter system is hypothesized to respond to conditioned stimuli for punishment and nonreward, as well as novelty and fear stimuli, to bring about passive avoidance and extinction. It is thought to be localized in the septohippocampal system, its noradrenergic afferents from the locus ceruleus and serotonergic inputs from the raphe nucleus, and in the frontal cortex, and recent data have also emphasized the influence of the amygdala and hypothalamus.

Another hypothesis connects BI with increased activation of hypothesized "withdrawal centers," including areas of the right frontal region, the amygdala, and the temporal polar region, and with deactivation of hypothesized "approach centers," including areas of the left dorsolateral prefrontal cortex, basal ganglia, amygdala, and projections to the hypothalamus (Davidson, 1994). Several small studies have suggested that high-reactive, inhibited, or shy children show increased right cerebral hemisphere or decreased left hemisphere activation (Calkins, Fox, & Marshall, 1996; Davidson, 1994; Schmidt, Fox, et al., 1999). These findings parallel observations of adults with mood and anxiety disorders (Davidson, 1992; Harris, Hoehn-Saric, Lewis, Pearlson, & Streeter, 1994; Reiman, Raichle, Butler, Hercovitch, & Robins, 1984).

Heritability

BI appears to have moderate heritability (DiLalla, Kagan, & Reznick, 1994; Emde et al., 1992; Matheny, 1989; Robinson et al., 1992). Matheny reported that at 18, 24, and 30 months monozygotic twin pairs were significantly more concordant than in dizygotic twins on inhibited behaviors (total $N = 130$). Moreover, changes in inhibited behaviors over time were more similar in monozygotic than in dizygotic twin pairs. These results were confirmed in the MacArthur Longitudinal Twin Study, in which the heritability of observed BI in twins ages 14, 20, and 24 months was estimated at .55, .41, and .51, respectively, based on observations of a child's response to novel or unusual toys and an unfamiliar adult (Plomin et al.,

1993; Robinson et al., 1992). As in the earlier study, the stability of BI between these two ages appeared genetically mediated (with the heritability of continuity estimated at .38). The heritability at 24 months, based on observations of children's behavior during play with an unfamiliar peer (N = 135), was estimated at .64 (DiLalla et al., 1994). Moderate genetic influence on continuity of BI was also observed. Additional analyses suggested that heritabilities were even higher when the sample was restricted to children extreme in BI or in uninhibition (e.g., > 70% at 2 years of age in children 1 SD above or below the mean); however, the accuracy of these estimates is limited by small sample size (DiLalla et al., 1994; Robinson et al., 1992).

The few candidate gene studies of BI or similar traits conducted to date have shown mainly negative findings (e.g., no associations with the adenosine A1A or A2A receptor or preproenkephalin or the serotonin transporter gene; Jorm et al., 1998, 2000; Smoller et al., 2001). However, among 72 children classified as inhibited based on behavioral observations of interaction with unfamiliar adults in Kagan's laboratory, Smoller and colleagues found modest evidence of an inverse association between BI and the glutamic acid decarboxylase gene (65-kDa isoform), which encodes an enzyme involved in GABA synthesis (Smoller et al., 2001). This isoform appears to respond to short-term changes in the demand for GABA, as might be needed in the face of novelty or threat, and a mouse knockout of this gene has been shown to exhibit increased BI.

Associated Constructs

Other constructs that capture similar variation in child temperament or behavior include *shyness, social fearfulness,* and *social withdrawal.* Various researchers have defined *shyness* as discomfort, inhibition, and awkwardness in social settings; a tendency to avoid or fail to participate appropriately in social situations; a reluctance to approach people or enter situations in which one cannot avoid the attention of others; a fear of negative evaluation accompanied by emotional distress or inhibition that interferes with social or occupational functioning; or timid or withdrawn behavior in response to new people (as reviewed by St. Lorant, Henderson, & Zimbardo, 2000). Therefore, it appears to refer to initial reticence or anxiety in social settings. It differs from BI in its narrower scope, pertaining to novel social situations only, and also perhaps in its duration within a given social encounter, because shyness is often used to refer to initial behavior with an unfamiliar person, whereas BI is sustained over the course of an entire 30- to 60-minute interaction with an unfamiliar examiner (Kagan, Reznick, & Snidman, 1988) and may persist longer (for example, into the school year in a kindergarten classroom; Gersten, 1989). *Social fearfulness* is a scale on some child-temperament inventories; it differs from BI both in its range (anxiety in social situations) and in its focus on experienced or articulated fear rather than on behaviorally observed indicators. *Social withdrawal* or *isolation* refers to the observed tendency of some children to spend a substantial proportion of their free-play time apart from other children, engaged in watchful behavior or noninteractive play. BI children have been observed to be more solitary (Gersten, 1989), but whereas there may be overlap between inhibition and social isolation, children may present as isolated in their peer groups for other reasons (e.g., low sociability, peer rejection, depression). Despite their incomplete overlap, studies of these other constructs may contribute to our understanding of BI. Therefore, in the sections that follow, studies of shy or withdrawn children will also be mentioned where they are applicable.

Animal Models

The temperamental tendency to exhibit distress and restraint in unfamiliar situations has been observed in a broad range of other mammalian species, including rats, cats, dogs (Adamec & Stark-Adamec, 1989; Mineka & Zinbarg, 1995), and primates (Suomi, 1986, 1987, 1997). In their review of the ethological literature, Mineka and Zinbarg (1995) conclude that animals bred for timidity or fear tend to exhibit inhibition to nonsocial and social novelty, social anxiety, and submissiveness, suggesting that inhibition may be linked more broadly to general anxiety proneness (Mineka & Zinbarg, 1995). Suomi and colleagues have observed that a subset of about 20% of rhesus monkeys, termed "high reactive," are much more prone to develop anxiety syndromes in response to environmental perturbations such as repeated maternal separations (Suomi, 1986, 1987, 1997). The monkeys most likely to succumb show persistent heritable characteristics similar to those of BI children, such as withdrawal and diminished exploration in unfamiliar situations, hesitancy to approach unfamiliar peers, and markers of increased limbic–sympathetic arousal. The presence of BI in other species is consistent with hypotheses linking it to central nervous system structures that developed early in mammalian evolution.

Environmental Influences on Inhibited Temperament

Although BI is moderately heritable, it is also influenced by nongenetic factors. Investigations that model genetic and environmental variance suggest that nonshared environmental influences contribute more to BI than do factors shared by siblings within a family. It has been hypothesized that BI may be decreased by socialization (e.g., parental encouragement to be more outgoing). Indirect support accrues from several studies that find that preservation of extreme inhibition is more common among girls than boys (Hirshfeld et al., 1992; Kerr et al., 1994), suggesting that parents, teachers, and peers may find BI more objectionable in boys and may exert more pressure on boys to be more bold. However, no direct evidence has supported this hypothesis.

The suggestion that BI may be modified environmentally derives from primate studies of similar behaviors. For example, in a cross-fostering study, selectively bred high-reactive rhesus infants fostered by highly nurturant rhesus mothers (i.e., less physically punishing, more nurturant, and more promoting of independence) left their mothers earlier, explored more, and became more socially adept than high-reactive infants fostered by normal mothers and even than nonreactive monkeys (Suomi, 1997). Another primate study suggested that sustained long-term inhibited behaviors and their physiological correlates may be elicited by environmental adversity (Rosenblum et al., 1994): When monkey mothers were periodically and unpredictably required to work several hours per day to obtain full food rations and therefore did not engage in the usual compensatory behaviors following periods of disturbance in the mother–infant connection, their infants exhibited increased timidity, clinging in novel situations, hesitancy to explore, susceptibility to separation distress, and changes in noradrenergic functioning.

Two small studies in humans address the issue of parental influences on BI. Arcus (1991) conducted naturalistic home observations of a small sample of infants in the Boston area classified as high reactive at 4 months and found that maternal responsivity to fretting or crying (holding the infant proportionately more often) at ages 5–7 months was positively associated with higher BI at age 14 months, whereas limit setting (issuing firm prohibitions and removing objects) at ages 9–13 months was associated negatively with BI. She hypothesized that by requiring infants to undergo mild stress or frustration, mothers may have facilitated their developing coping strategies. It is also possible that other factors in this naturalistic study (e.g., maternal anxiety, maternal behaviors elicited by stable infant tendencies) may have accounted for the associations. In a larger study of 125 first-born white boys from intact middle- and working-class families in central Pennsylvania, Belsky, Hsieh, and Crnic (1998) measured positive and negative emotionality from parent reports at age 10 months and from laboratory observations at ages 12 and 13 months, observed parent–child interactions in four home visits from ages 15 to 33 months, and rated BI from laboratory observations at 36 and 37 months. Counterintuitively, they found that among children who showed negative affect in infancy, positive fathering (sensitivity, positive affect, cognitive stimulation, and absence of detachment) in the second year and less negative fathering (based on ratings of intrusiveness and negative affect) in the second and third years predicted BI at age 3 years, with parenting variables accounting for 27% of the variance in BI. They suggest that by pushing the child to change (thus appearing insensitive and intrusive to raters), fathers may have influenced sons to become less inhibited. They caution, however, that it is not known whether such fathering methods might have other negative influences. Moreover, because BI was not rated at ages earlier than 3 years, it is not known whether children's BI may have influenced or elicited fathers' behaviors.

Indeed, other studies have suggested that children's BI may elicit particular parental behaviors and that these behaviors may vary based on the cultural meaning of BI. For example, Hirshfeld, Biederman, Brody, Faraone, and Rosenbaum (1997) found that among children from the Boston area whose mothers had lifetime histories of anxiety disorder, BI was associated with criticism or dissatisfaction with the children, as coded from the Five-Minute Speech Sample of "expressed emotion." Another study found that among Canadian 2-year-olds, laboratory-observed BI was associated positively with mothers' punishment orientation and negatively with acceptance and encouragement (Chen et al., 1998). In contrast, the same study found opposite associations among 2-year-olds from the People's Republic of China, where BI was associated positively with warm and accepting attitudes and negatively with rejection and punishment orientation in the mother. These results suggest that BI is responded to differently by parents of different cultures.

Beyond parental influences, there is evidence that other social factors may influence BI. For example, Asendorpf (1994) found that preschool nonverbal IQ and teacher-rated social competence were inversely associated with the maintenance of laboratory and classroom inhibition 3 years later. He suggested that children who are better able to formulate coping strategies because of higher intelligence or better social competencies may be more competent at reducing their inhibited behavior.

Methodological Issue Concerning the Construct of Behavioral Inhibition

Whereas the evidence for the temperamental basis, moderate stability, and moderate heritability of BI is convincing, some issues require further study. First, the definition, scope, and operationalization of the construct itself could be better clarified. Different investigators have distinguished between inhibition to different novel stimuli, such as nonsocial novelty (objects or settings), novel adults, or novel peers (Kochanska, 1991; Rubin, Hastings, Stewart, Henderson, & Chen, 1997). Rubin and colleagues (1997) found that there was only a moderate tendency for unselected 2-year-olds to show cross-situational consistency to these three types of novelty. Moreover, even when investigators study a corresponding aspect of inhibition (e.g., adult social inhibition), they may operationalize the measures differently. For example, Rubin and colleagues (1997) measured inhibition toward a novel adult based on maintenance of contact with the mother and latencies to approach the adult and interact with her, whereas Kagan, Reznick, and Snidman (1988) also included counts of the child's crying, fretting, distress vocalizations, withdrawals, and absence of spontaneous interactions with the examiner across the battery. Moreover, some investigators include parent-report measures in their aggregates of BI, whereas others rely solely on observed interactions. It would be useful if investigators could agree on standard situations and sets of variables to rate (perhaps a maximally inclusive set to enable maximal examination of correlates of BI), so that findings could be better compared across studies. On the other hand, the general consistency of findings across studies with regard to the stability of BI and its correlates is impressive, given the variability in assessment methods used.

A second, related concern relates to the comparability of measures of BI at different ages. Investigators face the dilemma of keeping assessment protocols developmentally appropriate while capturing the same construct at different ages. Thus it is unclear whether the modest stability noted in BI is due to instability in the trait itself or to inexact correspondence in the observational measures used at different ages. As Turner and Beidel (1996) have observed, it would be helpful to develop batteries with established task equivalency from age to age.

Third, it is unclear how parent- or self-report measures of BI relate to observed measures of BI. Observational measures are objective and do not introduce interpretive biases or social desirability; moreover, they may be better indices of change over time (because they do not rely on an individual's stable perception of a "trait" quality). On the other hand, it might be argued that several brief laboratory observations may not be as accurate as observations summed over time, such as may be derived from the reports of parents, teachers, or peers. Studies that compare parent reports and laboratory measures of shyness or BI typically find low to moderate correlations, ranging from .41 to .60, using selected samples (Fordham & Stevenson-Hinde, 1999; Kagan, Reznick, Clarke, Snidman, & Garcia-Koll, 1984; Kerr et al., 1994) and from .28 to .52 in unselected samples (Asendorpf, 1990; Kerr et al., 1994; Stevenson-Hinde & Shouldice, 1995), with one study finding that agreement with regard to children extreme in inhibition or uninhibition was higher than among the unselected sample as a whole (.60 vs. .42; Kerr et al., 1994). Studies that compare two different constructs, such as parent-completed questionnaire measures of social fearfulness with laboratory observations of BI (Nachmias et al., 1996; Rubin et al., 1997) or parent-rated BI with observed unoccupied and onlooking behaviors during a dyadic peer play (social withdrawal; Asendorpf, 1991), find slightly lower correlations (.22–.33). Additionally, the overlap between BI and other constructs, such as shyness and social withdrawal or isolation, needs further assessment.

Longitudinal studies of BI and its outcomes would benefit from using a variety of multimethod assessments—including different novel stimuli, different means of operationalizing them, moderate length observations (1 hour, not 5–15 minutes), and a variety of observational and parent-, teacher-, or peer-report measures—and determining empirically which methods or combinations of methods afford the best predictive validity. Ideally, such studies would assess BI using task-equivalent comprehensive batteries at multiple ages and would assess related constructs, such as shyness, social isolation, withdrawal, and perhaps attachment quality, as well as hypothesized psychopathological outcome variables.

EVIDENCE FOR HYPOTHESIZED LINKS WITH ANXIETY DISORDERS

A growing number of studies over the past 15 years have suggested that BI represents a precursor to anxiety disorders in children. The evidence stems from studies of BI in children at risk for anxiety disorders, from studies of psychopathology in parents of inhibited children, from studies of psychiatric correlates or outcomes of children with BI, and from retrospective studies of childhood temperament in anxious adults.

Studies of At-Risk Offspring

Children of parents with anxiety disorders such as panic disorder or agoraphobia are known to be at increased risk for developing childhood anxiety disorders themselves (Beidel & Turner, 1997; Biederman, Faraone, et al., 2001; Biederman, Rosenbaum, Bolduc, Faraone, & Hirshfeld, 1991; Merikangas, Avenevoli, Dierker, & Grillon, 1999; Merikangas, Dierker, & Szatmari, 1998; Sylvester, Hyde, & Reichler, 1987; Turner, Beidel, & Costello, 1987; Weissman, Leckman, Merikangas, Gammon, & Prusoff, 1984). Because not all such offspring are affected, however, they represent a population at risk that may be studied for potential risk factors for onset of anxiety. In several studies, BI has been found to have increased prevalence among young offspring of parents with panic disorder and agoraphobia (PDA). In the first study to examine this issue, our research group found that rates of laboratory-observed behavioral inhibition were significantly higher among the 2- to 7-year-old offspring of parents with

PDA than among psychiatric controls ($N = 56$; Rosenbaum et al., 1988). In another small study, Battaglia and colleagues (1997) compared 19 children of parents with panic disorder and 16 children of parents without panic disorder (ages 4–8) on their behavior both during a free period in an unfamiliar room with two unfamiliar adults and while watching neutral and anxiogenic videotapes. The offspring of patients with panic disorder showed significantly longer latencies in making their first spontaneous comment, irrespective of anxiety disorders in the children themselves, and displayed fewer prosocial and exploration behaviors, more distress behaviors, and higher heart rate during the anxiogenic film clips. In an uncontrolled study, Manassis, Bradley, Goldberg, Hood, and Swinson (1995) found high rates of observed BI (65%) in twenty 18- to 59-month-old children of eighteen mothers with panic disorder or other anxiety disorders. However, in a study that used a child self-report measure of BI in an older sample (ages 7–17 years), no differences between offspring of parents with anxiety disorders and comparison offspring were found (Merikangas et al., 1999). Most recently, in a controlled study of a large sample of 2- to 6-year-old children ($N = 284$), we replicated our initial finding of increased BI in the offspring of parents with panic disorder compared with offspring of nonreferred parents without mood or major anxiety disorders (Rosenbaum et al., 2000). In this sample, rates of BI were especially high among offspring of parents with comorbid panic disorder and depression. This study classified children as BI based on observed interactions with unfamiliar adults and toys in unfamiliar rooms, coded for variables that included distress to and avoidance of new toys among younger children and minimal vocalization and smiling at all ages.

Whereas these studies suggest that BI is associated with risk for panic disorder, questions remain as to the specificity of the link between BI and parental panic disorder. The possibility that BI may be linked to familial risk for disorders other than panic disorder has not been ruled out. For example, in our study (Rosenbaum et al., 2000), lifetime history of parental depression was also significantly associated with BI in offspring. Similarly, Kochanska (1991) compared rates of BI (to an unfamiliar setting and unfamiliar female examiner) in eighty-eight 2–3½-year-old children of parents with unipolar and bipolar depression with those in offsping of nondepressed comparisons and found significantly higher rates among children of mothers with unipolar depression, with rates of BI highest among mothers who had been recently depressed. However, in a subsequent study of an expanded sample ($N = 127$) of children assessed at age 5 for inhibition in a 50-minute dyadic peer-play interaction, rates of BI did not differ between offspring of depressed and nondepressed mothers (Kochanska & Radke-Yarrow, 1992). Moreover, one small study ($N = 36$) also found a link to alcoholism, with BI in 4- to 6-year-olds (observed during multiple dyadic peer plays) more prevalent among the offspring of parents with multi-generational, high-density-alcoholism pedigrees than among children from control families (Hill, Lowers, Locke, Snidman, & Kagan, 1999). This sample was highly unusual in that there were virtually no comorbid lifetime anxiety (0%) or depressive (11%) disorders among the parents from the alcohol-abusing families. In contrast, when we restratified the large (N = 284) Rosenbaum and colleagues (2000) sample of offspring of parents with panic disorder and depression and nonclinical comparison offspring, we found no association between BI and parental alcoholism, even in the nonclinical comparison group, despite adequate power to detect differences (Biederman, Hirshfeld-Becker, Rosenbaum, Perenick, et al., 2001).

"Bottom-Up" Studies

In complementary fashion, studies have examined psychopathology among parents of inhibited or shy children. Thus we assessed parents of inhibited children from one of the nonclinical samples followed longitudinally by Kagan, Reznick, and Snidman (1988) and compared them with parents of uninhibited children and of normal nonpsychiatrically ill control children. We found that parents of inhibited children had increased rates of social phobia, retrospectively reported childhood anxiety disorders (mainly overanxious and avoidant disorders), and anxiety disorder history that persisted from childhood to adulthood (Rosenbaum, Biederman, Hirshfeld, Faraone, et al., 1991). Similarly, investigators from another group found that child BI (based upon dyadic peer plays at age 30 months) was associated with low extroversion and sociability and high shyness and avoidance in mothers (Rickman & Davidson, 1994). In a related study, shyness among 4-year-olds (N = 43), based on mother or teacher report, was associated with maternal anxiety disorder in general and social phobia in particular (Cooper & Eke, 1999). Shy children who had no other comorbid problems had mothers with a nearly eightfold increase in lifetime social phobia compared with normal control children. Because children are presumably at heightened risk for the anxiety disorders shown by their parents, these three studies are consistent with the hypothesis that childhood BI may be associated with risk for social anxiety that persists to adulthood.

Studies of Outcome in Children with Behavioral Inhibition

The hypothesis linking BI to anxiety disorders has also been tested in studies that assess inhibited children themselves. For example, our group (Biederman et al., 1990) conducted blind structured clinical interviews (using the Diagnostic Interview for Children and Adolescents—Parent Version

[DICA-P]) about children ages 5–8 years from both the sample of offspring of patients with panic disorder we had studied earlier (Rosenbaum et al., 1988) and the longitudinal cohort studied by Kagan and colleagues from age 21 months on (Garcia-Coll et al., 1984). The inhibited children showed significantly more multiple (≥ 2) DSM-III anxiety disorders, mainly overanxious disorder, avoidant disorder, and phobic disorders. Although the DICA-P did not distinguish between social and specific phobias, the most common feared situations included speaking in class, strangers, and crowds. The association between BI and multiple (≥ 2) anxiety disorders was stronger among children who also had parents with multiple anxiety disorders (Rosenbaum et al., 1992). Furthermore, when the same samples were reassessed at 3-year follow-up, BI prospectively predicted the onset of multiple (≥ 2) anxiety disorders, separation anxiety disorder, and avoidant disorder (Biederman et al., 1993). Stability of BI throughout early childhood (Hirshfeld et al., 1992) in the Kagan and colleagues longitudinal cohort (Garcia-Koll et al., 1984) appeared to increase the risk that an inhibited child would develop anxiety disorders, as well as the chance that the child's parents had a history of anxiety disorders.

In a subsequent follow-up of both this latter (age 21 months) cohort (Garcia-Koll et al., 1984) and a similar one initially ascertained at age 31 months (total N = 79) (Kagan, 1994), children were assessed at age 13 by direct psychiatric interview using modules adapted from the Diagnostic Interview Schedule for Children (DISC) to assess specific fears, separation anxiety, performance anxiety, and generalized social anxiety (Schwartz, Snidman, & Kagan, 1999). Although the authors did not apply DSM-IV criteria, youngsters who had been classified as inhibited as toddlers (at ages 21 or 31 months) were found to have significantly higher rates of current general social anxiety than uninhibited youngsters. No other types of anxiety, including performance anxiety, differed between groups. Generalized social anxiety associated with impairment was significantly higher in inhibited than in uninhibited youngsters (34% vs. 9%, $p < .05$), with the effect more pronounced for girls (44% vs. 6%, $p < .05$).

Assessment of children from our new large sample of children at risk for panic disorder and children of comparison parents, discussed previously (Rosenbaum et al., 2000) has supported the association between BI and social anxiety disorder (Biederman, Hirshfeld-Becker, Rosenbaum, Friedman, et al., 2001). In this sample, although we assessed temperament at ages 2–6 years, we conducted diagnostic assessments (Schedule for Affective Disorders and Schizophrenia for School-Age Children, Epidemiological Version [K-SADS-E] with mothers with DICA–P supplement to assess avoidant disorder), blind to temperamental data, on all children who reached the age of 5 years within the 5-year initial study period. Thus approximately half of the children were assessed within a year of their temperamental observation, and half were evaluated later than that. Despite the limitation of the inclusion of cross-sectional data, the study revealed that BI was significantly and specifically associated with social anxiety (defined as either social phobia or avoidant disorder) and with avoidant disorder alone. Rates of other anxiety disorders did not differ between inhibited and noninhibited children. Although the interaction between temperament and parental diagnostic status in predicting child social anxiety disorder was not significant, the association between BI and avoidant disorder was noted only among the offspring of parents with panic disorder and/or depression.

Hayward, Killen, Kraemer, and Taylor (1998) studied the predictive ability of BI in a longitudinal sample of more than 2,000 high school students recruited in ninth grade and diagnostically interviewed for depression and social phobia at yearly intervals for the next 4 years. Because the study began when children were in ninth grade, BI was assessed retrospectively at that point, using the Retrospective Self-Report of Inhibition (RSRI), which asks about behaviors recalled from grades 1–6 and can be used to derive factors relating to inhibition (Reznick, Hegeman, Kaufman, Woods, & Jacobs, 1992). In this sample, three inhibition scales were derived by factor analysis: fearfulness, social avoidance, and illness behavior. In both males and females, social avoidance was significantly associated with social phobia but not depression, and fearfulness was significantly associated with both social phobia and depression. When the analysis was restricted to participants who had new onset of social phobia during follow-up, participants who scored in the top 15th percentile on both social avoidance and fearfulness were found to have a greater than fivefold increase of developing social phobia than participants who were high on neither. Although the study is limited by the absence of early childhood observations of BI, its results suggest that retrospectively reported BI among ninth graders can predict onset of social phobia during high school. Taken together, these studies cautiously support the hypothesis of a prospective association between BI in early childhood and generalized social phobia in later childhood or early adolescence.

Concurrent Self-Report Studies of Shy or Inhibited Children

Other studies have found that the symptomatic correlates of self-reported BI or shyness in children include a broader range than simply social anxiety. For example, Muris, Merckelbach, Wessel, and van de Ven (1999) examined correlates of self-reported BI in 152 twelve- to fifteen-year-old children in the Netherlands. BI was assessed by using four items querying about shyness, communication, fearfulness, and smiling when talking to "an unfamiliar person" and also by providing the children with descriptions of high-, middle-, and low-inhibited children (based on interactions with an unfamiliar person) and asking them to classify which best described them. Symptoms were assessed with the Screen for Child Anxiety Related Emotional Disorders (SCARED), the Penn State Worry Questionnaire for Children (PSWQ-C), and the Depression Questionnaire for Children (DQC). Eleven percent of children rated themselves as high inhibited. Compared with others, they scored much higher on the SCARED scale measuring social phobia and also scored significantly higher on worries (PSWQ-C), depression (DPQ), and SCARED total score and scales measuring panic disorder, generalized anxiety disorder, social phobia, separation anxiety disorder, obsessive–compulsive disorder (OCD), and blood–injection phobia.

Psychopathological Correlates or Outcome of Shyness and Social Withdrawal in Children

The literature on shyness and social withdrawal in children adds to the conclusion that these qualities may be associated with dysfunction or impairment. For example, among 126 preschoolers in Cambridge, England (ages 4 to 4½ years), high shyness, rated by mothers and observers, was significantly related to concurrent negative mood, fears and worries, and problem behaviors (Stevenson-Hinde & Glover, 1996). In a prospective study, children's composite observed ratings of global shyness, based on observed verbal responsiveness and nonverbal anxiety at ages 4½, 7, and 10 years, were significantly associated at age 10 with lower global self-worth on the Harter Self-Perception Profile and with higher trait anxiety on the State–Trait Anxiety Inventory for Children (Fordham & Stevenson-Hinde, 1999). Similarly, Hymel, Rubin, Rowden, and LeMare (1990) found, among 87 children in the Waterloo Longitudinal Project, that peer-rated social isolation in grade 2 predicted teacher-rated shy–anxious behavior in grade 5, with passive–anxious children showing significantly higher depression and loneliness (Rubin & Mills, 1988). Prior, Smart, Sanson, and Oberklaid (2000) used data from the Australia Temperament Project ($N = 2,443$) to test associations between shyness (approach–sociability) and anxiety disorders in children followed from age 4 months to 14 years. Parent-reported shyness at each age, from 3–4 years up, increased the risk of anxiety problems at ages 13–14 at least twofold. Stability of shyness was associated with higher risk for anxiety, with the most persistently shy children (those who had been in the upper 15% of the sample at 6 or more points) having a 41.5% rate of anxiety problems (anxiety–withdrawal scores on the Revised Behavior Problem Checklist > 1 SD above the mean); children intermediate in persistence of shyness having lower rates (2–3 points, 26.1%; 4–5 points, 21%); and children never or rarely shy having an 11.7% rate.

In contrast, Caspi, Moffitt, Newman, and Silva (1996), in their study of the birth cohort from Dunedin, New Zealand, described earlier, found that children rated by examiners as inhibited at age 3 were significantly more likely than 3-year-olds rated as well adjusted to have depression at age 21 (using the Diagnostic Interview Schedule for DSM-III-R) but had no excess risk for anxiety disorders. This study rated current, but not lifetime, disorders.

Temperamental Correlates of Childhood Anxiety Disorders

In a cross-sectional study, Merikangas, Swendsen, Preisig, and Chazan (1998) and Merikangas and colleagues (1999) found that high-risk children ages 7–17 who had diagnosable DSM-III-R anxiety disorders had higher self-reported symptoms of BI on Reznick's Concurrent Self-Report of Child Inhibition (Reznick et al., 1992) than nonclinical children.

Retrospective Studies of Adults

The association between childhood BI and social phobia in adulthood has also been supported in studies using the RSRI (Reznick et al., 1992). Mick and Telch (1998) found that undergraduates with social anxiety (with or without generalized anxiety) scored significantly higher on total RSRI scores and on the Social Inhibition subscale than those with generalized anxiety or with minimal social anxiety. Moreover, the total RSRI score was significantly correlated with the Social Phobia and Anxiety Inventory (SPAI; Mick & Telch, 1998). In contrast, in a study that did not include a nonanxious control group, van Ameringen and colleagues found no significant differences in RSRI scores among clinic patients with social phobia, panic disorder, and OCD (van Ameringen, Mancini, & Oakman, 1998). Similarly, Reznick and colleagues (1992) administered the RSRI to adults in treatment for panic disorder or depression, as well as to nonclinical controls, and found that both clinical groups had significantly higher RSRI scores than controls.

Methodological Issues Concerning Behavioral Inhibition as a Risk Factor for Anxiety Disorders

The studies summarized previously provide compelling evidence for an association between childhood BI and social anxiety disorders; however, several methodological questions remain to be studied. The first concerns the specificity of the association between BI and social phobia. Whereas multiple studies using different methodologies found clear associations between

BI and social anxiety disorder (Biederman, Hirshfeld-Becker, Rosenbaum, Friedman, et al., 2001; Hayward et al., 1998; Rosenbaum, Biederman, Hirshfeld, Faraone, et al., 1991; Schwartz et al., 1999), other studies have suggested links between BI and panic disorder (Battaglia et al., 1997; Manassis et al., 1995; Reznick et al., 1992; Rosenbaum et al., 1988, 2000), other anxiety disorders in general (Biederman et al., 1990, 1993; Muris et al., 1999), and major depression (Caspi et al., 1996; Kochanska, 1991; Muris et al., 1999; Reznick et al., 1992; Rosenbaum et al., 2000). Considering the significant comorbidity between social phobia and panic disorder (DeRuiter, Rijkin, & Garssen, 1989; Mannuzza, Fyer, Liebowitz, & Klein, 1990; Turner & Beidel, 1989) and the earlier mean age of onset of social phobia, it has been hypothesized that BI may represent an early manifestation of a general anxiety diathesis, which presents as social phobia later in childhood or adolescence and may predispose an individual to panic disorder as the life cycle progresses (Rosenbaum, Biederman, Hirshfeld, Bolduc, & Chaloff, 1991; Rosenbaum et al., 1993; Rosenbaum, Biederman, Pollock, & Hirshfeld, 1994). A similar argument might be made for a general anxiety–depression diathesis, given the clear high comorbidity between social phobia and major depression and the observation that social phobia onset precedes onset of depression (Kessler, Stang, Wittchen, Stein, & Walters, 1999; Regier, Rae, Narrow, Kaelber, & Schatzberg, 1998; Stein, Fuetsch, et al., 2001).

Second, as discussed previously, childhood BI may not be a unitary construct. Inhibition responses to unfamiliar adults, unfamiliar peers, and novel objects or settings are not always correlated and may have different predictive associations with dysfunction (Kochanska, 1991; Kochanska & Radke-Yarrow, 1992; Rubin et al., 1997). Some studies suggest that inhibition to both social and nonsocial stimuli reflects the highest anxiety proneness. For example, Rubin and colleagues (1997) found that toddlers observed to be consistently inhibited in three distinct contexts (nonsocial, adult-social, and peer-social situations) were rated most fearful by their mothers and showed the most distress during observed maternal separations. In contrast, other studies suggest that social inhibition is associated with the greatest dysfunction and impairment (van Ameringen et al., 1998) or that social and nonsocial inhibition lead to differing outcomes (Hayward et al., 1998). Our high-risk studies that found links to parental panic and childhood avoidant disorders mainly measured inhibition in adult-social contexts. To best evaluate hypotheses about the risk conferred by BI, prospective longitudinal studies ought to be conducted using differing observational measures of BI in childhood.

Third, only a minority of children classified as inhibited in early childhood actually developed social anxiety disorder in the studies conducted to date (for example, 43% of early adolescent girls and 22% of boys

[Schwartz et al., 1999]; 17% of 5- to 6-year-old children [Biederman, Hirshfeld-Becker, Rosenbaum, Friedman, et al., 2001]). Moreover, some individuals who were not initially inhibited also developed social anxiety. Therefore, BI is neither a sufficient nor a necessary factor in the development of social phobia, consistent with the recognition by developmental psychopathologists that any given developmental outcome may come about through multiple diverse pathways (the principle of equifinality) and that varied outcomes can result from a common starting point (the principle of multifinality). Research is needed to better understand the moderating factors that might influence which inhibited children develop debilitating social anxiety and which do not. One hypothesis (Biederman, Hirshfeld-Becker, Rosenbaum, Friedman, et al., 2001; Rosenbaum et al., 1992) is that the combination of parental anxiety disorders and BI might put children at risk for social anxiety disorder.

Fourth, BI is not the only candidate for a temperamental precursor to anxiety disorder (Smoller & Tsuang, 1998). Studies of adults have described several anxiety-related traits and temperaments, including neuroticism (Eysenck, 1967), harm avoidance (Cloninger, 1986), trait anxiety, and anxiety sensitivity (McNally, 1996; Reiss, Peterson, Gursky, & McNally, 1986). For example, several studies have suggested that anxiety sensitivity, the tendency to fear anxiety-related sensations and interpret them as signals of impending physical or social catastrophe, increases the likelihood of onset of panic attacks in adults (Schmidt, Lerew, & Jackson, 1999) and adolescents (Hayward, Killen, Kraemer, & Taylor, 2000). Similarly, elevated harm avoidance (the tendency to exhibit anticipatory worry, passive avoidant behaviors, and rapid fatigue) has been observed among first-degree relatives of social phobics (Stein, Chartier, Lizak, & Jang, 2001). Further studies are needed to explore associations between these traits and BI and to explore whether traits other than BI can be measured validly early in childhood and represent precursors to disorder.

RESEARCH DIRECTIONS

As discussed elsewhere (Ollendick & Hirshfeld-Becker, 2002), several different lines of research would be helpful in elucidating the association between BI and anxiety disorders. Longitudinal prospective controlled studies of at-risk children, including large numbers of offspring of parents with social phobia, panic disorder, major depression, and other disorders that might be tested for links to BI (e.g., alcohol use disorders) would be useful to assess associations with parental disorders and course of psychopathology in children. Ideally, such studies would begin in infancy or toddlerhood and would periodically assess children temperamentally and diagnostically (observing inhibited responses to a variety of contexts and supplementing observations with parent, teacher, and perhaps peer reports), as well as monitoring the course of parental symptoms, parenting behaviors, and peer and sibling influences. To understand the genetic risk conferred by BI and its association with risk for anxiety disorders, it would be helpful to conduct twin studies that would assess both BI and DSM-IV childhood anxiety disorders and model associations between these factors (Goldsmith & Lemery, 2000). To best understand the effects of environmental moderators on the course and outcome of BI, one would ideally conduct adoption studies of at-risk children (i.e., either children with biological parents known to have anxiety or mood disorders or children with BI) in which biological and adoptive parents, as well as children, could be assessed temperamentally and diagnostically and adoptive family environment variables could also be assessed. The increase in open adoptions might potentially make such a study more feasible. Additionally, our understanding of both the malleability of BI and its link to social anxiety disorder could be enhanced through intervention studies with at-risk offspring with BI, in which factors thought to contribute to onset of social phobia were targeted and intervened with and child outcome measured. Although intervention studies cannot clarify etiology, they can shed light on maintaining factors and on ways to prevent or mitigate the course of social anxiety. Intervention approaches might include behavioral or psychopharmacological interventions with the children themselves (Beidel, Turner, & Morris, 2000; Kendall & Southam-Gerow, 1996; Silverman et al., 1999), parental anxiety management (Cobham, Dadds, & Spence, 1998), parental coaching in helping the young child manage BI and social anxiety (currently under study by Rapee and colleagues and by Hirshfeld-Becker and colleagues), peer modeling (Beidel et al., 2000), or dyadic peer interventions. In addition, researchers ought to develop creative ways to operationalize and observe other trait-like anxiety precursors, including neuroticism, harm avoidance, and anxiety sensitivity in young children, so that these constructs can be compared for overlap with BI and can be tested as precursors to other anxiety disorders. It may well be that BI predisposes to social phobia and possibly to subsequent comorbid conditions (such as depression and panic disorder), whereas other prodromes are linked to other anxiety conditions.

CLINICAL IMPLICATIONS

Parents and clinicians should recognize that some toddlers and preschoolers with BI, particularly those with family history of anxiety disorders and stable inhibition, may carry increased risk for anxiety disorders, in particular social phobia. These children should be monitored, and early intervention should be considered in cases in which anxiety symptoms impair functioning. Intervention could include advice to parents on anxiety management strategies, on promoting child coping and graduated exposure to feared situations, and on not facilitating avoidant coping. Trials of such approaches are underway, with the hope that manualized preventive interventions for young inhibited youngsters will ultimately be available.

ACKNOWLEDGMENTS

We acknowledge Sara Calltharp, Lynette Dufton, and Jennifer Gilbert for their assistance with this chapter.

REFERENCES

Adamec, R., & Stark-Adamec, C. (1989). Behavioral inhibition and anxiety: Dispositional, developmental and neural aspects of the anxious personality of the domestic cat. In J. Reznick (Ed.), *Perspectives on behavioral inhibition* (pp. 93–124). Chicago: University of Chicago Press.

Arcus, D. M. (1991). *The experiential modification of temperamental bias in inhibited and uninhibited children.* Unpublished doctoral dissertation, Harvard University.

Asendorpf, J. (1994). The malleability of behavioral inhibition: A study of individual developmental functions. *Developmental Psychology, 30*(6), 912–919.

Asendorpf, J. B. (1990). Development of inhibition during childhood: Evidence for situational specificity and a two-factor model. *Developmental Psychology, 26*(5), 721–730.

Asendorpf, J. B. (1991). Development of inhibited children's coping with unfamiliarity. *Child Development, 62*(6), 1460–1474.

Battaglia, M., Bajo, S., Strambi, L. F., Brambilla, F., Castronovo, C., Vanni, G., & Bellodi, L. (1997). Physiological and behavioral responses to minor stressors in offspring of patients with panic disorder. *Journal of Psychiatric Research, 31*(3), 365–376.

Beidel, D., & Turner, S. (1997). At risk for anxiety: I. Psychopathology in the offspring of anxious parents. *Journal of the American Academy of Child and Adolescent Psychiatry, 36*(7), 918–924.

Beidel, D. C., Turner, S. M., & Morris, T. L. (2000). Behavioral treatment of childhood social phobia. *Journal of Consulting and Clinical Psychology, 68*(6), 1072–1080.

Belsky, J., Hsieh, K.-H., & Crnic, K. (1998). Mothering, fathering, and infant negativity as antecedents of boys' externalizing problems and inhibition at age 3 years: Differential susceptibility to rearing experience? *Development and Psychopathology, 10*, 301–319.

Biederman, J., Faraone, S., Hirshfeld-Becker, D., Friedman, D., Robin, J., & Rosenbaum, J. (2001). Patterns of psychopathology and dysfunction in a large sample of high-risk children of parents with panic disorder and major depression: A controlled study. *American Journal of Psychiatry, 158*(1), 49–57.

Biederman, J., Hirshfeld-Becker, D. R., Rosenbaum, J. F., Friedman, D., Snidman, N., Kagan, J., & Faraone, S. V. (2001). Further evidence of association between behavioral inhibition and social anxiety in children. *American Journal of Psychiatry, 158*(10), 1673–1679.

Biederman, J., Hirshfeld-Becker, D. R., Rosenbaum, J. F., Perenick, S. G., Wood, J., & Faraone, S. V. (2001). Lack of association between parental alcohol or drug addiction and behavioral inhibition in children. *American Journal of Psychiatry, 158*(10), 1731–1733.

Biederman, J., Rosenbaum, J. F., Bolduc, E. A., Faraone, S. V., & Hirshfeld, D. R. (1991). A high-risk study of young children of parents with panic disorder and agoraphobia with and without major depression. *Psychiatry Research, 37,* 333–348.

Biederman, J., Rosenbaum, J. F., Bolduc-Murphy, E. A., Faraone, S. V., Chaloff, J., Hirshfeld, D. R., & Kagan, J. (1993). A 3–year follow-up of children with and without behavioral inhibition. *Journal of the American Academy of Child and Adolescent Psychiatry, 32*(4), 814–821.

Biederman, J., Rosenbaum, J. F., Hirshfeld, D. R., Faraone, S. V., Bolduc, E. A., Gersten, M., Meminger, S. R., Kagan, J., Snidman, N., & Reznick, J. S. (1990). Psychiatric correlates of behavioral inhibition in young children of parents with and without psychiatric disorders. *Archives of General Psychiatry, 47,* 21–26.

Broberg, A., Lamb, M., & Hwang, P. (1990). Inhibition: Its stability and correlates in sixteen- to forty-month-old children. *Child Development, 61,* 1153–1163.

Calkins, S. D., Fox, N. A., & Marshall, T. R. (1996). Behavioral and physiological antecedents of inhibited and uninhibited behavior. *Child Development, 67,* 523–540.

Caspi, A., Bem, D. J., & Elder, G. H. (1989). Continuities and consequences of interactional styles across the life course. *Journal of Personality, 57*(2), 375–406.

Caspi, A., Moffitt, T. E., Newman, D. L., & Silva, P. A. (1996). Behavioral observations at age 3 years predict adult psychiatric disorders. *Archives of General Psychiatry, 53*(11), 1033–1039.

Caspi, A., & Silva, P. A. (1995). Temperamental qualities at age 3 predict personality traits in young adulthood: Longitudinal evidence from a birth cohort. *Child Development, 66,* 486–498.

Chen, X., Hastings, P. D., Rubin, K. H., Chen, H., Cen, G., & Stewart, S. (1998). Child-rearing attitudes and behavioral inhibition in Chinese and Canadian toddlers: A cross-cultural study. *Developmental Psychology, 34*(4), 677–686.

Cloninger, C. (1986). A unified biosocial theory of personality and its role in the development of anxiety states. *Psychiatric Development, 3,* 167–226.

Cobham, V., Dadds, M., & Spence, S. (1998). The role of parental anxiety in the treatment of childhood anxiety. *Journal of Consulting and Clinical Psychology, 66*(6), 893–905.

Cooper, P. J., & Eke, M. (1999). Childhood shyness and maternal social phobia: A community study. *British Journal of Psychiatry, 174,* 439–443.

Davidson, R. (1992). Emotion and affective style: Hemispheric substrates. *Psychological Science, 3*(1), 39–43.

Davidson, R. (1994). Asymmetric brain function, affective style, and psychopathology: The role of early experience and plasticity. *Development and Psychopathology, 6,* 741–758.

DeRuiter, C., Rijkin, H., & Garssen, B. (1989). Comorbidity among the anxiety disorders. *Journal of Anxiety Disorders, 3,* 57–68.

Dettling, A. C., Gunnar, M. R., & Donzella, B. (1999). Cortisol levels of young children in full-day childcare centers: Relations with age and temperament. *Psychoneuroendocrinology, 24,* 519–536.

DiLalla, L. F., Kagan, J., & Reznick, J. S. (1994). Genetic etiology of behavioral inhibition among 2–year-old children. *Infant Behavior and Development, 17,* 405–412.

Emde, R. N., Plomin, R., Robinson, J., Corley, R., DeFries, J., Fulker, D. W., Reznick, J. S., Campos, J., Kagan, J., & Zahn-Waxler, C. (1992). Temperament, emotion, and cognition at fourteen months: The MacArthur Longitudinal Twin Study. *Child Development, 63,* 1437–1455.

Eysenck, H. (1967). *Biological bases of personality.* Springfield, IL: Thomas.

Fordham, K., & Stevenson-Hinde, J. (1999). Shyness, friendship quality, and adjustment during middle childhood. *Journal of Child Psychology and Psychiatry, 40*(5), 757–768.

Garcia-Coll, C., Kagan, J., & Reznick, J. S. (1984). Behavioral inhibition in young children. *Child Development, 55,* 1005–1019.

Gersten, M. (1989). Behavioral inhibition in the classroom. In J. Resnick (Ed.), *Perspectives on behavioral inhibition* (pp. 71–91). Chicago: University of Chicago Press.

Gest, S. D. (1997). Behavioral inhibition: Stability and associations with adaptation from childhood to early adulthood. *Journal of Personality and Social Psychology, 72*(2), 467–475.

Goldsmith, H. H., & Lemery, K. S. (2000). Linking temperamental fearfulness and anxiety symptoms: A behavior-genetic perspective. *Biological Psychiatry, 48*(12), 1199–1209.

Gray, J. (1982). *The neuropsychology of anxiety: An enquiry into the functions of the septohippocampal system.* Oxford, UK: Clarendon Press.

Gray, J. A. (1991). Neural systems, emotion and personality. In J. Madden IV (Ed.), *Neurobiology of learning, emotion, and affect* (pp. 273–306). New York: Raven Press.

Gray, J. A., & McNaughton, N. (1996). The neuropsychiatry of anxiety: Reprise. In D. Hope (Ed.), *Nebraska Symposium on Motivation: Vol. 43. Perspectives on anxiety, panic, and fear* (pp. 61–134). Lincoln: University of Nebraska Press.

Harris, G., Hoehn-Saric, R., Lewis, R., Pearlson, G., & Streeter, C. (1994). Mapping of SPECT regional cerebral perfusion abnormalities in obsessive–compulsive disorder. *Human Brain Mapping, 1,* 237–248.

Hayward, C., Killen, J., Kraemer, H. C., & Taylor, C. B. (1998). Linking self-reported childhood behavioral inhibition to adolescent social phobia. *Journal of the American Academy of Child and Adolescent Psychiatry, 37*(12), 1308–1316.

Hayward, C., Killen, J. D., Kraemer, H. C., & Taylor, C. B. (2000). Predictors of panic attacks in adolescents. *Journal of the American Academy of Child and Adolescent Psychiatry, 39*(2), 207–214.

Hill, S. J., Lowers, L., Locke, J., Snidman, N., & Kagan, J. (1999). Behavioral inhibition in children from families at high risk for developing alcoholism. *Journal of the American Academy of Child and Adolescent Psychiatry, 38*(4), 410–420.

Hirshfeld, D. R., Biederman, J., Brody, L., Faraone, S. V., & Rosenbaum, J. F. (1997). Expressed emotion toward children with and without behavioral inhibition: Associations with maternal anxiety disorders. *Journal of the American Academy of Child and Adolescent Psychiatry, 36,* 910–917

Hirshfeld, D. R., Rosenbaum, J. F., Biederman, J., Bolduc, E. A., Faraone, S. V., Snidman, N., Reznick, J. S., & Kagan, J. (1992). Stable behavioral inhibition and its association with anxiety disorder. *Journal of the American Academy of Child and Adolescent Psychiatry, 31*(1), 103–111.

Hymel, S., Rubin, K., Rowden, L., & LeMare, L. (1990). Children's peer relationships: Longitudinal prediction of internalizing and externalizing problems from middle to late childhood. *Child Development, 61,* 2004–2021.

Jorm, A. F., Henderson, A. S., Jacomb, P. A., Christensen, H., Korten, A. E., Rodgers, B., Tan, X., & Easteal, S. (1998). An association study of a functional polymorphism of the serotonin transporter gene with personality and psychiatric symptoms. *Molecular Psychiatry, 3*(5), 449–451.

Jorm, A. F., Prior, M., Sanson, A., Smart, D., Zhang, Y., & Easteal, S. (2000). Association of a functional polymorphism of the serotonin gene with anxiety-related temperament and behavior problems in children: A longitudinal study from infancy to the mid-teens. *Molecular Psychiatry, 5*(5), 542–547.

Kagan, J. (1994). *Galen's prophecy: Temperament in human nature.* New York: Basic Books.

Kagan, J., Arcus, D., Snidman, N., Feng, W. Y., Hendler, J., & Greene, S. (1994). Reactivity in infants: A cross-national comparison. *Developmental Psychology, 30,* 342–345.

Kagan, J., Reznick, J. S., Clarke, C., Snidman, N., & Garcia-Coll, C. (1984). Behavioral inhibition to the unfamiliar. *Child Development, 55,* 2212–2225.

Kagan, J., Reznick, J. S., & Snidman, N. (1988). Biological bases of childhood shyness. *Science, 240,* 167–171.

Kagan, J., Reznick, J. S., Snidman, N., Gibbons, J., & Johnson, M. O. (1988). Childhood derivatives of inhibition and lack of inhibition to the unfamiliar. *Child Development, 59*(6), 1580–1589.

Kagan, J., Snidman, N., Zetner, M., & Peterson, E. (1999). Infant temperament and anxious symptoms in school age children. *Development and Psychopathology, 11,* 209–224.

Kendall, P. C., & Southam-Gerow, M. A. (1996). Long-term follow-up of a cognitive-behavioral therapy for anxiety disordered youth. *Journal of Consulting and Clinical Psychology, 64*(4), 724–730.

Kerr, M., Lambert, W. W., Stattin, H., & Klackenberg-Larsson, I. (1994). Stability of inhibition in a Swedish longitudinal sample. *Child Development, 65,* 138–146.

Kessler, R. C., Stang, P., Wittchen, H. U., Stein, M., & Walters, E. E. (1999). Lifetime comorbidities between social phobia and mood disorders in the US National Comorbidity Survey. *Psychological Medicine, 29*(3), 555–567.

Kochanska, G. (1991). Patterns of inhibition to the unfamiliar in children of normal and affectively ill mothers. *Child Development, 62,* 250–263.

Kochanska, G., & Radke-Yarrow, M. (1992). Inhibition in toddlerhood and the dynamics of the child's interaction with an unfamiliar peer at age five. *Child Development, 63,* 325–335.

Manassis, K., Bradley, S., Goldberg, S., Hood, J., & Swinson, R. (1995). Behavioural inhibition, attachment and anxiety in children of mothers with anxiety disorders. *Canadian Journal of Psychiatry, 40,* 87–92.

Mannuzza, S., Fyer, A., Liebowitz, M., & Klein, D. (1990). Delineating the boundaries of social phobia: Its relationship to panic disorder and agoraphobia. *Journal of Anxiety Disorders, 4,* 41–59.

Marshall, P. J., & Stevenson-Hinde, J. (1998). Behavioral inhibition, heart period, and respiratory sinus arrythmia in young children. *Developmental Psychobiology, 33,* 283–292.

Matheny, A. P. (1989). Children's behavioral inhibition over age and across situations: Genetic similarity for a trait during change. *Journal of Personality, 57*(2), 215–235.

McNally, R. J. (1996). Anxiety sensitivity is distinguishable from trait anxiety. In R. M. Rapee (Ed.), *Current controversies in the anxiety disorders* (pp. 214–227). New York: Guilford Press.

Merikangas, K. R., Avenevoli, S., Dierker, L., & Grillon, C. (1999). Vulnerability factors among children at risk for anxiety disorders. *Biological Psychiatry, 46*(11), 1523–1535.

Merikangas, K. R., Dierker, L. C., & Szatmari, P. (1998). Psychopathology among offspring of parents with substance abuse and/or anxiety disorders: A high-risk study. *Journal of Child Psychology and Psychiatry, 39*(5), 711–720.

Merikangas, K. R., Swendsen, J. D., Preisig, M. A., & Chazan, R. Z. (1998). Psychopathology and temperament in parents and offspring: Results of a family study. *Journal of Affective Disorders, 51*(1), 63–74.

Mick, M., & Telch, M. (1998). Social anxiety and history of behavioral inhibition in young adults. *Journal of Anxiety Disorders, 12*(1), 1–20.

Mineka, S., & Zinbarg, R. (1995). Conditioning and ethological models of social phobia. In R. G. Heimberg, M. R. Liebowitz, D. A. Hope, & F. R. Schneier (Eds.), *Social phobia: Diagnosis, assessment, and treatment* (pp. 134–162). New York: Guilford Press.

Muris, P., Merckelbach, H., Wessel, I., & van de Ven, M. (1999). Psychopathological correlates of self-reported behavioural inhibition in normal children. *Behaviour Research and Therapy, 37*(6), 575–584.

Nachmias, M., Gunnar, M., Mangelsdorf, S., Hornik Parritz, R., & Buss, K. (1996). Behavioral inhibition and stress reactivity: The moderating role of attachment security. *Child Development, 67,* 508–522.

Ollendick, T. H., & Hirshfeld-Becker, D. R. (2002). The developmental psychopathology of social anxiety disorders. *Biological Psychiatry, 51,* 44–58.

Plomin, R., Emde, R., Braungart, J., Campos, J., Corley, R., Fulker, D., Kagan, J., Reznick, J., Robinson, J., Zahn-Waxler, C., & DeFries, J. (1993). Genetic change and continuity from fourteen to twenty months: The MacArthur Longitudinal Twin Study. *Child Development, 64,* 1354–1376.

Prior, M., Smart, D., Sanson, A., & Oberklaid, F. (2000). Does shy-inhibited temperament in childhood lead to anxiety problems in adolescence? *Journal of the American Academy of Child and Adolescent Psychiatry, 39*(4), 461–468.

Regier, D. A., Rae, D. S., Narrow, W. E., Kaelber, C. T., & Schatzberg, A. F. (1998). Prevalence of anxiety disorders and their comorbidity with mood and addictive disorders. *British Journal of Psychiatry, 34*(Suppl.), 24–28.

Reiman, E., Raichle, M., Butler, F., Hercovitch, P., & Robins, E. (1984). A focal brain abnormality in panic disorder, a severe form of anxiety. *Nature, 310,* 683–685.

Reiss, S., Peterson, R. A., Gursky, M., & McNally, R. J. (1986). Anxiety sensitivity, anxiety frequency, and the prediction of fearfulness. *Behaviour Research and Therapy, 24,* 1–8.

Reznick, J. S., Hegeman, I. M., Kaufman, E., Woods, S. W., & Jacobs, M. (1992). Retrospective and concurrent self-reports of behavioral inhibition and their relation to adult mental health. *Development and Psychopathology, 4,* 301–321.

Rickman, M., & Davidson, R. (1994). Personality and behavior in parents of temperamentally inhibited and uninhibited children. *Developmental Psychology, 30*(3), 346–354.

Robinson, J. L., Kagan, J., Reznick, J. S., & Corley, R. (1992). The heritability of inhibited and uninhibited behavior: A twin study. *Developmental Psychology, 28*(6), 1030–1037.

Rosenbaum, J., Biederman, J., Hirshfeld, D., Bolduc, E., & Chaloff, J. (1991). Behavioral inhibition in children: A possible precursor to panic disorder or social phobia. *Journal of Clinical Psychiatry, 52*(11, Suppl.), 5–9.

Rosenbaum, J. F., Biederman, J., Bolduc, E. A., Hirshfeld, D. R., Faraone, S. V., & Kagan, J. (1992). Comorbidity of parental anxiety disorders as risk for child-onset anxiety in inhibited children. *American Journal of Psychiatry, 149,* 475–478.

Rosenbaum, J. F., Biederman, J., Bolduc-Murphy, E. A., Faraone, S. V., Chaloff, J., Hirshfeld, D. R., & Kagan, J. (1993). Behavioral inhibition in childhood: A risk factor for anxiety disorders. *Harvard Review of Psychiatry, 1,* 2–16.

Rosenbaum, J. F., Biederman, J., Gersten, M., Hirshfeld, D. R., Meminger, S. R., Herman, J. B., Kagan, J., Reznick, J. S., & Snidman, N. (1988). Behavioral inhibition in children of parents with panic disorder and agoraphobia: A controlled study. *Archives of General Psychiatry, 45,* 463–470.

Rosenbaum, J. F., Biederman, J., Hirshfeld, D. R., Faraone, S. V., Bolduc, E. A., Kagan, J., Snidman, N., & Reznick, J. S. (1991). Further evidence of an association between behavioral inhibition and anxiety disorders: Results from a family study of children from a non-clinical sample. *Journal of Psychiatric Research, 25*(25), 49–65.

Rosenbaum, J. F., Biederman, J., Hirshfeld-Becker, D. R., Kagan, J., Snidman, N., Friedman, D., Nineberg, A., Gallery, D. J., & Faraone, S. V. (2000). A controlled study of behavioral inhibition in children of parents with panic disorder and depression. *American Journal of Psychiatry, 157*(12), 2002–2010.

Rosenbaum, J. F., Biederman, J., Pollock, R. A., & Hirshfeld, D. R. (1994). The etiology of social phobia. *Journal of Clinical Psychiatry, 55*(Suppl.), 10–16.

Rosenblum, L., Coplan, J., Friedman, S., Bassoff, T., Gorman, J., & Andrews, M. (1994). Adverse early experiences affect noradrenergic and serotonergic functioning in adult primates. *Biological Psychiatry, 35,* 221–227.

Rubin, K., Hastings, P., Stewart, S., Henderson, H., & Chen, X. (1997). The consistency and concomitants of inhibition: Some of the children, all of the time. *Child Development, 68*(3), 467–483.

Rubin, K., & Mills, R. (1988). The many faces of social isolation in childhood. *Journal of Consulting and Clinical Psychology, 56*(6), 916–924.

Scarpa, A., Raine, A., Venables, P., & Mednick, S. (1995). The stability of inhibited/uninhibited temperament from ages 3 to 11 years in Mauritian children. *Journal of Abnormal Child Psychology, 23*(5), 607–618.

Schmidt, L. A., Fox, N. A., Rubin, K. H., Sternberg, E. M., Gold, P. W., Smith, C. C., & Schulkin, J. (1997). Behavioral and neuroendocrine responses in shy children. *Developmental Psychobiology, 30,* 127–140.

Schmidt, L. A., Fox, N. A., Schulkin, J., & Gold, P. W. (1999). Behavioral and psychophysiological correlates of self-presentation in temperamentally shy children. *Developmental Psychobiology, 35,* 119–135.

Schmidt, N. B., Lerew, D. R., & Jackson, R. J. (1999). Prospective evaluation of anxiety sensitivity in the pathogenesis of panic: Replication and extension. *Journal of Abnormal Psychology, 108*(3), 532–537.

Schwartz, C., Snidman, N., & Kagan, J. (1999). Adolescent social anxiety as an outcome of inhibited temperament in childhood. *Journal of the American Academy of Child and Adolescent Psychiatry, 38*(8), 1008–1015.

Silverman, W. K., Kurtines, W. M., Ginsburg, G. S., Weems, C. F., Lumpkin, P. W., & Carmichael, D. H. (1999). Treating anxiety disorders in children with group cognitive-behavioral therapy: A randomized clinical trial. *Journal of Consulting and Clinical Psychology, 67*(6), 995–1003.

Smoller, J. W., Rosenbaum, J. F., Biederman, J., Susswein, L. S., Kennedy, J., Kagan, J., Snidman, N., Laird, N., Tsuang, M. T., Faraone, S. V., Schwarz, A., & Slaugenhaupt, S. A. (2001). Genetic association analysis of behavioral inhibition using candidate loci from mouse models. *American Journal of Medical Genetics (Neuropsychiatric Genetics), 105,* 226–235.

Smoller, J. W., & Tsuang, M. T. (1998). Panic and phobic anxiety: Defining phenotypes for genetic studies. *American Journal of Psychiatry, 155*(9), 1152–1162.

St. Lorant, T. A., Henderson, L., & Zimbardo, P. G. (2000). Comorbidity in chronic shyness. *Depression and Anxiety, 12,* 232–237.

Stein, M. B., Chartier, M. J., Lizak, M. V., & Jang, K. L. (2001). Familial aggregation of anxiety-related quantitative traits in generalized social phobia: Clues to understanding "disorder" heritability? *American Journal of Medical Genetics (Neuropsychiatric Genetics), 105*(1), 79–83.

Stein, M. B., Fuetsch, M., Muller, N., Hofler, M., Lieb, R., & Wittchen, H. U. (2001). Social anxiety disorder and the risk of depression: A prospective community study of adolescents and young adults. *Archives of General Psychiatry, 58*(3), 251–256.

Stevenson-Hinde, J., & Glover, A. (1996). Shy girls and boys: A new look. *Journal of Child Psychology and Psychiatry, 37*(2), 181–187.

Stevenson-Hinde, J., & Shouldice, A. (1995). 4.5 to 7 years: Fearful behavior, fears and worries. *Journal of Child Psychology and Psychiatry, 36*(6), 1027–1038.

Suomi, S. (1987). Genetic and maternal contributions to individual differences in rhesus monkey biobehavioral development. In N. A. Krasnegor, E. M. Blass, M. A.

Hofer, & W. P. Smotherman (Eds.), *Perinatal development: A psychobiological perspective* (pp. 397–419). New York: Academic Press.

Suomi, S. J. (1986). Anxiety-like disorders in young nonhuman primates. In R. Gittelman (Ed.), *Anxiety disorders of childhood* (pp. 1–23). New York: Guilford Press.

Suomi, S. J. (1997). Early determinants of behaviour: Evidence from primate studies. *British Medical Bulletin, 53*(1), 170–184.

Sylvester, C. E., Hyde, T. S., & Reichler, R. J. (1987). The Diagnostic Interview for Children and Personality Inventory for Children in studies of children at risk for anxiety disorders or depression. *Journal of the American Academy of Child and Adolescent Psychiatry, 26*(5), 668–675.

Tout, K., de Haan, M., Campbell, E. K., & Gunnar, M. R. (1998). Social behavior correlates of adrenocortical activity in daycare: Gender differences and time-of-day effects. *Child Development, 69*, 1247–1262.

Turner, S., & Beidel, D. (1989). Social phobia: Clinical syndrome, diagnosis and comorbidity. *Clinical Psychology Review, 9*, 3–18.

Turner, S., & Beidel, D. (1996). Is behavioral inhibition related to the anxiety disorders? *Clinical Psychology Review, 16*(2), 157–172.

Turner, S. M., Beidel, D. C., & Costello, A. (1987). Psychopathology in the offspring of anxiety disorders patients. *Journal of Consulting and Clinical Psychology, 55*(2), 229–235.

van Ameringen, M., Mancini, C., & Oakman, J. (1998). The relationship of behavioral inhibition and shyness to anxiety disorder. *Journal of Nervous and Mental Disease, 186*, 425–431.

Weissman, M. M., Leckman, J. F., Merikangas, K. R., Gammon, G. D., & Prusoff, B. A. (1984). Depression and anxiety disorders in parents and children: Results from the Yale family study. *Archives of General Psychiatry, 41*, 845–852.

Chapter 3

Social Development

TRACY L. MORRIS

Social factors related to the development of anxiety disorders in children have received renewed research attention over the past decade. Publications addressing the influence of parents and peers on the development and maintenance of anxiety have been appearing with ever increasing frequency in recent years. In this time frame we have also witnessed the growing prominence of *developmental psychopathology* (Cicchetti & Cohen, 1995). Kazdin (1989) described developmental psychopathology as "the study of clinical dysfunction over the course of development" (p. 180). The developmental psychopathology perspective constitutes a guiding framework through which information from diverse fields (e.g., behavior genetics, learning theory, developmental psychology, etc.) may be integrated to provide a more complete conceptualization of the origin and course of disorders across the lifespan. The perspective stresses the assumptions of multicausality and multifinality—essentially the notion that there are multiple entry points (i.e., risk factors) that may place a child on the path toward anxiety disorder and, conversely, multiple points at which a child may be diverted from the path (i.e., protective factors). Importantly, associations are not all considered linear, and the possibility of multiple entry points allows for tremendous diversity in individual etiological pathways.

By way of illustration, one potential pathway to social anxiety disorder would be that of a behaviorally inhibited infant being reared by an anxious parent who is unable to appropriately attend to the child's needs in a warm and responsive fashion. Poor fit between parent and child temperament styles may result in diminished quality of infant–caregiver attachment (Thomas & Chess, 1977). As the parent–child relationship serves as the model on which all other social relationships are formed, this inhibited and poorly attached child may have difficulty initiating and maintaining successful peer interactions. Social withdrawal and isolation from peers further restricts the child's opportunities for establishing and practicing effective social skills. This process serves to increase the child's inhibition and discomfort in social settings, thus perpetuating a vicious cycle.

Although issues of multicausality present a methodological challenge to our understanding of the etiology of anxiety disorders, we must keep in mind that multicausality also allows for multiple opportunities for intervention at virtually any developmental stage. However, given that the effects of risk factors tend to compound over time, interventions provided earlier in an individual's life course may have a greater likelihood for success.

This chapter provides a brief overview of the relevant literature with respect to the primary influences on children's social development: parents and peers. For a more extended discussion of processes related to the development of anxiety, the reader is referred to Vasey and Dadds (2001) and to other chapters in this volume.

PARENT–CHILD INTERACTION

Attachment

Children's earliest social interactions occur with their primary caregivers. Parent–child attachment has been the focus of much theoretical and empirical inquiry. Ainsworth, Blehar, Waters, and Wall (1978) identified three specific patterns of infant–caregiver attachment—secure, insecure–ambivalent, and insecure–avoidant—based on responses to the classic "Strange Situation" laboratory task. The "Strange Situation" entails observation of the infant or toddler's behavior during a series of separations and reunions with the caregiver, as well as his or her interactions with a stranger both in the presence and in the absence of the caregiver (Ainsworth, Bell, & Stayton, 1972). A considerable body of research has demonstrated associations between insecure infant–child attachment and later development of psychiatric disorders (e.g., Erickson, Sroufe, & Egeland, 1985; Kobak, Sudler, & Gamble, 1991; Muris & Meesters, 2002). For example, Warren, Huston, Egeland, and Sroufe (1997) evaluated 172 adolescents who had participated in the Strange Situation 16 years earlier (i.e., at 12 months of age). Not surprisingly anxious–resistant attachment style in infancy was associated with increased risk for anxiety disorders in childhood and adolescence (28% of the anxious–resistant infants, 16% of the avoidant infants, and 11% of securely attached infants met criteria for an anxiety disorder). Furthermore, attachment classification predicted anxiety disorder over and above measures of maternal anxiety and infant temperament. Although most of the attachment literature has focused on infant–caregiver attachment, increased attention is being paid to parent–adolescent attachment and to adult romantic attachment (Armsden & Greenberg, 1987; Berman, Heiss, & Sperling, 1994; Hazan & Shaver, 1987; Van IJzendoorn & Bakermans-Kranenburg, 1996).

Parenting Style

Childhood anxiety has been associated with parenting styles characterized by limited expressions of care and warmth and extreme displays of control and overprotection (e.g., Duggan, Sham, Minne, Lee, & Murray, 1998; Wiborg & Dahl, 1997). Although most of the research in this area has been retrospective in nature (e.g., Arrindell, Emmelkamp, Monsma, & Brilman, 1983; Arrindell et al., 1989), the observational studies of parent–child interaction conducted to date have yielded similar results (e.g., Hudson & Rapee, 2001; Hummel & Gross, 2001). Krohne and Hock (1991) observed mother–child dyads working together on a puzzle task and found mothers of high-anxious girls to be more controlling than were mothers of low-anxious girls. Dumas, LaFreniere, and Serketich (1995) found a pattern of bidirectional influence, with mothers of anxious children attempting to control their children by being coercive and unresponsive and anxious children trying to manage their mothers by being resistant and coercive. Similarly, Greco and Morris (2002) observed that fathers of highly socially anxious children exhibited more controlling behavior during an origami task than fathers of children who evinced low levels of social anxiety. Notably, children in the high-social-anxiety versus low-social-anxiety groups did not differ from one another in their responses toward their fathers during the task.

Family Sociability

Developmentalists have established a strong foundation of research related to parental influence on children's social development (Booth, Rose-Krasnor, McKinnon, & Rubin, 1994; Cohn, Patterson, & Christopoulos, 1991; Darling & Steinberg, 1993; Profilet & Ladd, 1994; Russell & Finnie, 1990). Young children are almost entirely dependent on their parents in terms of opportunities for social interaction (Bhavnagri & Parke, 1991; Bryant & DeMorris, 1992; Ladd, Profilet, & Hart, 1992; Putallaz &

Hefflin, 1990). That being the case, it is not a far reach to propose that parents who are anxious in social situations may be less likely to facilitate their children's social engagement. Indeed, parental reports of their own social networks have been found to be associated with the extent of their children's social networks (e.g., number of playmates, quality of after-school activities, self-reported loneliness). Adults with social phobia characterize their parents as less socially engaged and more socially avoidant than do normal controls (Bruch & Heimberg, 1994; Bruch, Heimberg, Berger, & Collins, 1989; Rapee & Melville, 1997).

It is commonly accepted that children of parents with anxiety disorders are themselves at risk for the development of anxiety disorders. Parents with anxiety disorders inevitably model poor coping strategies and engage in behavior that may promote heightened states of arousal and hypervigilance. Dadds, Barrett, and colleagues have conducted a series of investigations that provide support for the role of parental influence in the development of anxiety. In these studies, parents of anxious children were more likely to model threat interpretations to ambiguous cues and to provide and reinforce avoidant solutions in response to hypothetical social scenarios than were parents of aggressive or nonclinical control children (Barrett, Rapee, Dadds, & Ryan, 1996; Dadds, Barrett, & Rapee, 1996; Dadds, Barrett, Rapee, & Ryan, 1996). Continued work in laboratory and natural contexts is needed to expand our knowledge base with respect to potential causal factors in the development of social anxiety, as well as to provide information that may assist in the development of intervention programs that incorporate the family (see Barrett, Dadds, & Rapee, 1996, for a discussion of family anxiety management).

PEER RELATIONSHIPS

Children's interactions with peers are crucial for the optimal development of social and emotional competency (see Berndt & Ladd, 1989; Hartup, 1979). Peer interaction not only supplements familial influences but also contributes unique variance to the child's social and intellectual functioning (Hartup, 1979). The literature on adult and child psychopathology is replete with references to relations between social withdrawal and psychological impairment (e.g., Bellack & Hersen, 1979; Cowen, Pederson, Babigian, Izzo, & Trost, 1973; McFall, 1982; Roff, 1961).

Importantly, peer interaction provides opportunities for learning specific skills that are not attainable through adult–child interaction. Animal models have provided support for the developmental importance of peer interaction. For example, Suomi and Harlow (1975) found that monkeys reared in isolation from peers early in life failed to develop appropriate social interactive behavior. Suomi and Harlow suggest that play serves two important functions: (1) it provides opportunities to practice behaviors leading to appropriate adult functioning, and (2) it acts to mitigate social aggression through less aggressive behaviors exhibited in play.

Although most of the literature concerning peer relationships and psychopathology has focused on externalizing behavior problems (see Newcomb, Bukowski, & Pattee, 1993), the past decade has witnessed concerted efforts toward extension of this work to anxiety and depression. La Greca and colleagues have found peer acceptance to be inversely related to social anxiety in children and adolescents (La Greca, Dandes, Wick, Shaw, & Stone, 1988; La Greca & Lopez, 1998; La Greca & Stone, 1993). Morris (2001) reports the results of a 5-year longitudinal investigation to examine children's social relationships and the developmental progression of anxiety. Significant associations were found between children's peer status in first grade and self-reports of anxiety in fifth grade.

The role of social withdrawal in peer contexts is particularly relevant to discussions of developmental factors for anxiety. As noted previously, anxiety may lead to social withdrawal, and, conversely, social withdrawal may interfere with the development of social skills and interpersonal relationships, which may in turn lead to increased anxiety in social situations (e.g., Vernberg, Abwender, Ewell, & Beery, 1992).

Assessing Peer-Group Relations

Children's social relationships with peers have been examined at group and dyadic levels. At the group level, a child's peer status denotes his or her social standing within the peer group at large, whereas friendship is conceptualized as a dyadic relationship requiring mutual and voluntary selection between two specific individuals. As such, peer assessment conducted at both levels is likely to yield a more complete picture of the child's social world.

Peer Status

Group acceptance typically is assessed through nomination or rating methods. The standard sociometric nomination procedure involves having children nominate up to three classmates that he or she "likes the most" and three classmates that he or she "likes the least." Children are then classified into five social status groups (i.e., popular, rejected, neglected, controversial, average) based on the extent to which each is liked or disliked by peers. Similarly, sociometric rating procedures involve asking children to rate their classmates on various dimensions of social acceptance using Likert-type scales. In the revised class play technique (Matsen, Morrison, & Pelligrini, 1985), children are asked to assign peers to various roles in an imaginary play (e.g., which classmate is the most shy, bossy, smart, etc.).

Friendship Quality

Friendships vary greatly in terms of perceived closeness, social support, and conflict. Friendship quality most often is assessed using questionnaire measures, such as the Network of Relationships Inventory (Furman & Buhrmester, 1985), the Friendship Quality Questionnaire (Parker & Asher, 1993), and the Friendship Qualities Scale (Bukowski, Hoza, & Boivin, 1994). Qualitative aspects of children's close friendships also may be assessed through semistructured interviews (e.g., the Friendship Interview; Berndt & Perry, 1986).

Romantic Relationships

The formation and maintenance of romantic attachments often takes precedence over platonic friendships in adolescence. This may be a particularly painful transition for anxious adolescents, as elevated levels of anxiety interfere with the development of close, intimate bonds. Although a small body of research is available on dating and interpersonal functioning among anxious adults, empirical information for adolescents is scant at best.

Social Cognition

School-age children become increasingly adept at anticipating future events, including developing elaborate schemas concerning potential harm and catastrophic outcome (Magnusson, 1985; Piaget & Inhelder, 1966; Vasey & Borkovec, 1992; Vasey, Crnic, & Carter, 1994). As such, expressions of anxiety become increasingly characterized by social evaluative concerns and generalized worry. During this developmental period, children and adolescents become highly sensitive to issues of social acceptance and peer-group conformity. Self-awareness, self-consciousness, and the perceived subjective import of peer relationships increase throughout middle childhood, with the latter reaching its zenith in adolescence (Flavell, 1977; Panella & Henggeler, 1986). Short, Barrett, Dadds, and Fox (2001) examined the influence of parent behavior on the social cognitions of 101 children with anxiety disorders. Consistent with their previous research, the authors found that anxious children were more likely to interpret ambiguous hypothetical social scenarios as threatening. Further, many of these children's parents actually promoted avoidant responses during family discussion of the hypothetical scenarios.

INCORPORATING SOCIALIZATION AGENTS IN THE TREATMENT PROCESS

Including important socialization agents (parents, classmates, friends) in the treatment process may enhance generalizability and social validity of treatment gains. In cases in which parents also suffer from anxiety, it may be necessary to solicit their active participation throughout the course of therapy if one hopes to make substantive progress in remediating anxious behavior in child clients.

Family Therapy

Recognizing the impact of anxiety on the family system and the potential for family members to inadvertently reinforce anxious behavior, efforts toward incorporating parents in treatment are becoming more common (Barrett et al., 1996; Spence, Donovan, & Brechman-Toussaint, 2000; Toren et al., 2000). Family anxiety management (Dadds, Heard, & Rapee, 1992) is based on behavioral family intervention strategies proven effective in the treatment of disruptive behavior disorders (Sanders & Dadds-Markie, 1992). In family anxiety management, parents are trained in principles of reinforcement, child management, and selective inattention to their children's anxious behavior. Contingency management strategies are utilized to enhance communication and problem-solving skills within the family.

Peer-Mediated Treatment

Peer-pairing interventions involve strategically matching clients with popular, socially skilled peers and instructing them to engage in various activities together, including special free-play time or completion of tasks that require cooperation in service of a superordinate goal. In contrast, peer-helper interventions involve training of peers to initiate, model, and reinforce appropriate social behavior on the part of target children and to serve as role-play partners in social skills training sessions. In general, peer-pairing techniques are less time-consuming than peer-helper interventions, as specialized training of peers is not necessary prior to implementation of the treatment program (Morris, Messer, & Gross, 1995). Research suggests that both types of interventions lead to improved social status, increased rates of positive interaction, and decreased rates of solitary behavior.

CONCLUDING COMMENTS

Research on social development and its relation to anxiety in children and adolescents is advancing rapidly. Even so, this accumulating body of work is but a drop in a pond in comparison with what remains to be learned. This bold frontier presents an exciting challenge for researchers and clinicians. Each incremental gain in our understanding of causal factors allows for the possibility of more targeted delivery of intervention and prevention efforts. Explication of developmental pathways undoubtedly will enhance our ability to provide effective intervention across all stages of the lifespan. At this point, however, it appears safe to draw a general conclusion that incorporating relevant members of children's social networks into the therapeutic process enhances acquisition, generalization, and maintenance of treatment gains, and we strongly encourage practitioners to explore creative solutions in this regard.

ACKNOWLEDGMENTS

Preparation of this chapter was supported in part by Grant No. MH-61518 from the National Institutes of Health.

REFERENCES

Ainsworth, M. D., Bell, S. V., & Stayton, D. J. (1972). Individual differences in the development of some attachment behaviors. *Merill–Palmer Quarterly, 18,* 123–143.

Ainsworth, M. D. S., Blehar, M. C., Waters, E., & Wall, S. (1978). *Patterns of attachment: A psychological study of the Strange Situation.* Hillsdale, NJ: Erlbaum.

Armsden, G. C., & Greenberg, M. T. (1987). The inventory of parent and peer attachment: Individual differences and their relationship to well-being. *Journal of Youth and Adolescence, 16,* 427–454.

Arrindell, W. A., Emmelkamp, P. M. G., Monsma, A., & Brilman, E. (1983). The role of perceived parental rearing practices in the etiology of phobic disorders: A controlled study. *British Journal of Psychiatry, 155,* 526–535.

Arrindell, W. A., Kwee, M. G., Methorst, G. J., van der Ende, J., Pol, E., & Moritz, B. J. (1989). Perceived parenting styles of agoraphobic and socially phobic inpatients. *British Journal of Psychiatry, 155,* 526–535.

Barrett, P. M., Dadds, M. R., & Rapee, R. M. (1996). Family treatment of childhood anxiety: A controlled trial. *Journal of Consulting and Clinical Psychology, 64,* 333–342.

Barrett, P.M., Rapee, R. M., Dadds, M. M., & Ryan, S. M. (1996). Family enhancement of cognitive style in anxious and aggressive children. *Journal of Abnormal Child Psychology, 24,* 187–203.

Bellack, A. S., & Hersen, M. (Eds.). (1979). *Research and practice in social skills training*. New York: Plenum Press.

Berman, W. H., Heiss, G. E., & Sperling, M. B. (1994). Measuring continued attachment to parents: The Continued Attachment Scale—Parent Version. *Psychological Reports, 75*, 171–182.

Berndt, T. J., & Ladd, G. W. (Eds.). (1989). *Peer relationships in children's development*. New York: Wiley.

Berndt, T. J., & Perry, T. B. (1986). Children(s perceptions of friendships as supportive relationships. *Developmental Psychology, 22*, 640–648.

Bhavnagri, N. P., & Parke, R. D. (1991). Parents as direct facilitators of children's peer relationships: Effects of age of child and sex of parent. *Journal of Social and Personal Relationships, 8*, 423–440.

Booth, C. L., Rose-Krasnor, L., McKinnon, J., & Rubin, K. H. (1994). Predicting social adjustment in middle childhood: The role of preschool attachment security and maternal style. *Social Development, 3*, 189–204.

Bruch, M. A., & Heimberg, R. G. (1994). Difference in perceptions of parental and personal characteristics between generalized and nongeneralized social phobics. *Journal of Anxiety Disorders, 8*, 155–168.

Bruch, M. A., Heimberg, R. G., Berger, P., & Collins, T. M. (1989). Social phobia and perceptions of early parental and personal characteristics. *Anxiety Research, 2*, 57–65.

Bryant, B. K., & DeMorris, K. A. (1992). Beyond parent–child relationships: Potential links between family environments and peer relations. In R. D. Parke & G. W. Ladd (Eds.), *Family–peer relationships* (pp. 159–189). Hillsdale, NJ: Erlbaum.

Bukowski, W. M., Hoza, B., & Boivin, M. (1994). Measuring friendship quality during pre- and early adolescence: The development and psychometric properties of the Friendship Qualities Scale. *Journal of Social and Personal Relationships, 11*, 471–484.

Cicchetti, D., & Cohen, D. J. (1995). Perspectives on developmental psychopathology. In D. Cicchetti & D. Cohen (Eds.), *Developmental psychopathology: Vol. 1. Theory and methods* (pp. 3–20). New York: Wiley.

Cohn, D. A., Patterson, C. J., & Christopoulos, C. (1991). The family and children's peer relations. *Journal of Social and Personal Relationships, 8*, 315–346.

Cowen, E. L., Pederson, A., Babigian, H., Izzo, L. D., & Trost, M. A. (1973). Long-term follow-up of early detected vulnerable children. *Journal of Consulting and Clinical Psychology, 41*, 438–446.

Dadds, M. R., Barrett, P. M., & Rapee, R. M. (1996). Family process and child anxiety and aggression: An observational analysis. *Journal of Abnormal Child Psychology, 24*, 715–734.

Dadds, M. R., Barrett, P. M., Rapee, R. M., & Ryan, A. (1996). Family process and child anxiety and aggression: An observational analysis. *Journal of Abnormal Child Psychology, 24*, 715–734.

Dadds, M. R., Heard, P. M., & Rapee, R. M. (1992). The role of family intervention in the treatment of child anxiety disorders: Some preliminary findings. *Behaviour Change, 9*, 171–177.

Darling, N., & Steinberg, L. (1993). Parenting style as context: An integrative model. *Psychological Bulletin, 113*, 487–496.

Duggan, C., Sham, P., Minne, C., Lee, A., & Murray, R. (1998). Quality of parenting and vulnerability to depression: Results from a family study. *Psychological Medicine, 28,* 185–191.

Dumas, J. E., LaFreniere, P. J., & Serketich, W. J. (1995). Balance of power: A transactional analysis of control in mother–child dyads involving socially competent, aggressive, and anxious children. *Journal of Abnormal Psychology, 104,* 104–113.

Erickson, M. F., Sroufe, L. A., & Egeland, B. (1985). The relationship between quality of attachment and behavior problems in a high-risk sample. *Monographs of the Society for Research in Child Development, 50*(1–2 Serial No. 209), 147–166.

Flavell, J. H. (1977). *Cognitive development.* Englewood Cliffs, NJ: Prentice-Hall.

Furman, W., & Buhrmester, D. (1985). Children's perceptions of the personal relationships in their social networks. *Developmental Psychology, 21,* 1016–1022.

Greco, L. A., & Morris, T. L. (2002). Paternal child-rearing style and child social anxiety: Investigation of child perceptions and actual father behavior. *Journal of Psychopathology and Behavioral Assessment, 24,* 259–267.

Hartup, W. W. (1979). Peer relations and the growth of social competence. In M. W. Kent & J. E. Rolf (Eds.), *Primary prevention of psychopathology* (pp. 150–170). Hanover, NH: University Press of New England.

Hazan, C., & Shaver, C. (1987). Romantic love conceptualized as an attachment process. *Journal of Personality and Social Psychology, 52,* 511–524.

Hudson, J. L., & Rapee, R. M. (2001). Parent–child interactions and anxiety disorders: An observational study. *Behaviour Research and Therapy, 39,* 1411–1427.

Hummel, R. M., & Gross, A. M. (2001). Socially anxious children: An observational study of parent–child interaction. *Child and Family Behavior Therapy, 23,* 19–41.

Kazdin, A. E. (1989). Developmental psychopathology: Current research, issues, and directions. *American Psychologist, 44,* 180–187.

Kobak, R., Sudler, N., & Gamble, W. (1991). Attachment and depressive symptoms in adolescence: A developmental pathways analysis. *Development and Psychopathology, 3,* 461–474.

Krohne, H. W., & Hock, M. (1991). Relationships between restrictive mother–child interactions and anxiety of the child. *Anxiety Research, 4,* 109–124.

Ladd, G. W., Profilet, S. M., & Hart, C. H. (1992). Parents' management of children's peer relations: Facilitating and supervising children's activities in the peer culture. In R. D. Ross & G. W. Ladd (Eds.), *Family–peer relationships: Modes of linkage* (pp. 215–253). Hillsdale, NJ: Erlbaum.

La Greca, A. M., Dandes, S. K., Wick, P., Shaw, K., & Stone, W. L. (1988). Development of the Social Anxiety Scale for Children: Reliability and concurrent validity. *Journal of Clinical Child Psychology, 17,* 84–91.

La Greca, A. M., & Lopez, N. (1998). Social anxiety among adolescents: Linkages with peer relations and friendships. *Journal of Abnormal Child Psychology, 29,* 83–94.

La Greca, A. M., & Stone, W. L. (1993). Social Anxiety Scale for Children—Revised: Factor structure and concurrent validity. *Journal of Clinical Child Psychology, 22,* 17–27.

Magnusson, D. (1985). Situational factors in research in stress and anxiety: Sex and age differences. In P. B. Defares (Ed.), *Stress and anxiety* (Vol. 9, pp. 69–78). Washington, DC: Hemisphere.

Matsen, A. S., Morrison, P., & Pelligrini, D. S. (1985). A revised class play method of peer assessment. *Developmental Psychology, 21,* 523–533.

McFall, R. M. (1982). A review and reformulation of the concept of social skills. *Behavioral Assessment, 4,* 1–33.

Morris, T. L. (2001). Social phobia. In M. W. Vasey & M. R. Dadds (Eds.), *The developmental psychopathology of anxiety* (pp. 435–458). New York: Oxford University Press.

Morris, T. L., Messer, S. C., & Gross, A. M. (1995). Enhancement of the social interaction and status of neglected children: A peer-pairing approach. *Journal of Clinical Child Psychology, 25,* 11–20.

Muris, P., & Meesters, C. (2002). Attachment, behavioral inhibition, and anxiety disorder symptoms in normal adolescents. *Journal of Psychopathology and Behavioral Assessment, 24,* 97–106.

Newcomb, A. F., Bukowski, W. M., & Pattee, L. (1993). Children's peer relations: A meta-analytic review of popular, rejected, neglected, controversial, and average sociometric status. *Psychological Bulletin, 113,* 99–128.

Panella, D., & Henggeler, S. W. (1986). Peer interactions of conduct-disordered, anxious-withdrawn, and well-adjusted black adolescents. *Journal of Abnormal Child Psychology, 14,* 1–11.

Parker, J. G., & Asher, S. R. (1993). Friendship and friendship quality in middle childhood: Links with peer group acceptance and feelings of loneliness and social dissatisfaction. *Developmental Psychology, 29,* 611–621.

Piaget, J., & Inhelder, B. (1966). *The early growth of logic in the child.* New York: Harper & Row.

Profilet, S. M., & Ladd, G. W. (1994). Do mothers' perceptions and concerns about preschoolers' peer competence predict their peer-management practices? *Social Development, 3,* 205–221.

Putallaz, M., & Hefflin, A. H. (1990). Parent–child interaction. In S. R. Asher & J. D. Coie (Eds.), *Peer rejection in childhood* (pp. 189–216). New York: Cambridge University Press.

Rapee, R. M., & Melville, L. F. (1997). Recall of family factors in social phobia and panic disorder: Comparison of mother and offspring reports. *Depression and Anxiety, 5,* 7–11.

Roff, M. (1961). Childhood social relations and young adult bad conduct. *Journal of Abnormal and Social Psychology, 65,* 333–337.

Russell, A., & Finnie, V. (1990). Preschool children's social status and maternal instructions to assist group entry. *Developmental Psychology, 26,* 603–611.

Sanders, M. R., & Dadds-Markie, R. (1992). Toward a technology of prevention of disruptive behaviour patterns: The role of behavioural family intervention. *Behaviour Change, 9,* 186–200.

Short, A. L., Barrett, P. M., Dadds, M. R., & Fox, T. (2001). The influence of family and experimental context on cognition in anxious children. *Journal of Abnormal Child Psychology, 29,* 585–598.

Spence, S. H., Donovan, C., & Brechman-Toussaint, M. (2000). The treatment of childhood social phobia: The effectiveness of a social skills training-based, cognitive-behavioural intervention, with and without parental involvement. *Journal of Child Psychology and Psychiatry and Allied Disciplines, 41,* 713726.

Suomi, S., & Harlow, H. F. (1975). Effects of differential removal from group on social development of rhesus monkeys. *Journal of Child Psychology and Psychiatry, 16,* 149–164.

Thomas, A., & Chess, S. (1977). *Temperament and development.* New York: Brunner/Mazel.

Toren, P., Wolmer, L., Rosental, B., Eldar, S., Koren, S., Lask, M., Weizman, R., & Laor, N. (2000). Case series: Brief parent–child group therapy for childhood anxiety disorders using a manual-based cognitive-behavioral technique. *Journal of the American Academy of Child and Adolescent Psychiatry, 39,* 1309–1312.

van IJzendoorn, M. H., & Bakermans-Kranenburg, M. J. (1996). Attachment representations in mothers, fathers, adolescents, and clinical groups: A meta-analytic search for normative data. *Journal of Consulting and Clinical Psychology, 64,* 8–21.

Vasey, M. W., & Borkovec, T. D. (1992). A catastrophizing assessment of worrisome thoughts. *Cognitive Therapy and Research, 16,* 505–520.

Vasey, M. W., Crnic, K. A., & Carter, W. G. (1994). Worry in childhood: A developmental perspective. *Cognitive Therapy and Research, 18,* 529–549.

Vasey, M. W., & Dadds, M. R. (Eds.). (2001). *The developmental psychopathology of anxiety.* New York: Oxford University Press.

Vernberg, E. M., Abwender, D. A., Ewell, K. K., & Beery, S. H. (1992). Social anxiety and peer relationships in early adolescence: A prospective analysis. *Journal of Clinical Child Psychology, 21,* 189–196.

Warren, S. L., Huston, L., Egeland, B., & Sroufe, L. A. (1997). Child and adolescent anxiety disorders and early attachment. *Journal of the American Academy of Child and Adolescent Psychiatry, 36,* 637–644.

Wiborg, I. M., & Dahl, A. A. (1997). The recollection of parental rearing styles in patients with panic disorder. *Acta Psychiatrica Scandinavica, 96,* 58–63.

Chapter 4

Behavioral Genetics

THALIA C. ELEY
ALICE M. GREGORY

Anxiety is common in children and adolescents. Although all children experience anxiety to some extent, approximately 10% are considered to have an anxiety disorder (Bird, Canino, & Rubio-Stipect, 1988; Costello & Angold, 1988). As well as causing discomfort, anxiety has been associated with more serious consequences, such as poor academic functioning (Ialongo, Edelsohn, Werthamer Larsson, Crockett, & Kellam, 1994) and suicide (Statham, Heath, & Madde, 1998). Given the seriousness of the condition, it is essential that the origins of childhood anxiety are unraveled so that risk factors can be identified and preventative methods and treatments developed.

Behavioral genetic research has provided a wealth of information concerning the origins of childhood anxiety. This chapter begins by outlining the key findings in respect to the etiology of childhood anxiety. It then explores some sources of heterogeneity in estimations of heritability. These include differences between studies in terms of phenotype, treatment of comorbidity, age and sex, and rater. Exciting directions for research investigating childhood anxiety are outlined, including the search for specific genes and studies that investigate genetic influence on environmental measures. It is hoped that with a greater understanding of the genetics of childhood anxiety, preventative methods and individually targeted and tailored treatments can be developed.

FAMILY STUDIES

Early work investigating the etiology of anxiety in children explored the co-occurrence of anxiety within families. A range of designs were used in such studies. These included "top-down" designs, in which the children of adults with anxiety disorders were studied (e.g., Biederman, Rosenbaum, Bolduc, Faraone, & Hirshfeld, 1991; Weissman, Leckman, Merikangas, Gammon, & Prusoff, 1984; Weissman, Warner, Wickramaratne, Moreau, & Olfson, 1997); "bottom-up" designs, in which the adult relatives of child probands were studied (e.g., Last, Hersen, Kazdin, Orvaschel, & Perrin, 1991; Livingston, Nugent, Rader, & Smith, 1985); and sibling studies, whereby aggregation within sibling pairs was investigated (e.g., Rende, Warner, Wickramaratne, & Weissman, 1999).

All such studies have demonstrated the high familiality of anxiety. For example, a classic top-down study compared symptoms of anxiety and fear in children (ages 7–12) from four groups: children of probands with anxiety disorders; children of probands with dysthymia; children of parents who were never mentally ill; and normal school children (Turner, Beidel, & Costello, 1987). The children of the anxiety probands reported (on self-report questionnaires) higher levels of anxiety and fear symptoms than both the children of normal controls and the normal schoolchildren. The children of parents with anxiety disorders were seven times more likely to attract a diagnosis of anxiety disorder than the control group children and twice as likely as the children of the dysthymic group.

Although such studies have been valuable in highlighting the aggregation of anxiety symptoms and disorders in families, they are unable to provide information as to whether environmental influences shared by family members or shared genes account for family resemblance.

TWIN AND ADOPTION STUDIES

Twin and adoption studies, in contrast, provide a means for disentangling genetic and environmental influences. Twin studies are able to disentangle genetic and environmental influences by comparing within-pair similarity for groups of monozygotic (MZ) twins, who are genetic clones, and dizygotic (DZ) twins, who share only half their segregating genes (see Plomin, DeFries, McClearn, & McGuffin, 2001). The comparison of biologically related and biologically unrelated siblings or parent–child pairs in adoption studies similarly allows the comparison of environmental and genetic influences on the phenotype of interest. Additionally, twin and adoption studies are able to distinguish shared environmental effects (which make family members resemble one another) from nonshared environmental effects (which make family members differ from one another).

In the standard twin design, variance in the phenotype (V_p) is divided into three latent factors described as heritability or additive genetics (A), common or shared environment (C), and nonshared environment (E; i.e., $V_p = A + C + E$). Resemblance within MZ twin pairs is due to genes and shared environment (i.e., $r_{MZ} = A + C$), whereas resemblance in DZ pairs is due to sharing half their genes and their shared environment (i.e., $r_{DZ} = \frac{1}{2}A + C$). From these equations it is possible to estimate heritability as twice the difference between the MZ and DZ correlations (i.e., $A = 2[r_{MZ} - r_{DZ}]$) and shared environment as the difference between the MZ correlation and the heritability (i.e., $C = r_{MZ} - A$). Twin data can also be used to estimate the effects of genetic dominance. However, dominance is rarely seen in data on anxiety and is not discussed further here (for more detail of dominance, see Plomin et al., 2001).

Although twin studies have been described as "the perfect natural experiment" (Martin, Boomsma, & Machin, 1997), they are not without limitations. One such limitation includes the possibility that MZ twins experience more-similar environments than DZ twins, the occurrence of which would artificially inflate estimates of heritability. Despite this possibility, a series of studies using a variety of methods have demonstrated that the more-similar environments experienced by MZ pairs are due to their own genetic similarity, which leads them to elicit or produce more similar environments (e.g., Kendler, Neale, Kessler, Heath, & Eaves, 1993). A further criticism leveled toward twin studies concerns chorionicity. Whereas two-thirds of MZ twins are monochorionic (share one sac within the placenta), all DZ twins are dichorionic (have separate sacs within the placenta). The increased similarity of gestational environment in monochorionic MZ twins could artificially inflate heritability. This problem is reduced by the finding that monochorionicity is likely to lead to more birth problems than dichorionicity (e.g., Martin et al., 1997), which would reduce predicted heritability.

Adoption studies have a different set of limitations. Three main difficulties have been highlighted (Plomin et al., 2001). First, it is possible that families involved in adoption are not representative of the general population. Second, biological mothers provide the child's environment for 9 months, which could increase their similarity beyond that produced by genetic factors. Third, selective placement occurs, whereby adoptive families are matched on certain characteristics (e.g., socioeconomic status, height, coloring, etc.) to biological parents. Although selective placement would artificially inflate estimations of shared environment, there is little evidence that this occurs (Plomin et al., 2001).

Twin and adoption studies have been fairly consistent in showing that anxiety is heritable and that both shared and nonshared environmental factors have important effects on anxiety. Typically, genetic influences account for roughly 30%, shared environment 20%, and nonshared environment the remaining 50% of the variance in childhood anxiety. The finding that shared environmental influences are important is particularly exciting given the rarity with which this parameter has been found to be significant for most other behavioral disorders among both children and adults. In particular, adult studies of anxiety disorders have been notable for the lack of significant influence of shared environment (e.g., Kendler, Neale, Kessler, Heath, & Eaves, 1992). This finding emphasizes the need for separate research into anxiety disorders in children and adolescents among whom the shared environment has been demonstrated to be a significant influence.

Despite these general findings, estimations of genetic and environmental influences have fluctuated greatly between studies, suggesting heterogeneity in the phenotype. The most obvious reason for this heterogeneity is the fact that there are many manifestations of anxiety, as can be seen from the varied diagnoses within classification systems, and associated clusters of anxiety symptoms, resulting in phenotypic heterogeneity. As a result of the co-occurrence of subtypes of anxiety, several investigators have taken a "vulnerability" or "trait" approach to anxiety. The co-occurrence of depression with anxiety has also been explored, as have age, sex, and rater effects.

EXPLORING SOURCES OF HETEROGENEITY

Anxiety Subtypes

Studies investigating childhood anxiety have considered a range of phenotypes. Anxiety can be seen as an umbrella term encompassing a number of subtypes—including separation anxiety disorder (SAD), overanxious disorder (OAD), general anxiety symptoms, and phobia or fear symptoms. Furthermore, given the common co-occurrence of anxiety with depression, some studies have investigated a phenotype of combined anxiety–depression. This section describes some of the work investigating subtypes of anxiety.

Separation Anxiety Disorder

A number of reports from the large-scale Virginia Twin Study of Adolescent Behavioral Development (VTSABD) present data on SAD (Eaves et al., 1997; Silberg, Rutter, & Eaves, 2001; Topolski et al., 1997). These articles have come from a variety of reporters and have shown rather mixed results. For example, one report, which looked only at child measures, found variance in SAD to be due to shared and nonshared environment only

(Topolski et al., 1997). A further article investigating mothers', fathers', and children's self-reports explained the variance of anxiety reported by all three raters by additive genetic and nonshared factors only (Eaves et al., 1997). There are no clear reasons for the discrepancy between children's self-reports in these two studies, and one can only speculate that different formulations of the diagnosis of SAD were used in the different analyses.

Despite these differences, the majority of investigations have found that both genetic and shared environmental influences play a role in SAD (see Table 4.1). The influence of shared environment is particularly interesting, given that most other phenotypes are not influenced by this factor.

Overanxious Disorder

A further phenotype to be considered is OAD, which was looked at only in the VTSABD (Eaves et al., 1997; Silberg, Rutter, & Eaves, 2001; Topolski et al., 1997). As shown in Table 4.1, the results for OAD are more similar across the studies than those for SAD and indicate only additive genetics and nonshared environment as significant influences on OAD in children and adolescents, for mother-, father-, and self-reported data.

Anxiety Symptoms

The etiology of anxiety symptoms has been explored in a number of studies (Eaves et al., 1997; Eley & Stevenson, 1999a; Thapar & McGuffin, 1995; Topolski et al., 1997). These studies show a modest influence of shared environment and a moderate influence of additive genetic and nonshared environmental factors (see Table 4.1). The heritability of different types of anxiety symptoms may also vary. This possibility was investigated in a study of self-reported anxiety among 326 seven-year-old twin pairs in which behavioral genetic analyses on both total scores and subscale scores were conducted (Warren, Schmitz, & Emde, 1999). This study found that the level of genetic influence varied for the three subscales, accounting for 30% and 34% of the variance in physiological and social anxiety but none of the variance in worry. In contrast, shared environment accounted for 30% of the variance in worry score. Interestingly, this finding contrasts with the general finding in behavioral genetics that shared environment is important in explaining the etiology of social anxiety.

Fear and Phobia Symptoms

Other studies have investigated fear and phobia symptoms (see Table 4.1). These studies typically show that variance in these phenotypes is due to additive genetic, shared, and nonshared environmental factors. Despite this

TABLE 4.1. Summary of Results from Studies Exploring Different Subtypes of Anxiety in Children and Adolescents

Study	Number of subjects	Age range (yr)	Measure	A		C		E	
				Male	Female	Male	Female	Male	Female
			Separation anxiety disorder (SAD)						
Eaves et al. (1997)	1,412 twin pairs	8–16	SAD: Mother interview	.04	.74	—	—	.96	.26
			SAD: Father interview	.00	.74	—	—	1.0	.27
			SAD: Child interview	.19	.31	—	—	.81	.69
Feigon et al. (in press)	2,043 same-sex twin pairs	3–18	SAD	.14	.50	.51	.21	.35	.29
Silberg et al. (2001)	609 female twin pairs		SAD: Self-report						
		8–13	8- to 13-year-olds		—		.14		.86
		14–17	14- to 17-year-olds		—		.23		.77
Silove et al. (1995)	200 same-sex twin pairs	17–66	*Retrospective SAD symptoms*	.00	.57	.27	.02	.73	.41
Topolski et al. (1997)	1,412 same-sex twin pairs	8–16	SAD: Child interview	.04		.40		.56	
			Overanxious disorder (OAD)						
Eaves et al. (1997)	1,412 twin pairs	8–16	OAD: Mother interview	.31	.66	—	—	.69	.34
			OAD: Father interview	.54	.59	—	—	.46	.41
			OAD: Child interview	.30	.46	—	—	.70	.54
Silberg et al. (2001)	609 female twin pairs		OAD: Self-report						
		8–13	8- to 13-year-olds		.14		—		.86
		14–17	14- to 17-year-olds		.12		.07		.81
Topolski et al. (1997)	1,412 same-sex twin pairs	8–16	OAD: Child interview	.37		.11		.52	
			General anxiety symptoms						
Eaves et al. (1997)	1,412 twin pairs	8–16	Mother-report factor	.57	.52	—	—	.43	.48
			Father-report factor	.72	.69	—	—	.28	.31
			Child-report factor	.00	.37	.33	.08	.67	.55

Study	Sample	Age	Measure						
Eley & Stevenson (1999b)	395 same-sex twin pairs	8–16	Child-report factor	.10				.39	.51
Thapar & McGuffin (1995)	376 same-sex twin pairs	8–16	RCMAS: Parent report	.59				.00	.41
		12–16	RCMAS: Self-report	.00				.55	.45
Topolski et al. (1997)	1,412 same-sex twin pairs	8–10	RCMAS	.15	.58	.14	.00	.71	.42
		11–13	RCMAS	.01	.40	.44	.03	.55	.57
		14–16	RCMAS	.01	.42	.22	.14	.77	.44
Warren et al. (1999)	326 same-sex twin pairs	7	RCMAS: Self-report						
			Physiology	.30			—		.70
			Worry	—			.30		.70
			Social	.34			—		.66
			Total	.25			.11		.64
Fear and phobia symptoms									
Lichtenstein & Annas (2000)	1,106 twin pairs	8–9	Fear of animals	.23	.56	.58	.32	.20	.12
			Situational fear	.58	.37	.23	.46	.18	.18
			Mutilation fear	.29	.38	.50	.45	.21	.17
			Any fear	.40	.32	.43	.49	.17	.19
Nelson et al. (2000)	1,344 female twin pairs	Mean = 18.2	Social phobia: diagnostic interview		.28				.72
Rose & Ditto (1983)	354 same-sex twin pairs	14–34	FSS-II: Fear of . . .						
			Negative social interaction	.44	.56				
			Social responsibility	.60	.40				
			Dangerous places	.58	.42				
			Small organisms	.66	.34				
			Deep water	.32	.68				
			Loved one's misfortune	.28	.72				
			Personal death	.72	.28				
Silberg et al. (2001)	609 female twin pairs	8–13	Social phobia: Self-report — 8- to 13-year-olds	.10	—				.90
		14–17	14- to 17-year-olds	.09	.05				.86

(continued)

TABLE 4.1. (*continued*)

Study	Number of subjects	Age range (yr)	Measure	A Male	A Female	C Male	C Female	E Male	E Female
Stevenson et al. (1992)	319 same-sex twin pairs	8–18	Normal range						
			Fear of failure		.12	.51			.37
			Fear of unknown		.46	.29			.25
			Fear of injury and animals		.46	.23			.31
			Fear of danger		.34	.39			.27
			Fear of medical		.14	.39			.47
			1 SD extreme group[a]						
			Fear of failure	-.03			.59		.22
			Fear of unknown	.50			.21		.29
			Fear of injury and animals	.60			.10		.30
			Fear of danger	.47			.15		.38
			Fear of medical	.14			.36		.50
Combined anxiety and depression									
Deater-Deckard et al. (1997)	720 sibling pairs (wave 1) 395 sibling pairs (wave 2: 3 yr later)	9–18	CBCL: A/D Normal range						
			Mother wave 1		.62		.04		.34
			Mother wave 2		.52		.08		.40
			Father wave 1		.52		.25		.23
			Father wave 2		.59		.07		.34
			1 SD extreme group[a]						
			Mother wave 1		.38		.09		.53
			Mother wave 2		.24		.34		.42
			Father wave 1		.40		.28		.32
			Father wave 2		.39		.26		.35
Edelbrock, Rende, Plomin, & Thompson (1995)	181 same-sex twin pairs	7–15	CBCL: A/D		.34		.30		.36

Study	Sample	Age	Measure					
Eley (1996)	395 same-sex twin pairs	8–16	CBCL: A/D	.49	.05		.46	
Gjone & Stevenson (1997)	915 twin pairs	5–15	CBCL: A/D Ages 5–9 Ages 12–15	.44 .26	.25 .50	.34 .45	.31 .24	.29 .21
van den Oord, Boomsma, & Verhulst (1994)	332 adopted siblings	10–15	CBCL: A/D	.13		.31	.59	
van den Oord et al. (1996)	1,377 twin pairs	3	CBCL: A/D	.72	—		.28	
van den Oord & Rowe (1997)	436 same-sex full siblings, 119 half siblings, 122 cousins	4–6 6–8 8–10	BPI: Anxious/depressed	.24 .28 .26	.16 .18 .18		.59 .53 .56	
van der Valk et al. (1998)	3,620 twin pairs	2–3	CBCL: A/D	.68	—		.32	
van der Valk et al. (2001a)	3,873 twin pairs 1,924 twin pairs	3 7	CBCL: A/D Wave 1 Wave 2	.59 .40	.10 .31		.31 .29	
van der Valk et al. (2001b)	1,940 twin pairs	7	CBCL: A/D Mothers Fathers	.38 .35	.32 .33		.30 .32	
van der Valk et al. (2001c)	3,501 twin pairs	3	CBCL: A/D Mothers Fathers	.69 .59	— .10		.31 .31	
van der Valk, Verhulst, et al. (2001d)	1,816 adoptees 1,309 adoptees	10–15 13–18	CBCL: A/D Wave 1 Wave 2	.16 .08	.30 .33		.54 .59	

Note. CBCL: A/D, the anxious/depressed subscale of the Child Behavior Checklist (Achenbach, 1991); BPI, Behavior Problem Index (Peterson & Zill, 1986); FSS-II, Fear Survey Schedule–II; RCMAS, Revised Children's Manifest Anxiety Scale (Reynolds & Richmond, 1979).

[a]These analyses considered the etiology of extreme groups (those scoring 1 standard deviation or more above or below mean).

general finding, the estimates for these factors vary considerably depending on the specific symptoms being investigated. For example, the heritability of fear of animals across the entire sample ($A = .58$) is considerably higher than that of fear of mutilation ($A = .28$; Lichtenstein & Annas, 2000). A further study found that nonshared environment was more important for fear of medical procedures than for other fears (Stevenson, Batten, & Cherner, 1992). The authors explain this finding by noting that experiences of medical procedures are in their nature generally child-specific—and therefore that nonshared environmental factors are more likely to elicit these fears. This study also found that fear of failure has a large shared-environment factor ($C = .51$) compared with other fear dimensions, such as fear of injury and of small animals ($C = .23$). This finding is consistent with the suggestion that fear of failure is learned in the family setting.

Combined Anxiety and Depression

Parents are rather poor at distinguishing between anxiety and depression in their children (Achenbach, 1991), so for this reason many studies have explored mixed anxiety–depression in parent-reported data. As illustrated in Table 4.1, a number of studies using different designs—namely, twin, adoption, and sibling–cousin designs—have reached the same conclusion: that additive genetic, shared, and nonshared environmental influences are important for this phenotype. Despite this general finding, further studies have found a negligible or nonexistent impact of shared environment on the etiology of anxiety–depression (e.g., Eley, 1996; van den Oord, Verhulst, & Boomsma, 1996; van der Valk, Verhulst, Stroet, & Boomsma, 1998). Clearly, further research is needed before a firm conclusion can be drawn concerning the influence of shared environmental factors on the anxious–depressed phenotype.

In summary, although the etiology of anxiety in children does not seem to differ according to the severity of anxiety, it does appear to differ somewhat according to other phenotypic issues. For example, although it is premature to draw clear distinctions between different subtypes of anxiety, some indications suggest that SAD may be more influenced by the family environment than OAD. This finding could perhaps be interpreted in the light of the role that attachment may have in SAD (Warren, Huston, Egeland, & Sroufe, 1997). However, it should be noted that the questionnaire measures also revealed significant influence of shared environment and that these questionnaires were designed to tap into the kinds of symptoms that would form the basis of a diagnosis such as OAD. This work highlights the need for precisely defined phenotypes to facilitate the search for genetic factors and to make research outcomes comparable.

Trait Approaches to Anxiety

In addition, a variety of approaches have been used to identify vulnerability for trait anxiety. These involve investigating the heritability of trait versus state anxiety, examining the heritability of aspects of temperament or personality related to anxiety, and considering whether vulnerability factors are the same for normal and abnormal or extreme anxiety.

Trait versus State Anxiety

Whereas most studies of anxiety symptoms attempt to measure an ongoing trait, studies investigating state (fluctuating) anxiety have found a rather different pattern of results. This was found to be the case in a study investigating anxiety in children and adolescents (Legrand, McGue, & Iacono, 1999). Trait anxiety symptoms were moderately heritable, with genes accounting for 45% of the variance; the rest of the variance was accounted for by nonshared environment and measurement error. State scores were, however, best explained without a genetic parameter, and shared environment was found to be large and significant (C was estimated before and after a morning of psychophysiological assessments at .39 and .19, respectively). The authors suggest that the results for state anxiety may be due to the anxiety-provoking situation—having to complete a questionnaire in an unfamiliar laboratory—overpowering genetic similarity. However, the differences reported here for the etiologies of trait and of state anxiety clearly warrant further investigation.

Temperament

Anxiety symptoms can be regarded as the extremity of anxious temperament or personality. Investigations of anxiety-related temperament have shown moderate to strong genetic influences for fearfulness (Goldsmith & Lemery, 2000), timidity (Mestel, 1994), behavioral inhibition (Robinson, Kagan, Reznick, & Corley, 1992) neuroticism (Boomsma, Koopmans, & Dolan, 1997; Thapar & McGuffin, 1996b), and shyness and emotionality (Saudino, Cherny, & Plomin, 2000). Interestingly, studies investigating temperament have found discrepancies in estimates for the heritability of temperament between twin and adoption studies. For example, although one adoption study reported no evidence for the heritability of temperament (including emotionality) in children between ages 1 and 7 (Plomin, Coon, Carey, DeFries, & Fulker, 1991), a great deal of support exists from twin studies for genetic influence of various personality traits and temperaments, including neuroticism (e.g., Plomin et al., 2001). However, more recent adoption studies have provided evidence for the heritability of temperaments, including emotionality (Schmitz, Saudino, Plomin, Fulker, & DeFries, 1996).

Extreme Anxiety

Differences in the severity of anxiety among participants in different studies may provide a further explanation of different results, as the causes of variation within the whole range of anxiety may differ from those between the extremes of anxiety and the rest of the population. In this review we have covered behavioral genetic analyses of anxiety disorders, as well as anxiety within the normal range. In order to assess the possibility that severe anxiety may be qualitatively rather than quantitatively different from anxiety that falls within the normal range, a number of different studies looking at temperament and anxiety have compared the heritability of normal and extreme anxiety (Deater-Deckard, Reiss, Hetherington, & Plomin, 1997; Goldsmith & Lemery, 2000; Robinson et al., 1992; Stevenson et al., 1992). These studies have failed to show etiological differences for normal and extreme anxiety, suggesting that vulnerability factors for anxiety operate along a continuum and that anxiety disorders may simply be the extremes of quantitative traits. However, it should be noted that many of these studies have used small samples (e.g., Goldsmith & Lemery, 2000; Robinson et al., 1992) and so may not have the power to detect modest differences.

Comorbidity

Anxiety commonly co-occurs with depression (Angold, Costello, & Erkanli, 1999; Brady & Kendall, 1992). Studies have dealt with the issue of comorbidity in different ways, which may further explain the inconsistent pattern of results coming from behavioral genetic studies of anxiety in children. The majority of studies have not addressed the issue of comorbidity (e.g., Feigon, Waldman, Levy, & Hay, 2001; Stevenson et al., 1992; Thapar & McGuffin, 1995; Topolski et al., 1999) or have used measures that group the symptoms of anxiety and depression together, as described previously (Eley, 1996; Gjone & Stevenson, 1997; van der Valk et al., 1998). Other studies have distinguished between anxiety and depression and addressed the origin of the correlation between anxiety and depression within a behavioral genetic design. These studies show that most of the covariation between anxiety and depression can be explained by genetic factors (Eley & Stevenson, 1999b; Thapar & McGuffin, 1997).

A number of studies investigating the relationship between different anxiety syndromes and a range of other comorbid phenotypes have also highlighted the importance of shared genetic factors in comorbidity between syndromes. For example, one recent study demonstrated shared genetic vulnerability between social phobia and major depressive disorder (genetic correlation = 1) and moderate shared genetic vulnerability between social phobia and alcohol dependence (genetic correlation = .5; Nelson et al., 2000). Furthermore, a multivariate longitudinal analysis of anxiety, neuroticism, and depression was conducted in adolescent and young adult twin pairs (Boomsma et al., 1997), with all genetic covariance between measures attributed to a common genetic factor. In contrast, another study found that the covariance between internalizing and externalizing disorders was mainly due to shared environmental factors (Gjone & Stevenson, 1997).

In addition to investigating a range of different anxiety syndromes and comorbid conditions, we must consider development when addressing comorbidity. Most studies have investigated concurrent comorbidity (comorbidity within an episode of psychiatric illness). However, comorbidity may also be successive (i.e., may occur during different stages of the life course). For example, anxious children may become depressed as adolescents (Angold, Costello, & Workman, 1998; Hankin et al., 1998; McGee, Feehan, Williams, & Anderson, 1992; Silberg et al., 1999, Velez, Johnson, & Cohen, 1989). The extent to which the shift from anxiety in childhood to depression in adolescence is due to a shared etiological vulnerability was considered in a recent study from the VTSABD using 609 female twin pairs ages 8–13 and 14–17 years old (Silberg, Rutter & Eaves, 2001). The results of multivariate genetic model fitting suggest that depression before the age of 14 has a distinct etiology as compared with depression after the age of 14, which shares genetic vulnerability with OAD and simple phobia. The final model included one shared genetic factor that influenced just OAD and simple phobia (but not major depression) during middle childhood and early adolescence and OAD, simple phobia, *and* major depression (MD) in middle adolescence. There were two shared environmental factors—one influencing early adolescent SAD and major depressive disorder (MDD) and later simple phobia; the other influencing early SAD and later OAD, SAD, and MD. Interestingly, although strong genetic continuity existed across time for OAD and simple phobia, depression in early adolescence was not influenced by genetic factors. This finding suggests that the genetic vulnerability to depression manifests as anxiety disorders, including OAD and simple phobia, early in adolescence and plays a role in depression only during middle to late adolescence.

Studies investigating comorbidity between anxiety and depression suggest that the two syndromes share genetic influence but that environmental influences are largely specific. This finding is helpful in directing the search for genes, suggesting that genes for anxiety may be the same as those for depression.

Age and Sex

Different studies have used children of different ages and sexes, and these differences may provide a further explanation for the heterogeneous results.

Studies that have directly tested for age effects typically show that heritability increases with age (e.g., Eley & Stevenson, 1999a; Feigon et al., 2001; Silberg, Rutter & Eaves, 2001; Topolski et al., 1997). For example, a study of SAD found an increase in heritability with age (Feigon et al., 2001). It should be noted, however, that other studies have not found significant age effects (e.g., Eaves et al., 1997; Legrand et al., 1999; Thapar & McGuffin, 1995). One study has found a decrease in heritability with age. Maternal ratings on the Child Behavior Checklist (CBCL) in 3,873 twin pairs at age 3 and then at age 7 showed that for internalizing problems genetic influence decreased over time, whereas shared environmental influences increased (van der Valk, Van den Oord, Verhulst, & Boomsma, 2001c).

Etiological differences have also been found in studies investigating sex effects, with consistent reports of higher heritability in girls than in boys (e.g., Eaves et al., 1997; Eley & Stevenson, 1999a; Feigon et al., in press; Lichtenstein & Annas, 2000; Silove, Manicavasagar, O'Connell, & Morris-Yates, 1995; Topolski et al., 1999). One study, illustrating gender differences in SAD, reported a genetic influence of $A = .50$ for girls and $A = .14$ for boys (Feigon et al., in press).

A number of studies have investigated both age and gender effects, showing an interaction between the two (Eley & Stevenson, 1999a; Topolski et al., 1997). In a study of child-reported anxiety symptoms, heritability was higher in adolescents (12–16 years) than in children (8–11 years), particularly for the females (Eley & Stevenson, 1999a).

Further studies have explored genetic and environmental influences on the stability of anxiety (Silberg, Rutter, Neale, & Eaves, 2001; Topolski et al., 1999; van der Valk et al., 2001a; van der Valk, Verhulst, Neale, & Boomsma, 2001). Estimations of genetic and environmental influences on stability differ between twin and adoption studies and between phenotypes and raters. For example, for parent-reported symptoms of anxiety, more than half the continuity across time was due to genetic continuity, whereas in the child-reported data continuity was largely influenced by shared environment (around 50%) and less so by genes (20%; Topolski et al., 1999). Overall, these studies demonstrate that stability is due to familial factors (either genes or shared environment), with parent-reported data tending to show genetic stability and child reports tending to show shared environmental stability.

Rater Effects

The use of different raters to assess childhood anxiety provides another explanation for the varied results from behavioral genetic studies of anxiety in children. Some studies exclusively report data provided by children themselves, whereas others have relied on parent reports. Parent reports are particularly valuable in studies assessing anxiety in children under the age of 8, because children may not have adequate self-awareness to respond reliably to questions regarding mood. Several studies to date have assessed both children's self-reports and parent reports of childhood anxiety, providing opportunities to compare such data within the same sample.

There are a number of differences in the conclusions that can be drawn from data provided by children as compared with those from parents. Overall, analyses of data provided by both children and parents suggest that genetic and shared environmental factors account for around half of the variance in anxiety, with the other half accounted for by nonshared environment and error. Differences include the suggestion from child-reported data that shared environment is slightly more important than genetic influence, whereas parent-reported data suggest that genetic influence is slightly greater than that of the shared environment. A study highlighting differences between self-reports and parental reports involved 376 pairs of twins aged 8 to 16 years (Thapar & McGuffin, 1994). In this study a parent-report anxiety questionnaire was completed for the whole sample, and the adolescents (ages 12–16 years) also completed a self-report version. The results from these two data sets were very different. The parent report of anxious symptomatology was found to have an estimated heritability of 59% with no age effect, whereas the adolescent self-report measure showed no significant genetic component. The shared-environment factor showed the reverse pattern, being large and significant for the adolescent self-report measures only. These results have since been replicated in a number of studies (e.g., Eaves et al., 1997), and it has been hypothesized that the reason for this discrepancy is that parents rate enduring traits, whereas children report current states.

In order to test this hypothesis, repeated assessments were made of parent- and self-rated anxiety in children (Topolski et al., 1999). Although overall the prediction that children were rating states and parents rating traits was largely disconfirmed, the study highlighted a number of interesting differences between the components that contribute to temporal stability between different informants. For example, whereas the stability of anxiety assessed by children's self-reports was largely due to environmental factors (genetic effects = 20%), stability assessed using parent reports was primarily due to genetic factors. Furthermore, important gender differences were reported, with parent reports showing higher heritability than boys' self-reports and lower heritability than girls' self-reports. Additionally, whereas the genetic covariance between parental reports and their sons' self-reports of anxiety was near zero, genetic covariation between mother reports and their daughters' self-reports was high and similar to that between mother and father reports of their daughters' anxiety. This pattern of results suggests that whereas parents are reporting different aspects of anxiety from those reported by their sons, they are reporting the same genetically influenced aspects of anxiety as their daughters.

The finding that parent-reported data indicate that genetic influences are slightly greater than those of shared environment is particularly interesting considering that rater effects due to one parent rating two children tends to inflate the shared environment rather than the genetic parameter (it would tend to inflate both MZ and DZ correlations). This result suggests that parents and children may be rating somewhat different phenomena, although at present the nature of these differences is unclear.

In addition to the distinction between children and parents as raters, differences in conclusions can be drawn from data provided by mothers and fathers. For example, parental ratings of temperament in twins have produced an unusual pattern of results whereby MZ correlations are typically moderate and DZ correlations are very low or negative—a phenomenon referred to as the "too low" DZ correlation (Neale & Stevenson, 1989; Plomin et al., 1993; Stevenson & Fielding, 1985). This pattern of results is consistent with rater biases whereby parents exaggerate differences between DZ twins (contrast effects) or accentuate similarity between MZ twins (assimilation effects). It is also consistent with dominant genetic variance. In order to examine which of these effects explain the too-low DZ correlation, one study applied model-fitting procedures to parent reports of temperaments, including emotionality and shyness, in 196 twin pairs ages 14–36 months (Saudino et al., 2000). It was found that a model that included contrast effects provided the best fit to the data. Another interesting finding concerning rater effects is that there may be differences between parents' reports in that, although both parents assess the same behavior in the child, each parent also assesses a unique aspect of the child's behavior (the psychometric model). This hypothesis was tested against the alternative hypothesis that both parents assess exactly the same behavior in the child (the rater-bias model; van der Valk, Van den Oord, Verhulst, & Boomsma, 2001c). Mother and father reports were obtained for 3,501 three-year-old twin pairs using the CBCL and support was found for the psychometric model. Interestingly, common factors (influencing similarity of assessment between parents) were more important than unique factors (influenced behaviors assessed by just one parent). These findings have since been replicated in a sample of 7-year-old twins (van der Valk, Van den Oord, Verhulst, & Boomsma, 2001b). It is unclear why parents should be influenced by contrast effects when rating their children's temperaments but not when rating their anxiety-related symptoms, and this issue requires further exploration.

CURRENT DIRECTIONS IN GENETIC RESEARCH ON CHILDHOOD ANXIETY

Molecular Genetics and Anxiety

Quantitative genetic studies have consistently shown important genetic influences on anxiety. Molecular genetic techniques are now being harnessed, with the eventual aim of using molecular genetics to influence diagnosis, treatment, and prevention of anxiety. The main techniques used to identify gene–trait or gene–disorder relationships are linkage and association. Linkage refers to a within-family technique in which the presence of a trait or disease is traced through a family alongside a particular version of DNA (allele), the trait or disease being less likely in individuals without the risk allele. This technique lacks statistical power in cases in which multiple genes (or quantitative trait loci, QTL) are involved in the trait or disorder and no one gene is necessary or sufficient to cause the disorder (Risch & Merikangas, 1996). Association provides a more powerful technique for identifying QTLs (Plomin, Owen, & McGuffin, 1994; Risch & Merikangas, 1996). This method compares allele frequencies in cases and controls, with a significant difference implying that the genotype is related to the disorder differentiating the cases and controls.

There are few linkage studies for anxiety, and those that have been conducted tend to focus on panic disorder (PD). One such study suggested linkage at two locations on chromosomes 16 and 6 (Crowe, Noyes, Persico, Wilson, & Elston, 1988), but these findings were not replicated in a subsequent study by the same group.

Association studies have provided more data exploring the relationship between specific genes and anxiety. The major focus of molecular genetic association studies in anxiety has been markers in the serotonin (5HT) system, which contributes to variation in many physiological functions such as food intake, sleep, motor activity, and reproductive activity, in addition to emotional states such as mood and anxiety, and which is the target of uptake-inhibiting antidepressant and antianxiety drugs. An early finding in this area was an association between the short form of a marker in the promoter region of the serotonin transporter (5-HTTLPR) and the emotional triad of anxiety, depression, and neuroticism (Lesch et al., 1996).

Despite positive replications of this finding (e.g., Katsuragi et al., 1999; Osher, Hamer, & Benjamin, 2000), several attempts to replicate this finding have failed (e.g., Ball et al., 1997; Flory et al., 1999; Gustavsson, Nothen, & Jonsson, 1999; Mazzanti et al., 1998). Interestingly, however, research examining the temperament of infants age 2 months found an association between high scores on negative emotionality and distress to limitations and short 5-HTTLPR (Auerbach, Geller, & Lezer, 1999). These findings led to the examination of the association between 5-HTTLPR and anxiety-related temperament and behavioral problems in children from infancy to mid-teens (Jorm et al., 2000). This investigation did not support the association between 5-HTTLPR and anxiety-related traits in early life; however, it did highlight the importance of developmental stage in assessing the relationship between genetic influence and anxiety. Although no significant associations were found during early childhood, between the ages of 13 and 16 the long/long genotype *was* associated with higher anxiety. This finding complements the quantitative work outlined previously, which suggests that genetic factors appear to have the greatest influence on anxiety in adolescent girls.

Several other markers related to the serotonin system have also been associated with anxiety (Bengel et al., 1999; McDougle, Epperson, Price, & Gelernter, 1998; Mundo, Richter, Sam, Macciardi, & Kennedy, 2000; Ohara, Suzuki, Ochiai, Tsukamoto, & Tani, 1999). In addition, markers within the dopamine system have been explored, particularly in relation to obsessive–compulsive disorder (Billett et al., 1998; Cruz et al., 1997) and within the gene for catechol-O-methyltransferase (COMT), an enzyme involved in the inactivation of catecholamines from both the serotonin and dopamine pathways (Camarena, Cruz, de la Fuente, & Nicolini, 1998; Karayiorgou et al., 1997, 1999). (For a more comprehensive review of molecular genetic research in anxiety, see Eley, Collier, & McGuffin, 2002).

Environment

Perhaps surprisingly, a key finding from behavioral genetic studies concerns the environment—many environmental measures are genetically influenced (gene–environment correlation). There are three types of gene–environment correlations: passive, evocative, and active (Plomin, DeFries, & Lochlin, 1977; see also Scarr & McCartney, 1983). The passive type refers to the fact that children gain both their genes and their environments from their parents, resulting in the two being correlated. Evocative gene–environment correlations occur when certain reactions are evoked from others due to characteristics influenced by genetic propensities. Finally, the active type involves individuals selecting and adapting experiences correlated with their genotypes. Such gene–environment correlations result in influences that were previously thought of as purely environmental, now being considered to have a heritable component. For example, studies have demonstrated that many traditional "environmental" measures are influenced by genetic factors, including life events (Thapar & McGuffin, 1996b) and parenting behaviors (O'Connor, Caspi, DeFries, & Plomin, 2000; Pike, McGuire, Hetherington, Reiss, & Plomin, 1996). In addition to these measures of the environment being heritable, there are also genetic influences on the association between these environmental measures and outcomes. Although no such studies exist to date in which the outcome measures include anxiety, one study has explored the association between depressive symptoms and parental negativity (Pike et al., 1996). It found a substantial genetic influence on the association between parental negativity and adolescent depression, which the authors interpreted as likely to result from an evocative gene–environment correlation, with adjustment problems influenced by genetic propensities leading to negative reactions from others.

In addition to gene–environment correlations, genetic factors can influence individual sensitivity to the environment (gene–environment interaction). Research showing that stressful environments have a greater effect on those who are at genetic risk highlights gene–environment interactions. For example, one study investigated subjective and physiological responses to inhalations of 35% carbon dioxide in a community sample comprising individuals with variations in the serotonin transporter gene (5-HTT; Schmidt, Storey, Greenberg, Santiago, & Murphy, 2000). As predicted, it was found that the group of individuals homozygous for the long allele showed greater fear of the inhalations. However, it was also found that individuals who expressed high fear of arousal symptoms and who have long alleles showed decreased heart rate variability in response to the challenge. These results need to be considered in the context of the small sample of 72 used in this investigation.

Along with evidence for gene–environment interactions in humans, animal studies, in which it is possible to control genes and environment, have the potential to be informative. Preliminary research of this nature has shown that genetically fearful infant rats show greater distress when separated from their mothers than infant rats that are not genetically fearful (Insel & Hill, 1987).

CONCLUSION

The proliferation of genetically sensitive studies of anxiety disorders and symptoms in children and adolescents over the past decade has provided a wealth of new data. These studies have demonstrated that genes account for around one-third of the variance for most measures of anxiety, that there is significant shared environmental influence on many definitions of anxiety in children and adolescents, and that individual-specific factors also play a substantial and significant role in the etiology of anxiety. However, substantial heterogeneity exists in these data, and the roles of age, sex, and rater on the etiology of anxiety has begun to be explored. Furthermore, finding that the definition of anxiety influences heritability estimates highlights the need for clearer definitions of anxiety.

Quantitative genetics is also moving beyond simply quantifying genetic influence on anxiety and beginning to explore the mechanisms by which genes have their effect. Such studies are able to shed light on fundamental questions concerning childhood anxiety. For example, these studies have the power to assess the developmental changes in genetic effects, as well as the relationship between nature and nurture, the specificity of different subtypes of anxiety, and links between normal and abnormal anxiety.

The search is now on for genes that affect anxiety. Genes need to be specified and their products characterized. Quantitative genetic study is informative in directing this search, having shown that genetic factors appear to have the greatest influence on anxiety in adolescent girls and that genes found for anxiety are likely to be associated with depression. Molecular research may also help us understand developmental changes in anxiety, by assessing, for example, whether the effects of genes change during development.

The next stage of research in this area will be to begin to identify the mechanisms by which genes and the environment interact and mediate risks for anxiety. With increased knowledge of the processes involved in the development of anxiety comes promise of developing methods of prevention and treatment for anxiety and its potentially severe consequences.

REFERENCES

Achenbach, T. M. (1991). *Manual for the Child Behavior Checklist and 1991 profile.* Burlington: University of Vermont, Department of Psychiatry.

Angold, A., Costello, E. J., & Erkanli, A. (1999). Comorbidity. *Journal of Child Psychology and Psychiatry, 40*(1), 57–87.

Angold, A., Costello, E. J., & Worthman, C. M. (1998). Puberty and depression: The roles of age, pubertal status and pubertal timing. *Psychological Medicine, 28*(1), 51–61.

Auerbach, J., Geller, V., Lezer, S., Shinwell, E., Belmaker, R. H., Levine, J., & Ebstein, R. (1999). Dopamine D4 receptor (DRD4) and serotonin transporter promoter (5–HTTLPR) polymorphism in the determination of temperament in 2-month-old infants. *Molecular Psychiatry, 4,* 369–373.

Ball, D. M., Hill, L., Freeman, B., Eley, T. C., Strelau, J., Riemann, R., Spinath, F. M.,

Angleitner, A., & Plomin, R. (1997). The serotonin transporter gene and peer-rated neuroticism. *NeuroReport, 8*,1301–1304.

Bengel, D., Greenberg, B. D., Cora-Locatelli, G., Altemus, M., Heilis, A., Li, Q., & Murphy, D. L. (1999). Association of the serotonin transporter promoter regulatory region polymorphism and obsessive–compulsive disorder. *Molecular Psychiatry 4*, 463–466.

Biederman, J., Rosenbaum, J. F., Bolduc, E. A., Faraone, S. V., & Hirshfeld, D. R. (1991). A high risk study of young children of parents with panic disorder and agoraphobia with and without comorbid major depression. *Psychiatry Research, 37*, 333–348.

Billett, E. A., Richter, M. A., Sam, F., Swinson, R. P., Dai, X. Y., King, N., Badri, F., Sasaki, T., Buchanan, J. A., & Kennedy, J. L. (1998). Investigation of dopamine system genes in obsessive–compulsive disorder. *Psychiatric Genetics, 8*, 163–169.

Bird, H. R., Canino, G., Rubio-Stipec, M., Gould, M. S., Ribera, J., Sesman, M., Woodbury, M., Huertas-Goldman, S., Pagan, A., Sanchez-Lacay, A., et al. (1988). Estimates of the prevalence of childhood maladjustment in a community survey in Puerto Rico. *Archives of General Psychiatry 45*, 1120–1126.

Boomsma, D. I., Koopmans, J. R., Dolan, C. V. (1997). Genetic longitudinal analysis of anxiety, neuroticism, and depression in adolescent and young-adult Dutch twins [Abstract]. *Behavior Genetics, 27*(6), 584.

Brady, E. U., & Kendall, P. C. (1992). Comorbidity of anxiety in children and adolescents. *Psychological Bulletin, 111*, 244–255.

Camarena, B., Cruz, C., de la Fuente, J., & Nicolini, H. (1998). A higher frequency of a low activity-related allele of the MAO-A gene in females with obsessive–compulsive disorder. *Psychiatric Genetics, 8*, 255–257.

Costello, A., & Angold, A. (1988). Scales to assess child and adolescent depression: Checklists, screens, and nets. *Journal of the American Academy of Child and Adolescent Psychiatry, 27*, 726–737.

Crowe, R. R., Noyes, R., Persico, T., Wilson, A. F., & Elston, R. C. (1988). Genetic studies of panic disorder and related conditions. In D. L. Dunnel, E. S. Gershon, & J. E. Barrett (Eds.), *Relatives at risk for mental disorders* (pp 73–85). New York: Raven Press.

Cruz, C., Camarena, B., King, N., Paez, F., Sidenberg, D., de la Fuente, J. R., & Nicolini, H. (1997). Increased prevalence of the seven-repeat variant of the dopamine D4 receptor gene in patients with obsessive–compulsive disorder with tics. *Neuroscience Letters, 231*, 1–4.

Deater-Deckard, K., Reiss, D., Hetherington, E. M., & Plomin, R. (1997). Dimensions and disorders of adolescent adjustment: A quantitative genetic analysis of unselected samples and selected extremes. *Journal of Child Psychology and Psychiatry, 38*, 515–525.

Eaves, L. J., Silberg, J. L., Meyer, J. M., Maes, H. H., Simonoff, E., Pickles, A., Rutter, M., Neale, M. C., Reynolds, C. A., Erickson, M. T., Heath, A. C., Loeber, R., Truett, K. R., & Hewitt, J. K. (1997). Genetics and developmental psychopathology: 2. The main effects of genes and environment on behavioral problems in the Virginia Twin Study of Adolescent Behavioral Development. *Journal of Child Psychology and Psychiatry 38*, 965–980.

Edelbrock, C., Rende, R., Plomin, R., & Thompson, L. A. (1995). A twin study of competence and problem behavior in childhood and early adolescence. *Journal of Child Psychology and Psychiatry and Allied Disciplines, 36,* 775–785.

Eley, T. C. (1996). *The etiology of emotional symptoms in children and adolescents: Depression and anxiety in twins.* Unpublished doctoral dissertation, University of London.

Eley, T. C., Collier, D., & McGuffin, P. (2002). Anxiety and eating disorders. In P. McGuffin, M. J. Owen, & I. I. Gottesman (Eds.), *Psychiatric genetics and genomics* (pp. 303–340). Oxford, UK: Oxford University Press.

Eley, T. C., & Stevenson, J. (1999a). Exploring the covariation between anxiety and depression symptoms: A genetic analysis of the effects of age and sex. *Journal of Child Psychology and Psychiatry and Allied Disciplines, 40(8),* 1273–1282.

Eley, T. C., & Stevenson, J. (1999b). Using genetic analyses to clarify the distinction between depressive and anxious symptoms in children. *Journal of Abnormal Child Psychology, 27,* 105–114.

Feigon, S. A., Waldman, I. D., Levy, F., & Hay, A. D. (2001). Genetic and environmental influences on separation anxiety disorder symptoms and their moderation by age and sex. *Behavior Genetics, 31,* 403–411.

Flory, J. D., Manuck, S. B., Ferrell, R. E., Dent, K. M., Peters, D. G., & Muldoon, M. F. (1999). Neuroticism is not associated with the serotonin transporter (5-HTTLPR) polymorphism. *Molecular Psychiatry, 4,* 251–257.

Gjone, H., & Stevenson, J. (1997). The association between internalizing and externalizing behavior in childhood and early adolescence: Genetic or environmental common influences. *Journal of Abnormal Child Psychology, 54,* 277–286.

Goldsmith, H. H., & Lemery, K. S. (2000). Linking temperamental fearfulness and anxiety symptoms: A behavior-genetic perspective. *Biological Psychiatry, 48,* 1199–1209.

Gustavsson, J. P., Nothen, M. M., Jonsson, E. G., Neidt, H., Forslund, K., Rylander, G., Mattilda-Evenden, M., Sedvall, G. C., Propping, P., & Asberg, M. (1999). No association between serotonin transporter gene polymorphism and personality traits. *American Journal of Medical Genetics, 88,* 430–436.

Hankin, B. L., Abramson, L. Y., Moffitt, T. E., Silva, A., McGee, R., & Angell, K. E. (1998). Development of depression from preadolescence to young adulthood: Emerging gender differences in a 10-year longitudinal study. *Journal of Abnormal Psychology, 107,* 128–140.

Ialongo, N., Edelsohn, G., Werthamer-Larsson, L., Crockett, L., & Kellam, S. (1994). The significance of self-reported anxious symptoms in first grade children. *Journal of Abnormal Child Psychology, 22,* 441–455.

Insel, T. R., & Hill, J. L. (1987). Infant separation distress in genetically fearful rats. *Biological Psychiatry, 22,* 786–789.

Jorm, A. F., Henderson, A. S., Jacomb, P. A., Christensen, H., Korten, A. E., Rodgers, B., Tan, X., & Easteal, S. (2000). Association of a functional polymorphism of the monoamine oxidase A gene promoter with personality and psychiatric symptoms. *Psychiatric Genetics, 10,* 87–90.

Karayiorgou, M., Altemus, M., Galke, B. L., Goldman, D., Murphy, D. L., Ott, J., & Gogos, J. A. (1997). Genotype determining low catechol-O-methyltransferase activity as a risk factor for obsessive–compulsive disorder. *Proceedings of the National Academy of Sciences of the United States of America, 94,* 4572–4575.

Karayiorgou, M., Sobin, C., Blundell, M. L., Galke, B. L., Malinova, L., Goldberg, P., Ott, J., & Gogos, J. A. (1999). Family-based association studies support a sexually dimorphic effect of COMT and MAOA on genetic susceptibility to obsessive–compulsive disorder. *Biological Psychiatry, 45,* 1178–1189.

Katsuragi, S., Kunugi, H., Sano, A., Tsutsumi, T., Isogawa, K., Nanko, S., & Akiyoshi, J. (1999). Association between serotonin transporter gene polymorphism and anxiety-related traits. *Biological Psychiatry, 45,* 368–370.

Kendler, K. S., Neale, M. C., Kessler, R. C., Heath, A. C., & Eaves, L. J. (1992). The genetic epidemiology of phobias in women: The interrelationship of agoraphobia, social phobia, situational phobia, and simple phobia. *Archives of General Psychiatry, 49,* 273–281.

Kendler, K. S., Neale, M. C., Kessler, R. C., Heath, A. C., & Eaves, L. J. (1993). Major depression and phobias: The genetic and environmental sources of comorbidity. *Psychological Medicine, 23,* 361–371.

Last, C. G., Hersen, M., Kazdin, A. E., Orvaschel, H., & Perrin, S. (1991). Anxiety disorders in children and their families. *Archives of General Psychiatry, 48,* 928–934.

Legrand, L. N., McGue, M., & Iacono, W. G. (1999). A twin study of state and trait anxiety in childhood and adolescence. *Journal of Child Psychology and Psychiatry, 40,* 953–958.

Lesch, K. P., Bengel, D., Heils, A., Zhang Sabol, S., Greenburg, B. D., Petri, S., Benjamin, J., Müller, C. R., Hamer, D. H., & Murphy, D. L. (1996). Association of anxiety-related traits with a polymorphism in the serotonin transporter gene regulatory region. *Science, 274,* 1527–1531.

Lichtenstein, P., & Annas, P. (2000). Heritability and prevalence of specific fears and phobias in childhood. *Journal of Child Psychology and Psychiatry, 41,* 927–937.

Livingston, R., Nugent, H., Rader, L., & Smith, G. R. (1985). Family histories of depressed and severely anxious children. *American Journal of Psychiatry, 142,* 1497–1499.

Martin, N., Boomsma, D. I., & Machin, G. (1997). A twin-pronged attack on complex trait. *Nature Genetics, 17,* 387–392.

Mazzanti C. M., Lappalainen, J., Long, J. C., Bengel, D., Naukkarinen, H., Eggert, M., Virkkunen, M., Linnoila, M., & Goldman, D. (1998). Role of the serotonin transporter promoter polymorphism in anxiety-related traits. *Archives of General Psychiatry, 55,* 936–940.

McDougle, C. J., Epperson, C. N., Price, L. H., & Gelernter, J. (1998). Evidence for linkage disequilibrium between serotonin transporter protein gene (SLC6A4) and obsessive–compulsive disorder. *Molecular Psychiatry, 3,* 270–273.

McGee, R., Feehan, M., Williams, . S, & Anderson, J. C. (1992). DSM-III disorders from age 11 to age 15 years. *Journal of the American Academy of Child and Adolescent Psychiatry, 31,* 50–59.

Mestel, R. (1994). The fearful gene in our children's make-up. *New Scientist, 141,* 10.

Mundo, E., Richter, M. A., Sam, F., Macciardi, F., & Kennedy, J. L. (2000). Is the 5–HT(1Dbeta) receptor gene implicated in the pathogenesis of obsessive–compulsive disorder? *American Journal of Psychiatry, 157,* 1160–1161.

Neale, M. C., & Stevenson, J. (1989). Rater bias in the EASI temperament scales: A twin study. *Journal of Personality and Social Psychology, 56*, 446–455.

Nelson, E. C., Grant, J. D., Bucholz, K. K., Glowinski, A., Madden, P. A. F., Reich, W., & Heath, A. C. (2000). Social phobia in population-based female adolescent twin sample: Comorbidity and associated suicide-related symptoms. *Psychological Medicine, 30*, 797–804.

O'Connor, T. G., Caspi, A., DeFries, J. C., & Plomin, R. (2000). Are associations between parental divorce in children's adjustment genetically mediated ? An adoption study. *Developmental Psychology, 36*, 429–437.

Ohara, K., Suzuki, Y., Ochiai, M., Tsukamoto, T., & Tani, K. (1999). A variable-number-tandem-repeat of the serotonin transporter gene and anxiety disorders. *Progress in Neuro-Psychopharmacology and Biological Psychiatry, 23*, 55–65.

Osher, Y., Hamer, D., & Benjamin, J. (2000). Association and linkage of anxiety-related traits with a functional polymorphism of the serotonin transporter gene regulatory region in Israeli sibling pairs. *Molecular Psychiatry, 5*, 216–219.

Peterson, J. L., & Zill, N. (1986). Marital disruption, parent–child relationship, and behavior problems in children. *Journal of Marriage and the Family, 48*, 295–307.

Pike, A., McGuire, S., Hetherington, E. M., Reiss, D., & Plomin, R. (1996). Family environment and adolescent depressive symptoms and antisocial behavior: A multivariate genetic analysis. *Developmental Psychology, 32*, 590–603.

Plomin, R., Coon, H., Carey, G., DeFries, J. C., & Fulker, D. W. (1991). Parent–offspring and sibling adoption analyses of parental ratings of temperament in infancy and childhood. *Journal of Personality, 59*, 705–732.

Plomin, R., DeFries, J. C., & Loehlin, J. C. (1977). Genotype–environment interaction and correlation in the analysis of human behavior. *Psychological Bulletin, 85*, 309–322.

Plomin, R., DeFries, J. C., McClearn, G. E., & McGuffin, P. (2001). *Behavioral genetics* (4th ed.). New York: Worth.

Plomin, R., Emde, R. N., Braungart, J. M., Campos, J., Corley, R., Fulker, D. W., Kagan, J., Reznick, J. S., Robinson, J., Zahn-Waxler, C., & DeFries, J. C. (1993). Genetic change and continuity from fourteen to twenty months: The MacArthur Longitudinal Twin Study. *Child Development, 64*, 1354–1376.

Plomin, R., Owen, M. J., & McGuffin, P. (1994). The genetic basis of complex human behaviors. *Science, 264*, 1733–1739.

Rende, R., Warner, V., Wickramaratne, P., & Weissman, M. (1999). Sibling aggregation for psychiatric disorders in offspring at high and low risk for depression: 10-year follow-up. *Psychological Medicine, 29*, 1291–1298.

Risch, N., & Merikangas, K. R. (1996). The future of genetic studies of complex human diseases. *Science, 273*, 1516–1517.

Robinson, J. L., Kagan, J., Reznick, J. S., & Corley, R. (1992). The heritability of inhibited and uninhibited behavior: A twin study. *Developmental Psychology, 28*, 1030–1037.

Rose, R. J., & Ditto, W. B. (1983). A developmental-genetic analysis of common fears from early adolescence to early adulthood. *Child Development, 54*, 361–368.

Saudino, K. J., Cherny, S. S., & Plomin, R. (2000). Parent ratings of temperament in twins: Explaining the "too low" DZ correlations. *Twin Research, 3,* 224–233.

Scarr, S., & McCartney, K. (1983). How people make their own environments: A theory of genotype - environmental effects. *Child Development, 54,* 424–435.

Schmidt, N. B., Storey, J., Greenberg, B. D., Santiago, H. T., Li, Q., & Murphy, D. L. (2000). Evaluating gene x psychological risk factor effects in the pathogenesis of anxiety: A new model approach. *Journal of Abnormal Psychology, 109,* 308–320.

Schmitz, S., Saudino, K. J., Plomin, R., Fulker, D. W., & DeFries, J. C. (1996). Genetic and environmental influences on temperament in middle childhood: Analyses of teacher and tester ratings. *Child Development, 67,* 409–422.

Silberg, J., Pickles, A., Rutter, M., Hewitt, J., Simonoff, E., Maes, H., Carbonneau, R., Murrell, L., Foley, D., & Eaves, L. (1999). The influence of genetic factors and life stress on depression among adolescent. *Archives of General Psychiatry, 56,* 225–232.

Silberg, J. L., Rutter, M., & Eaves, L. (2001). Genetic and environmental influences on the temporal association between earlier anxiety and later depression in girls. *Biological Psychiatry, 49,* 1040–1049.

Silberg, J., Rutter, M., Neale, M., & Eaves, L. (2001). Genetic moderation of environmental risk for depression and anxiety in adolescent girls. *British Journal of Psychiatry, 179,* 116–121.

Silove, D., Manicavasagar, V., O'Connell, D., & Morris-Yates, A. (1995). Genetic factors in early separation anxiety: Implications for the genesis of adult anxiety disorders. *Acta Psychiatrica Scandinavica, 92,* 17–24.

Statham, D. J., Heath, A., & Madde, P. A. F. (1998). Suicidal behavior: An epidemiological and genetic study. *Psychological Medicine, 28*(4), 839–855.

Stevenson, J., Batten, N., & Cherner, M. (1992). Fears and fearfulness in children and adolescents: A genetic analysis of twin data. *Journal of Child Psychology and Psychiatry, 33,* 977–985.

Stevenson, J., & Fielding, J. (1985). Ratings of temperament in families of young twins. *British Journal of Developmental Psychology, 3,* 143–152.

Thapar, A., & McGuffin, P. (1994). A twin study of depressive symptoms in childhood. *British Journal of Psychiatry, 165,* 259–265.

Thapar, A., & McGuffin, P. (1995). Are anxiety symptoms in childhood heritable? *Journal of Child Psychology and Psychiatry, 36,* 439–447.

Thapar, A., & McGuffin, P. (1996a). Genetic influences on life events in childhood. *Psychological Medicine, 26,* 813–820.

Thapar, A., & McGuffin, P. (1996b). A twin study of antisocial and neurotic symptoms in childhood. *Psychological Medicine, 26,* 1111–1118.

Thapar, A., & McGuffin, P. (1997). Anxiety and depressive symptoms in childhood: A genetic study of comorbidity. *Journal of Child Psychology and Psychiatry, 38,* 651–656.

Topolski, T. D., Hewitt, J. K., Eaves, L., Meyer, J. M., Silberg, J. L., Simonoff, E., & Rutter, M. (1999). Genetic and environmental influences on ratings of manifest anxiety by parents and children. *Journal of Anxiety Disorders, 13,* 371–397.

Topolski, T. D., Hewitt, J. K., Eaves, L. J., Silberg, J. L., Meyer, J. M., Rutter, M.,

Pickles, A., & Simonoff, E. (1997). Genetic and environmental influences on child reports of manifest anxiety and symptoms of separation anxiety and over-anxious disorders: A community-based twin study. *Behavioral Genetics, 27*, 15–28.

Turner, S. M., Beidel, D. C., & Costello, A. (1987). Psychopathology in the offspring of anxiety disordered patients. *Journal of Consulting and Clinical Psychology, 55*, 229–235.

van den Oord, E. J., Boomsma, D. I., & Verhulst, F. C. (1994). A study of problem behaviors in 10- to 15-year-old biologically related and unrelated international adoptees. *Behavioral Genetics, 24*, 193–205.

van den Oord, E. J., Verhulst, F. C., & Boomsma, D. I. (1996). A genetic study of maternal and paternal ratings of problem behaviors in 3-year-old twins. *Journal of Abnormal Psychology, 105*, 349–357.

Van den Oord, J. C. G., & Rowe, D. C. (1997). Continuity and change in children's social maladjustment: A developmental behavior genetic study. *Developmental Psychology, 33*, 319–332.

van der Valk, J. C., Van den Oord, E. J. C. G., Verhulst, F. C., & Boomsma, D. I. (2001a). Genetic and environmental contributions to continuity and change of internalizing and externalizing problems during childhood. In J. C. van der Valk (Ed.), *The genetic and environmental contributions to children's problem behaviors: A developmental approach* (pp. 95–113). Enschede, The Netherlands: FEBO Druk.

van der Valk, J. C., Van den Oord, E. J. C. G., Verhulst, F. C., & Boomsma, D. I. (2001b). Using common and unique parental views to study the etiology of 7-year-old twins' internalizing and externalizing problems. In J. C. van der Valk (Ed.), *The genetic and environmental contributions to children's problem behaviors: A developmental approach* (pp. 73–94). Enschede, The Netherlands: FEBO Druk.

van der Valk, J. C., Van den Oord, E. J. C. G., Verhulst, F. C., & Boomsma, D. I. (2001c). Using parental ratings to study the etiology of 3-year-old twins' problem behaviors: Different views or rater bias? In J. C. van der Valk (Ed.), *The genetic and environmental contributions to children's problem behaviors: A developmental approach* (pp. 49–71). Enschede, The Netherlands: FEBO Druk.

van der Valk, J. C., Verhulst, F. C., Neale, M. C., & Boomsma, D. I. (2001). Longitudinal genetic analysis of problem behaviors in biologically related and unrelated adoptees. In J. C. van der Valk (Ed.), *The genetic and environmental contributions to children's problem behaviors: A developmental approach* (pp. 115–142). Enschede, The Netherlands: FEBO Druk.

van der Valk, J. C., Verhulst, F. C., Stroet, T. M., & Boomsma, D. I. (1998). Quantitative genetic analysis of internalizing and externalizing problems in a large sample of 3-year-old twins. *Twin Research, 1*, 25–33.

Velez, C. N., Johnson, J., & Cohen, P. (1989). A longitudinal analysis of selected risk factors for childhood psychopathology. *Journal of the American Academy of Child and Adolescent Psychiatry, 28*(6), 861–865.

Warren, S. L., Huston, L., Egeland, B., & Sroufe, A. (1997). Child and adolescent anxiety disorders and early attachment. *Journal of the American Academy of Child and Adolescent Psychiatry, 36*, 637–644.

Warren, S. L., Schmitz, S., & Emde, R. (1999). Behavioral genetic analyses of self-reported anxiety at 7 years of age. *Journal of the American Academy of Child and Adolescent Psychiatry, 38*(11), 1403–1408.

Weissman, M. M., Leckman, J. F., Merikangas, K. R., Gammon, G. D., & Prusoff, B. A. (1984). Depression and anxiety disorders in parents and children: Results from the Yale Family Study. *Archives of General Psychiatry, 41*, 845–852.

Weissman, M. M., Warner, V., Wickramaratne, P., Moreau, D., & Olfson, M. (1997). Offspring of depressed parents: 10 years later. *Archives of General Psychiatry, 54*, 932–942.

Chapter 5

Assessment

LAURIE A. GRECO
TRACY L. MORRIS

The reliable and valid assessment of child and adolescent anxiety faces numerous challenges, including high comorbidity within anxiety disorder categories and between anxiety and depression (Anderson, 1994; Kovacs & Devlin, 1998; Manassis, 2000). Low congruence among parent, child, and teacher reports further complicates accurate assessment and diagnosis (e.g., Epkins, 1996; Epkins & Meyers, 1994). Self-report is essential to assessing the internal and subjective nature of anxiety; however, young children's ability to identify and effectively report cognitions and physiological–somatic sensations has been called into question (Quay & La Greca, 1986; Stone & Lemanek, 1990).

Despite such challenges, the past decade has witnessed advances in the development of psychometrically sound, clinically useful measures of child and adolescent anxiety (see Barrios & Hartmann, 1997; Langley, Bergman, & Piacentini, 2002; Schniering, Hudson, & Rapee, 2000; Wood, Piacentini, Bergman, McCracken, & Barrios, 2002). Such progress can be attributed in part to improvements in the standardized nomenclature, with anxiety disorder categories undergoing significant revision and enhanced clarification in the fourth edition of the *Diagnostic and Statistical Manual of Mental Disorders* (DSM-IV; American Psychiatric Association, 1994). Moreover, the increasing focus on empirically supported treatments has necessitated the development and refinement of global and syndrome-specific measures of anxiety and related disorders. In this chapter, we address general issues in assessment and describe instruments commonly used with children and adolescents. The utility of conducting behavioral observations across important developmental domains and exploring current limitations in assessment research are also discussed.

GENERAL ISSUES IN ASSESSMENT

Given the multifaceted nature of anxiety, it is important to assess cognitive, overt behavioral, and somatic responding across multiple contexts such as home and school environments. Ideally, several methods should be used (e.g., interview, questionnaire, and behavioral observation), with information obtained from multiple sources (e.g., parents, teachers, and peers). The collective findings should then be used to guide case conceptualization and to identify pertinent information such as symptom frequency and severity, potential fear-eliciting stimuli, and exacerbating and/or mitigating factors.

When working with children and adolescents, it is important to select measures that are culturally and developmentally relevant and sensitive to children's understanding of emotion and level of self-awareness (Schniering et al., 2000). Most of the earlier instruments used to assess anxiety were adapted from adult measures. Although useful, these instruments generally were based on adult models of anxiety and were not considered ideal for measuring the structural and functional presentation of this construct in childhood and adolescence (Beidel & Stanley, 1993; Schniering et al., 2000). Over time, a trend has arisen toward enhanced developmental sensitivity and greater specificity with respect to the assessment of anxiety and related behavior in children.

Stallings and March (1995) proposed five important selection criteria for assessment instruments, recommending those that (1) provide reliable and valid information, (2) discriminate among symptom clusters, (3) evaluate the frequency and severity of target response(s), (4) incorporate multiple observations, and (5) are sensitive to treatment effects. The authors further recommend the integration of dimensional and categorical measures to provide information regarding anxiety symptomatology and diagnostic or group status. Both approaches have been used to inform treatment outcome research, and, when used in conjunction, they provide supplementary indices of anxiety symptoms and disorder. We now summarize commonly used measures of anxiety and provide examples of structured interview, parent, teacher, and self-report measures, and behavioral observation strategies.

SEMISTRUCTURED INTERVIEWS

The Anxiety Disorders Interview Schedule for DSM-IV—Child and Parent Version (ADIS-C/P; Silverman & Albano, 1996) is a semistructured interview developed specifically to assess child and adolescent anxiety disorders. The ADIS-C/P is administered separately to children and their parent(s), with the resulting information combined to facilitate differential diagnosis. Items on the ADIS-C/P assess cognitive, behavioral, and physiological responding across a range of potentially anxiety-inducing situations (e.g., interacting with peers, being apart from a parent). In addition, respondents are asked to rate symptom severity and interference with daily functioning using an 8-point Likert-type scale (0 = lowest severity/interference; 8 = highest severity/interference). Although the ADIS-C/P focuses primarily on anxiety disorders, interview questions screen for other conditions in childhood and adolescence, such as mood disorders, attention-deficit/hyperactivity disorder, developmental delays, and disruptive behavior disorders.

In general, research supports the psychometric properties and clinical utility of the ADIS-C/P. The anxiety disorder categories have excellent test–retest and interrater reliability (e.g., Rapee, Barrett, Dadds, & Evans, 1994; Silverman, Saavedra, & Pina, 2001) and appear sensitive to treatment-produced change (e.g., Barrett, Dadds, & Rapee, 1996; Kendall et al., 1997). Furthermore, research supports the concurrent validity of the Social Phobia, Separation Anxiety, and Panic Disorder scales on the ADIS-C/P, with strong correspondence found between these diagnoses and the empirically derived factor scores on the Multidimensional Anxiety Scale for Children (MASC; Wood et al., 2002).

Other structured and semistructured interviews have been used in research and practice to assess anxiety symptoms and disorder, including the Schedule for Affective Disorders and Schizophrenia for School-Aged Children (SADS; Kaufman et al., 1997), the National Institute of Mental Health Diagnostic Interview Schedule for Children—Version IV (DISC-IV; Shaffer et al., 2000), and the Diagnostic Interview for Children and Adolescents (DICA-R; Herjanic & Reich, 1997). The ADIS-C/P, however, is the only measure developed specifically to facilitate differential diagnosis of anxiety and related disorders and currently is considered the "gold standard" interview for assessing anxiety in youths. Strengths of the ADIS-C/P are the parallel parent and child versions, empirical support, and demonstrated clinical utility. In addition, the ADIS-C/P screens for symptom severity and level of interference, which are essential to assigning DSM-IV diagnoses and which may serve as indicators of adaptation and quality of life. Potential barriers to using the ADIS-C/P include the time-intensive nature of administration (approximately 1½ hours for each version) and the restricted focus on categorical (DSM-IV) information.

PARENT AND TEACHER REPORT MEASURES

In general, poor concordance has been found among parent, child, and teacher reports of child anxiety and related behavior (e.g., Sprafkin, Gadow, Salisbury, Schneider, & Loney, 2002). Most research suggests that child self-reports reveal higher levels of anxiety and depression than those obtained from third-party reports, whereas parents and teachers generally report higher levels of disruptive behavior than children will indicate for themselves (e.g., Edelbrock, Costello, Dulcan, Kalas, & Conover, 1985). Some findings, however, indicate the reverse, with children self-reporting more behavior problems and parents describing higher levels of internalizing symptoms (e.g., Earls, Reich, Jung, & Cloninger, 1988; Frick, Silverthorn, & Evans, 1994). Inconsistencies across reporters may be attributable to numerous factors, such as the child's developmental–cognitive ability and the level of social desirability and psychopathology experienced by the informant (Cole, Hoffman, Tram & Maxwell, 2000; Kashani, Orvaschel, Burk, & Reid, 1985). Another possibility is that children's cognitive and emotional states may be less evident to "outside" observers such as parents and teachers. Thus researchers and clinicians generally advocate the integration of parent, child, and teacher data to enhance our understanding of child functioning across unique perspectives (Cole et al., 2000).

Traditionally, parent and teacher report questionnaires have not been specific to child and adolescent anxiety per se. Instead, more general or "broadband" measures have been used to assess behavioral, social, and emotional problems exhibited at home and school. Given their widespread use in research and practice, we briefly present the Child Behavior Checklist (CBCL) and Teacher Report Form (TRF). Next, teacher and parent versions of the Child Symptom Inventory (CSI-4) and the Screen for Child Anxiety Related Emotional Disorders (SCARED; parent version) are discussed as more diagnostically relevant alternatives.

Child Behavior Checklist and Teacher Report Form

The CBCL and TRF (Achenbach, 1991a, 1991b; Achenbach & Rescorla, 2001) are used extensively in research and clinical settings to assess a broad range of internalizing and externalizing problems in childhood and adolescence. In addition to a Total Behavior Problem score, these measures yield three empirically derived factor scores (i.e., Internalizing, Externalizing, and Social Competence) and nine narrow-band scales, including Anxious/Depressed, Withdrawn, and Somatic Complaints. In general, the CBCL and TRF have been successful in discriminating between clinically referred and nonreferred samples (e.g., Achenbach, 1991a, 1991b). However, concerns have been raised regarding the limited correspondence among empirically derived scales on the CBCL and TRF and the DSM-IV diagnostic categories (e.g., Compas & Oppedisano, 2000). Thus, although the Internalizing and Anxious/Depressed subscales correlate positively with measures of general and syndrome-specific anxiety, no compelling data currently support the discriminative validity of the CBCL or the TRF in assessing anxiety as defined in the DSM-IV. Rather, the Internalizing and Anxious/Depressed scales appear to measure a more global construct (i.e., negative affect) common to both mood and anxiety disorders (Chorpita, Albano, & Barlow, 1998; Chorpita & Daleiden, 2002).

Child Symptom Inventory — Fourth Revision

The CSI-4 (Gadow & Sprafkin, 1994) is a behavior rating scale completed by parents (97 items) or teachers (77 items). Items on the CSI-4 correspond to DSM-IV categories, with two scoring procedures available to yield (1) categorical and/or (2) dimensional indices of adjustment. On the CSI-4, three scales screen for common child and adolescent anxiety disorders; that is, generalized anxiety disorder (GAD; eight items); social phobia (SP; four items); and separation anxiety disorder (SAD; eight items). In addition, single items screen for simple phobias, obsessions, and compulsions.

Parent and teacher versions of the CSI-4 generally converge and diverge in a theoretically expected pattern with respective scales of the CBCL, TRF, and diagnostic semistructured interviews (Gadow & Sprafkin, 2002). Additionally, GAD ratings on the CSI-4 (parent and teacher versions) have demonstrated moderate to high sensitivity and specificity when compared with clinician-reported psychiatric diagnoses (Gadow & Sprafkin, 1994, 2002). Similarly, moderate correlations have been found between parent ratings on the CSI-4 and corresponding DSM-IV categories derived from a structured interview (GAD, $r = .49$; SP, $r = .44$; and SAD, $r = .63$; Sprafkin et al., 2002). Thus, relative to the CBCL and TRF, the CSI-4 appears to provide categorical and dimensional ratings specific to child and adolescent anxiety. More research is needed, however, to document further the reliability, validity, and clinical utility of the anxiety disorder scales on this measure.

Screen for Child Anxiety Related Emotional Disorders

The parent version of the SCARED (Birmaher et al., 1997) screens for DSM-IV anxiety disorders in children and adolescents 9 to 18 years old. This measure consists of 38 items that are grouped into five factor domains: Panic/Somatic, Separation Anxiety, General Anxiety, Social Phobia, and School Phobia. Birmaher and colleagues have reported excellent internal consistency and good test–retest reliability. Adequate discriminative validity also has been documented, with the SCARED distinguishing between anxiety and related disorders (e.g., mood and disruptive behavior disorders). Overall, preliminary data suggest that the SCARED may be a promising parent-report measure of child anxiety. Additional research is needed to establish further the psychometric properties and clinical usefulness of this instrument.

GLOBAL SELF-REPORT MEASURES

Self-report questionnaires are used with grade-school children and adolescents to assess global and specific types of anxiety. Global measures provide a general or overall index of anxiety, whereas syndrome-specific instruments assess anxiety symptoms that are elicited by particular stimuli or experienced in certain contexts. Historically, researchers and clinicians have measured global anxiety using the Revised Children's Manifest Anxiety Scale (RCMAS; Reynolds & Richmond, 1978), Fear Survey Scale for Children—Revised (FSSC-R; Ollendick, 1983), and State-Trait Anxiety Inventory for Children (STAI-C; Spielberger, 1973). All three instruments are age-downward modifications of adult questionnaires developed prior to the publication of the DSM-IV. Consequently, these measures were based initially on adult models of anxiety; they do not reflect the most recent diagnostic taxonomy, and therefore they may have restricted clinical utility (Muris, Mayer, Bartelds, Tierney, & Bogie, 2001; Perrin & Last, 1992). Moreover, the RCMAS, FSSC-R, and STAI-C are good measures of global distress but generally do not distinguish between anxiety and related conditions such as depression, attention deficits, and hyperactivity (Hodges, 1990; Perrin & Last, 1992; Stark, Kaslow, & Laurent, 1993).

More thorough reviews of the RCMAS, FSSC-R, and STAI-C have been presented elsewhere (e.g., Langely et al., 2002; Stallings & March, 1995) and thus are not repeated here. Instead, we focus our discussion on more recently developed measures that have demonstrated greater specificity with respect to anxiety in children. The MASC, SCARED-R, and Spence Children's Anxiety Scale (SCAS) were published following the publication of the DSM-IV and have demonstrated promise in the evaluation of syndrome-specific and global indices of anxiety.

Multidimensional Anxiety Scale for Children

The MASC is a 45-item self-report instrument that screens for anxiety symptoms experienced by children and adolescents. The MASC yields a Total Anxiety Disorder Index and four main factor scores (with subfactor domains noted in parentheses as applicable): Social Anxiety (performance anxiety, humiliation), Physical Symptoms (tension–restlessness; somatic–automatic arousal), Harm/Avoidance (perfectionism, anxious coping), and Separation/Panic. Finally, six items yield an Inconsistency Index to identify careless or contradictory responding. Notably, the initial factor structure for the MASC has been replicated via confirmatory factor analyses in both community and clinical samples (March, 1998).

The MASC has become one of the most widely used measures of child and adolescent anxiety, with a growing empirical base supporting its use in research and practice (e.g., Langley et al., 2002). March, Parker, Sullivan, Stallings, and Conners (1997) reported excellent internal consistency and satisfactory to excellent test–retest reliability (r = .60–.93) across community and epidemiological samples. Moreover, findings support the concurrent validity of the MASC, with the Anxiety Disorder Index (ADI) and the four factor domains correlating in the expected direction with global and syndrome-specific measures, respectively (Greenhill, Pine, March, Birmaher, & Riddle, 1998; March et al., 1997; Wood et al., 2002). Finally, good discriminant validity (95% sensitivity) has been found for this measure, with the ADI discriminating between children with and without anxiety disorders using a gender-matched comparison group design (March, 1998). In summary, the MASC rapidly has become a preferred instrument in the assessment of child and adolescent anxiety, with increasing support found for its psychometric properties and clinical relevance.

Screen for Child Anxiety Related
Emotional Disorders – Revised

The SCARED-R (Birmaher et al., 1997; Muris, Merckelbach, Van Brakel, & Mayer, 1999) is a 66-item self-report instrument with subscales corresponding to the following DSM-IV categories: generalized anxiety disorder, social phobia, separation anxiety disorder, panic disorder, obsessive–compulsive disorder, traumatic stress disorder, and three types of specific phobias (blood–injection–injury, animal, environmental phobias). Using a 3-point Likert-type scale, children rate how frequently they experience each symptom. Scores are then summed across relevant items to yield a total anxiety score and six DSM-based subscale scores.

Parallel parent and child versions are available, and both versions have shown excellent internal consistency, good test–retest reliability, and moderate levels of parent–child agreement (Birmaher et al., 1997, 1999). For the child version, positive relations have been found between the total anxiety score and other widely used measures of global anxiety, including the RCMAS, FSSC-R, and STAI-C (e.g., Muris et al., 1999). Moreover, initial data support the validity of various domains measured by the SCARED-R, such as the traumatic stress disorder scale (Muris, Merckelbach, Koerver, & Meesters, 2000) and the social phobia scale (Muris, Merckelbach, & Damsma, 2000). Finally, results from outcome research supported the treatment sensitivity of this measure, with significant declines in scores reported following participation in either group or individual CBT for anxiety disorders (Muris et al., 2001). Overall, findings suggest that the SCARED-R is a promising new measure that can be used to assess global and syndrome-specific symptoms of anxiety in childhood and adolescence.

Spence Children's Anxiety Scale

The SCAS (Spence, 1997, 1998) consists of 45 items, 7 assessing social desirability and 38 corresponding to the following DSM-IV categories: generalized anxiety (GA), social anxiety (SOC), separation anxiety (SA), panic/agoraphobia (P/A), obsessions/compulsions (O/C), and fear of physical injury (FPI). The SCAS total score has demonstrated good internal consistency and test–retest reliability over a 6-month interval for Australian children 8–12 years of age (Spence, 1997). Moreover, preliminary findings support the convergent validity of this measure, with strong correlations found between the SCAS Total Anxiety Scale and the RCMAS (Chorpita, Yim, Moffitt, Umemoto, & Francis, 2000; Spence, 1998). Finally, an expected pattern of relations has been reported among the SCARED-R and SCAS subscale scores (Muris, Merckelbach, & Damsma, 2000; Muris, Schmidt, & Merckelbach, 2000).

Despite relatively high correspondence between the SCAS and relevant DSM-IV criteria, some concerns have been reported. For example, limited support has been found for the validity of the GAD scale, which appears to be a better indicator of negative affect and autonomic responding than of generalized anxiety (Spence, 1997). Similarly, the content validity of the GAD subscale has been questioned given that no items corresponded directly to excessive worry, a key feature of GAD in childhood and adolescence (Chorpita, Tracey, Brown, Collica, & Barlow, 1997). Chorpita and colleagues (1997; Chorpita et al., 2000) have taken an active role in further refining and testing clinically relevant modifications of this questionnaire, renaming it the Revised Child Anxiety and Depression Scales (RCADS). Seven items were added to measure hallmark features of GAD (e.g., worrying that bad things will happen, feeling shaky when one has a problem), and items reflecting DSM-III-R overanxious disorder were omitted. Acknowledging the high overlap between anxiety and depression, Chorpita and colleagues also added an 11-item depression scale (e.g., feeling sad or empty, feeling nothing is much fun, having problems with appetite). Preliminary data for the RCADS have been promising and support the factor structure, internal consistency, and concurrent validity of this revision (Chorpita et al., 2000).

In summary, well-known measures of anxiety such as the RCMAS, FSSC-R, and STAI-C are useful instruments in screening for general levels of distress and negative affect. Increased recognition of limitations of these measures has prompted the development and refinement of more syndrome-specific, and DSM-relevant, measurement strategies. A growing literature is investigating the psychometric properties of the MASC, SCARED-R, and SCAS/RCADS. Future research might focus on the relative strengths and incremental utility of these instruments. In addition, it is important to examine further the pattern of relations among general and syndrome-specific scales on the MASC, SCARED-R, and SCAS/RCADS and to document the relative strengths, limitations, and unique contributions of each measure. Finally, there is a clear need to develop parent- and teacher-report measures of child anxiety and related difficulties. A future direction, therefore, might be to develop and empirically test parent and teacher versions of these measures.

SYNDROME-SPECIFIC MEASURES

Social Anxiety Disorder (Social Phobia)

Social Anxiety Scale for Children – Revised

The SASC-R is a 22-item empirically derived instrument used to assess subjective (e.g., fear of negative evaluation) and behavioral (e.g., avoidance, withdrawal) indicators of social anxiety (La Greca, 1998; La Greca, Dandes, Wick, Shaw, & Stone, 1988; La Greca & Stone, 1993). Items on the SASC-R were developed to reflect a theoretically derived construct of social anxiety (Leary, 1983; Watson & Friend, 1969), and as a result they do not correspond fully to DSM criteria (Epkins, 2002; Morris & Masia, 1998). The SASC-R is composed of three factors: Fear of Negative Evaluation (FNE), Generalized Social Avoidance and Distress (SAD-G), and Social Avoidance and Distress with new or unfamiliar peers (SAD-New). The SASC-R has excellent internal consistency and test–retest reliability (La Greca, 1998; La Greca & Stone, 1993). Support also has been found for its concurrent validity (La Greca, 1998; La Greca & Stone, 1993). SASC-R total and factor scores, for example, have been associated with general anxiety, social competence, global self-worth, and peer relationship difficulties (e.g., La Greca & Stone, 1993; Strauss & Last, 1993). Finally, the SASC-R has successfully discriminated between children with and without a comorbid diagnosis in which social anxiety was the key criterion (Ginsburg, La Greca, & Silverman, 1998).

Social Phobia and Anxiety Inventory for Children

The SPAI-C (Beidel, Turner, & Morris, 1995, 1998) is a 26-item empirically derived measure that evaluates the range and frequency of social anxiety experienced by children and adolescents (8–14 years). Items on the SPAI-C reflect DSM-IV criteria for social anxiety disorder (social phobia), assessing relevant cognitions, behavior, and somatic responses across a range of potentially fear-eliciting situations (e.g., school plays, parties, eating in public). The SPAI-C also distinguishes among anxiety experienced in the presence of familiar peers, unfamiliar peers, and adults, with some items measuring anxious responding before and during social interaction and performance situations. Overall, the SPAI-C has demonstrated excellent internal consistency and high test–retest reliability, and scores have correlated moderately with general anxiety, fear of criticism, and parent-reported internalizing symptoms and social competence (Beidel et al., 1995). Support also has been found for the SPAI-C's external and discriminative validity (Beidel, Turner, & Fink, 1996; Beidel, Turner, Hamlin, & Morris, 2000). For example, SPAI-C scores have correlated positively with (1) observer ratings of children's anxiety and effectiveness during read-aloud and role-play tasks, and (2) children's self-reported distress during these tasks. Most notably, the SPAI-C has successfully discriminated between children with and without social phobia, as well as between those with social phobia and with other anxiety disorder diagnoses (Beidel et al., 2000).

Modest associations have been reported between the SASC-R and SPAI-C (e.g., Epkins, 2002; Morris & Masia, 1998). This imperfect correspondence is not surprising, given that these measures were developed to assess overlapping though distinct theoretical (SASC-R) and DSM-relevant (SPAI-C) constructs. The SASC-R and SPAI-C are empirically derived questionnaires with utility in research and practice. The relative merits of each depend largely on the goal of assessment and type of information to be obtained. Items assessing physiological–somatic symptoms, for example, are included on the SPAI-C but not the SASC-R. In contrast, the SASC-R provides a more thorough index of children's fear of negative evaluation. Future research is needed to evaluate further the differential utility of the SASC-R and SPAI-C.

Obsessive–Compulsive Disorder

Children's Yale–Brown Obsessive Compulsive Scale

Adapted from its adult version, the CY-BOCS (Goodman, Price, Rasmussen, Riddle, & Rapoport, 1991) is a semistructured clinical interview used to evaluate the severity of obsessive–compulsive symptoms among children and adolescents 6–17 years old. Obsessions and compulsions are rated separately by the clinician in areas such as time involved, subjective distress, functional interference, and control. Scahill and colleagues (1997) investigated the psychometric properties of the CY-BOCS and found the measure to have high internal consistency, good to excellent interrater agreement, and moderate discriminant and convergent validity.

Leyton Obsessional Inventory – Child Version

The LOI-CV (Berg, Whitaker, Davies, Flament, & Rapoport, 1988) is a 20-item scale for the assessment of frequency and severity of obsessions and related symptoms. Four factors have been identified: General Obsessive, Dirt/Contamination, Numbers/Luck, and School-Related Symptoms. Flament, Whitaker, and Rapoport (1988) reported acceptable sensitivity but poor specificity for the measure in an epidemiological investigation of OCD in adolescents. Recently, Bamber, Tamplin, Park, Kyte, and Goodyear (2002) have reported preliminary psychometric data on a new short form of the LOI-CV that demonstrated adequate discriminability of OCD and major depressive disorder across five groups of adolescents, including patient and community control samples.

Posttraumatic Stress Disorder

Child Post-Traumatic Stress Disorder Reaction Index

The 20-item CPTSD-RI (Frederick, 1985; Frederick, Pynoos, & Nader, 1992) is used to assess the presence and severity of posttraumatic stress symptoms among children and adolescents (ages 8–18 years). Using either an interview or questionnaire format, the CPTSD-RI assesses general levels of functioning and screens for trauma-related fears, memories, and avoidance grouped into three diagnostically relevant clusters: Re-experiencing (five items), Avoidance (four items), and Hyper-arousal (five items). Although consistent with PTSD diagnostic criteria, these clusters are not exhaustive and do not include all relevant traumatic stress symptoms specified in the DSM-IV (Foa, Johnson, Feeny, & Treadwell, 2001; Nader, 1997). The CPTSD-RI has been found to have excellent internal consistency and good interrater and test–retest reliability (Frederick, 1985; Pynoos & Nader, 1989). The concurrent validity for this instrument has been demonstrated, with associations consistently reported among the CPTSD-RI and other measures of posttraumatic stress, such as the Impact of Events Scale—Revised (IES-R; Horowitz, Wilner, & Alvarez, 1979) and PTSD scales on diagnostic interviews (Frederick, 1985; Pynoos & Nader, 1989).

Child PTSD Symptom Scale

The CPSS is a relatively new measure to assess traumatic stress symptoms among children and adolescents 8–18 years old (Foa et al., 2001). The CPSS is a 24-item age-downward modification of the Posttraumatic Diagnostic Scale for adults (PTDS; Foa, Cashman, Jaycox, & Perry, 1997). Items on the CPSS assess all 17 DSM-IV symptom criteria for PTSD, some of which are not considered by other instruments (e.g., CPTSD-RI and IES-R). The CPSS yields a Total Severity Score (17 items) and three empirically derived factor scores representing DSM-IV clusters B (Re-experiencing), C (Avoidance), and D (Arousal). In addition, a 7-item scale was included to assess trauma-related functional impairment across important life domains (e.g., family, friends, and school). Preliminary support has been provided for the psychometric properties of this measure. Evidence indicates moderate to excellent internal consistency, test–retest reliability, and concurrent validity for Total Severity, Functional Impairment, and three subscale scores. Results of discriminant functional analysis have demonstrated excellent sensitivity (95%) and specificity (96%), further supporting the utility of this measure in research and practice (Foa et al., 1997).

Anxiety Sensitivity

The increasing conceptual and empirical attention devoted to anxiety sensitivity (AS) in childhood and adolescence has motivated the development and refinement of a reliable, valid, and clinically useful measure of AS in youths (Silverman, Fleisig, Rabian, & Peterson, 1991; Silverman & Weems, 1999). Briefly, AS refers to the fear of a variety of anxiety symptoms and has been identified as a potential risk factor contributing to the development of panic attacks and numerous anxiety disorders (Mattis & Ollendick, 1997; Reiss, 1991; Reiss, Silverman, & Weems, 2001). The Childhood Anxiety Sensitivity Index (CASI; Silverman et al., 1991) is an 18-item self-report inventory that represents an age-downward modification of the Anxiety Sensitivity Index (ASI; Peterson & Reiss, 1987). The CASI has been used with children and adolescents (6–17 years) and was tailored after the ASI to assess fear of various anxiety-related symptoms and bodily sensations (e.g., "It scares me when I feel shaky," "It scares me when I feel nervous").

The CASI has demonstrated high internal consistency and test–retest reliability in both clinical and community samples (Silverman et al., 1991). The concurrent validity of this instrument also has been documented, with positive associations found between the CASI total score and panic symptoms, including the number and perceived severity of panic attacks and panic-related distress (e.g., Lau, Calamari, & Waraczynski, 1996). Research investigating the factor structure of the CASI indicated three or four first-order factors, including Physical Concerns, Mental Incapacitation Concerns, Control of anxiety symptoms, and Social Concerns (Silverman, Ginsburg, & Goedhart, 1999). As noted by these authors, future research is needed to assess the utility of distinguishing between the latter two factors (i.e., Control and Social Concerns). Finally, despite questions regarding the parsimony of an AS construct (e.g., Lilienfeld, Jacob, & Turner, 1989), research has supported the incremental validity of the CASI for grade-school children (Weems, Hammond-Laurence, Silverman, & Ginsburg, 1998) and adolescents (Chorpita, Albano, & Barlow, 1996; Weems et al., 1998).

BEHAVIORAL ASSESSMENT

The importance of incorporating behavioral observations into batteries for child and adolescent anxiety is increasingly being recognized (e.g., Barrios & Hartman, 1997; Kendall & Flannery-Schroeder, 1998; Vasey & Lonigan, 2000). Weaknesses of questionnaire and interview strategies include children's potential metacognitive limitations and informant susceptibility to response bias and social desirability (Barrios & Hartman, 1997). Moreover, some children and adolescents may underreport anxiety symptoms and overreport competencies to cope, perhaps due to heightened levels of self-presentational and evaluative concerns (Kendall & Flannery-Schroeder, 1998). Finally, low to moderate correspondence traditionally has been found among child, parent, and teacher reports of child anxiety (e.g., Epkins & Meyers, 1994). These shortcomings suggest that it may be important to incorporate standardized behavioral observations into research and practice (Vasey & Lonigan, 2000). In this section, we describe several strategies that have been used to assess overt manifestations of anxiety.

Behavioral Assessment Tests

Behavioral assessment tests (BATs) traditionally have been used in laboratory or clinic settings to assess children's behavior in the presence of phobic stimuli (e.g., animals, blood, or darkness) and/or across a range of fear-eliciting situations (see Barrios & Hartmann, 1997). BATs originally were used with children and adolescents who had a circumscribed fear or specific phobia and more recently have been used to assess responding in social and performance situations (Beidel & Turner, 1998). Children and adolescents who experience high levels of social anxiety, for example, have been asked to participate in a "read aloud" task, to give an impromptu speech in front of an audience, and/or to converse with a same- or opposite-gender peer (e.g., Beidel & Turner, 1998; Beidel, Turner, & Morris, 1999; Spence, Donovan, & Brechman-Toussaint, 1999). Irrespective of the type of anxiety, a wide range of responses can be coded, such as latency to respond, proximity to the feared stimulus, duration or frequency of a target behavior, and/or degree of behavioral distress during the task. The Revised Behavioral Assertiveness Test for Children (BAT-CR; Ollendick, 1981) is one example of a standardized behavioral assessment test used to assess assertiveness and social skill competency. The BAT-CR includes a series of role-play tasks, during which numerous responses are coded, including eye contact and latency and length of responding.

Documenting the clinical utility of BATs has been quite difficult, in large part due to the absence of standardized behavioral assessment and coding procedures and the associated challenges of conducting cross-study comparisons (Barrios & Hartmann, 1997). Moreover, the use of BATs in clinical research has declined considerably, perhaps reflecting the general shift in anxiety research from specific phobias and fears to more generalized and pervasive types of anxiety (Dadds, Rappee, & Barrett, 1994). Despite these barriers, research indicates good interrater reliability (e.g., Ollendick, Meader, & Villanis, 1986; Sheslow, Bondy, & Nelson, 1982) and temporal stability (Hamilton & King, 1991) for standardized BATs. Other findings support their concurrent validity, with moderate associations reported between the target behavior(s) and subjective (Evans & Harmon, 1981) or physiological (Eisen & Silverman, 1991) indicators of anxiety. Despite these findings, the external validity of BATs has been questioned on the basis of the highly controlled and often contrived nature of the tasks. Thus recommendations have been made for conducting *both* laboratory-based BATs and behavioral observations in more naturalistic environments, particularly in settings that are likely to evoke a range of anxiety-related behavior (Kendall & Flannery-Schroeder, 1998; Morris & Kratochwill, 1983).

School and Peer Observation

Peer relationships have been recognized as important contexts for social, emotional, and interpersonal growth and have been linked with short- and long-term indices of adjustment (e.g., Newcomb, Bukowski, & Pattee, 1993). Given the demonstrated link between peer relationship difficulties and anxiety (e.g., Ollendick, Weist, Borden, & Greene, 1992; Strauss, Frame, & Forehand, 1987), it may be useful to include one or more of the following measures in the assessment process: (1) standardized sociometric procedures that assess level of popularity or acceptance within the peer group at large (e.g., Inderbitzen, Walters, & Bukowski, 1997; La Greca & Stone, 1993; Ollendick et al., 1992); (2) measures of friendship quantity and quality (e.g., La Greca & Lopez, 1998; Vernberg, Abwender, Ewell, & Beery, 1992); and (3) behavioral observations conducted in laboratory-based (e.g., Beidel et al., 1999) and school settings (e.g., Morris, Messer, & Gross, 1995). Assessment of children's peer relations may be particularly useful in evaluating "social validity" and generalization of treatment effects. The potential value of peer reports and observation of peer interaction offsets the inherent difficulties in obtaining such information; consequently, we encourage researchers and clinicians to incorporate these strategies whenever possible.

Family Observation

The familial aggregation of anxiety is now well established, with evidence supporting both genetic (e.g., Eley, 2001) and environmental (e.g., Dadds & Roth, 2001) explanations. Relevant to this chapter, a growing literature supports the interactive, bidirectional associations among parental anxiety, child-rearing style, and child anxiety (see Gerlsma, Emmelkamp, & Arrindell, 1990; Masia & Morris, 1998; Rapee, 1997). Overall, observational research suggests that mothers and fathers of anxious children may (1) themselves experience heightened levels of anxiety, (2) demonstrate a parenting style marked by overprotection, intrusiveness, and control, and/or (3) model and reinforce perceived threat and anxiety-related avoidance (e.g., Barrett, Rapee, Dadds, & Ryan, 1996; Dadds, Barrett, Rapee, & Ryan, 1996). In light of these and similar findings, there has been a move to incorporate family members into the assessment and subsequent treatment of child and adolescent anxiety disorders (e.g., Barrett, Dadds, & Rapee, 1996; Dadds, Heard, & Rapee, 1992).

When assessing parent–child interactions, parent and child behaviors often are coded as the dyad engages in a joint task. Krohne and Hock (1991), for example, coded mother and child behavior during a 15-minute puzzle task. Focusing on "restrictive" maternal behavior, these authors reported that mothers of high- versus low-anxious girls were the most likely to intervene in an intrusive manner during the task. Similar results have been found for father–child interactions. In our work, we coded father and child behavior during a 10-minute origami task (Greco & Morris, 2002). Results indicated that fathers of high socially anxious children exhibited elevated levels of overt control (e.g., physical interruptions such as grabbing and taking over the task) relative to fathers of low socially anxious children. Interestingly, there was no difference in child behavior (e.g., child soliciting assistance, seeking reassurance, and following instructions) that were hypothesized to evoke relevant father behavior.

In general, family-based observational research has focused on children and their parents, and little attention has been devoted to the patterns and correlates of interactions among other immediate or extended family members. Recognizing this limitation, Fox, Barrett, and Shortt (2002) examined the sibling relationships of children with and without an anxiety disorder. Using observational coding, sibling interactions of children with anxiety disorders were characterized by less warmth and more conflict and control relative to the sibling interactions of children without anxiety disorders. Although preliminary, these findings suggested that sibling relationships may be characterized by similar interactional styles demonstrated within parent–child interactions.

SUMMARY AND FUTURE DIRECTIONS

We have provided a nonexhaustive summary of new or commonly used instruments and approaches for assessing anxiety and related behavior among children and adolescents. As evident in this brief review, a tremendous amount of growth has taken place in this area, with the development and refinement of reliable and valid assessment instruments. Moreover, researchers have moved to develop psychometrically sound measures that are keyed to the most recent nosological constructs, as exemplified by the MASC, SCARED, SPAI-C, and CPSS. Despite these recent advances, reliable and valid parent and teacher report instruments specific to anxiety and related behavior are still needed. In addition, more research is needed to document the clinical utility of incorporating behavioral observations into assessment batteries for children and adolescents.

Another consideration for future research is to expand our conceptualization and assessment of anxiety to include scales related to the functional importance of these symptoms. Assessment and intervention research traditionally has focused on symptom alleviation and elimination, as opposed to healthy adaptation (e.g., Levi & Drotar, 1998). To date, little has been done to incorporate indices of adaptive functioning or quality of life into more traditional symptom-focused measures. As we continue to develop and refine anxiety measures over the next decade, we must strive to include items that reflect the multidimensional conceptualization of *health* provided by the World Health Organization (1948): "a state of complete physical, mental, and social well being, and not merely the absence of disease or infirmity." We must develop scales that screen for anxiety-related interference across numerous life domains, such as education, family life, peer and romantic relationships, health, and physical functioning. In closing, we would be remiss if we did not also stress the need to look beyond "negative" symptoms and expand our assessment strategies to include aspects representative of resilience and positive adjustment.

REFERENCES

Achenbach, T. M. (1991a). *Manual for the Child Behavior Checklist/4–18 and 1991 Profile*. Burlington: University of Vermont, Department of Psychiatry.

Achenbach, T. M. (1991b). *Manual for the Teacher's Report Form and 1991 Profile*. Burlington: University of Vermont, Department of Psychiatry.

Achenbach, T. M., & Rescorla, L. A. (2001). *Manual for ASEBA School-Age Forms and Profiles*. Burlington: University of Vermont, Research Center for Children, Youth, and Families.

American Psychiatric Association. (1994). *Diagnostic and statistical manual of mental disorders* (4th ed.). Washington, DC: Author.

Anderson, J. C. (1994). Epidemiological issues. In T. H. Ollendick, N. J. King, & W. Yule (Eds.), *International handbook of phobic and anxiety disorders in children and adolescents* (pp. 43–66). New York: Plenum Press.

Bamber, D., Tamplin, A., Park, R. J., Kyte, Z. A., & Goodyear, I. M. (2002). Development of a Short Leyton Obsessional Inventory for children and adolescents. *Journal of the American Academy of Child and Adolescent Psychiatry, 41*, 1246–1252.

Barrett, P. M., Dadds, M. R., & Rapee, R. M. (1996). Family treatment of childhood anxiety: A controlled trial. *Journal of Consulting and Clinical Psychology, 64*, 333–342.

Barrett, P. M., Rapee, R. M., Dadds, M. R., & Ryan, S. (1996). Family enhancement of cognitive style in anxious and aggressive children. *Journal of Abnormal Child Psychology, 24*, 187–203.

Barrios, B. A., & Hartmann, D. P. (1997). Fears and anxieties. In E. J. Mash & L. G. Terdal (Eds.), *Assessment of childhood disorders* (3rd ed., pp. 230–327). New York: Guilford Press.

Beidel, D.C., & Stanley, M. A. (1993). Developmental issues in measurement of anxiety. In C. G. Last (Ed.), *Anxiety across the lifespan: A developmental perspective* (pp. 167–203). New York: Springer.

Beidel, D. C., & Turner, S. M. (1998). *Shy children, phobic adults: Nature and treatment of social phobia*. Washington, DC: American Psychiatric Association.

Beidel, D. C., Turner, S. M., & Fink, C. M. (1996). Assessment of childhood social phobia: Construct, convergent, and discriminant validity of the Social Phobia and Anxiety Inventory for Children (SPAI-C). *Psychological Assessment, 8*, 235–240.

Beidel, D. C., Turner, S. M., Hamlin, K., & Morris, T. L. (2000). The Social Phobia and Anxiety Inventory for Children (SPAI-C): External and discriminative validity. *Behavior Therapy, 31*, 75–87.

Beidel, D. C., Turner, S. M., & Morris, T. L. (1995). A new inventory to assess childhood social anxiety and phobia: The Social Phobia and Anxiety Inventory for Children. *Psychological Assessment, 7*, 73–79.

Beidel, D. C., Turner, S. M., & Morris, T. L. (1998). *Social Phobia and Anxiety Inventory for Children*. North Tonawanda, NY: Multi-Health Systems.

Beidel, D. C., Turner, S. M., & Morris, T. L. (1999). Psychopathology of social phobia. *Journal of the American Academy of Child and Adolescent Psychiatry, 38,* 643–650.

Berg, C. Z., Whitaker, A., Davies, M., Flament, M. F., & Rapoport, J. L. (1988). The survey form of the Leyton Obsessional Inventory—Child Version: Norms from an epidemiological study. *Journal of the American Academy of Child and Adolescent Psychiatry, 27,* 759–763.

Birmaher, B., Brent, D. A., Chiappetta, L., Bridge, J., Monga, S., & Baugher, M. (1999). Psychometric properties of the Screen for Child Anxiety Related Emotional Disorders (SCARED): A replication study. *Journal of the American Academy of Child and Adolescent Psychiatry, 38,* 1230–1236.

Birmaher, B., Khetarpal, S., Brent, D., Cully, M., Balach, L., Kaufman, J., & McKenzie Neer, S. (1997). The Screen for Child Anxiety Related Emotional Disorders (SCARED): Scale construction and psychometric characteristics. *Journal of the American Academy of Child and Adolescent Psychiatry, 36,* 545–553.

Chorpita, B. F., Albano, A. M., & Barlow, D. H. (1996). Child Anxiety Sensitivity Index: Considerations for children with anxiety disorders. *Journal of Clinical Child Psychology, 25,* 77–82.

Chorpita, B. F., Albano, A. M., & Barlow, D. H. (1998). The structure of negative emotions in a clinical sample of children and adolescents. *Journal of Abnormal Psychology, 107,* 74–85.

Chorpita, B. F., & Daleiden, E. L. (2002). Tripartite dimensions of emotion in a child clinical sample: Measurement strategies and implications for clinical utility. *Journal of Consulting and Clinical Psychology, 70,* 1150–1160.

Chorpita, B. F., Tracey, S. A., Brown, T. A., Collica, T. J., & Barlow, D. H. (1997). Assessment of worry in children and adolescents: An adaptation of the Penn State Worry Questionnaire. *Behaviour Research and Therapy, 35,* 569–581.

Chorpita, B. F., Yim, L., Moffitt, C., Umemoto, L. A., & Francis, S. E. (2000). Assessment of symptoms of DSM-IV anxiety and depression in children: A revised child anxiety and depression scale. *Behaviour Research and Therapy, 38,* 835–855.

Cole, D. A., Hoffman, K., Tram, J. M., & Maxwell, S. E. (2000). Structural differences in parent and child reports of children's symptoms of depression and anxiety. *Psychological Assessment, 12,* 174–185.

Compas, B. E., & Oppedisano, G. (2000). Mixed anxiety/depression in childhood and adolescence. In A. J. Sameroff & M. Lewis (Eds.), *Handbook of developmental psychopathology* (2nd ed., pp. 531–548). New York: Kluwer Academic/ Plenum Press.

Dadds, M. R., Barrett, P. M., Rapee, R. M., & Ryan, S. (1996). Family process and child anxiety and aggression: An observational analysis. *Journal of Abnormal Child Psychology, 24,* 715–734.

Dadds, M. R., Heard, P. M., & Rapee, R. M. (1992). The role of family intervention in the treatment of child anxiety disorders: Some preliminary findings. *Behaviour Change, 9,* 171–177.

Dadds, M. R., Rapee, R. M., & Barrett, P. M. (1994). Behavioral observations. In T.

H. Ollendick, N. J. King, & W. Yule (Eds.), *International handbook of phobic and anxiety disorders in children and adolescents* (pp. 349–364). New York: Plenum Press.

Dadds, M. R., & Roth, J. H. (2001). Family processes in the development of anxiety problems. In M. W. Vasey & M. R. Dadds (Eds.), *The developmental psychopathology of anxiety* (pp. 278–303). Oxford, UK: Oxford University Press.

Earls, F., Reich, W., Jung, K. G., & Cloninger, C. R. (1988). Psychopathology in children of alcoholic and antisocial parents. *Alcoholism: Clinical and Experimental Research, 12,* 481–487.

Edelbrock, D., Costello, A. J., Dulcan, M. K., Kalas, R., & Conover, N. C. (1985). Age differences in the reliability of the psychiatric interview of the child. *Child Development, 56,* 265–275.

Eisen, A. R., & Silverman, W. K. (1991). Treatment of an adolescent with bowel movement phobia using self-control therapy. *Journal of Behavior Therapy and Experimental Psychiatry, 22,* 45–51.

Eley, T. C. (2001). Contributions of behavioral genetics research: Quantifying genetic, shared environmental, and nonshared environmental influences. In M. W. Vasey & M. R. Dadds, (Eds.), *The developmental psychopathology of anxiety* (pp. 45–59). Oxford, UK: Oxford University Press.

Epkins, C. C. (1996). Parent ratings of children's depression, anxiety, and aggression: A cross-sample analysis of agreement and differences with child and teacher ratings. *Journal of Clinical Psychology, 52,* 599–608.

Epkins, C. C. (2002). A comparison of two self-report measures of children's social anxiety in clinic and community samples. *Journal of Clinical Child and Adolescent Psychology, 31,* 69–79.

Epkins, C. C., & Meyers, A. W. (1994). Assessment of childhood depression, anxiety, and aggression: Convergent and discriminant validity of self-, parent-, teacher-, and peer-report measures. *Journal of Personality Assessment, 62,* 364–381.

Evans, P. D., & Harmon, G. (1981). Children's self-initiated approach to spiders. *Behaviour Research and Therapy, 19,* 543–546.

Flament, M. F., Whitaker, A., & Rapoport, J. L. (1988). Obsessive–compulsive disorder in adolescence: An epidemiological study. *Journal of the American Academy of Child and Adolescent Psychiatry, 27,* 764–771.

Foa, E. B., Cashman, L., Jaycox, L., & Perry, K. (1997). The validation of a self-report measure of posttraumatic stress disorder: The Posttraumatic Diagnostic Scale. *Psychological Assessment, 9,* 445–451.

Foa, E. B., Johnson, K. M., Feeny, N. C., & Treadwell, K. R. H. (2001). The Child PTSD Symptom Scale: A preliminary examination of its psychometric properties. *Journal of Clinical Child Psychology, 30,* 376–384.

Fox, T. L., Barrett, P. M., & Shortt, A. L. (2002). Sibling relationships of anxious children: A preliminary investigation. *Journal of Clinical Child and Adolescent Psychology, 31,* 375–383.

Frederick, C. J. (1985). Selected foci in the spectrum of posttraumatic stress disorders. In J. Laube & S. A. Murphy (Eds.), *Perspectives on disaster recovery* (pp. 110–131). Norwalk, CT: Appleton-Century-Crofts.

Frederick, C. J., Pynoos, R., & Nader, K. (1992). *Childhood Posttrautmatic Stress Reaction Index* [Copyrighted instrument]. (Available from UCLA Department of

Psychiatry and Biobehavioral Sciences, 760 Westwood Plaza, Los Angeles, CA 90024).

Frick, P. J., Silverthorn, P., & Evans, C. (1994). Assessment of childhood anxiety using structured interviews: Patterns of agreement among informants and association with maternal anxiety. *Psychological Assessment, 6,* 372–379.

Gadow, K. D., & Sprafkin, J. (1994). *Child Symptom Inventories manual.* Stony Brook, NY: Checkmate Plus.

Gadow, K. D., & Sprafkin, J. (2002). *Child Symptom Inventory—4 screening and norms manual.* Stony Brook, NY: Checkmate Plus.

Gerlsma, C., Emmelkamp, P. M. G., & Arrindell, W. A. (1990). Anxiety, depression, and perception of early parenting: A meta-analysis. *Clinical Psychology Review, 10,* 251–277.

Ginsburg, G. S., La Greca, A. M., & Silverman, W. K. (1998). Social anxiety in children with anxiety disorders: Relation with social and emotional functioning. *Journal of Abnormal Child Psychology, 26,* 175–185.

Goodman, W., Price, L., Rasmussen, S., Riddle, M., & Rapoport, J. (1991). *Children's Yale–Brown Obsessive–Compulsive Scale* (CY-BOS). New Haven, CT: Yale University.

Greco, L. A., & Morris, T. M. (2002). Paternal child-rearing style and child social anxiety: Investigation of child perceptions and actual father behavior. *Journal of Psychopathology and Behavioral Assessment, 24,* 259–267.

Greenhill, L. L., Pine, D., March, J., Birmaher, B., & Riddle, M. (1998). Assessment measures in anxiety disorders research. *Psychopharmacology Bulletin, 34,* 155–164.

Hamilton, D. I., & King, N. J. (1991). Reliability of a behavioral avoidance test for the assessment of dog phobic children. *Psychological Reports, 69,* 18.

Herjanic, B., & Reich, W. (1997). Development of a structured psychiatric interview for children: Agreement between child and parent on individual symptoms. *Journal of Abnormal Child Psychology, 25,* 21–31.

Hodges, K. (1990). Depression and anxiety in children: A comparison of self-report questionnaires to clinical interview. *Psychological Assessment, 2,* 376–381.

Horowitz, M., Wilner, N., & Alvarez, W. (1979). Impact of Events Scale: A measure of subjective stress. *Psychosomatic Medicine, 41,* 209–218.

Inderbitzen, H. M., Walters, K. S., & Bukowski, A. L. (1997). The role of social anxiety in adolescent–peer relations: Differences among sociometric status groups and rejected subgroups. *Journal of Clinical Child Psychology, 26,* 338–348.

Kashani, J., Orvaschel, H., Burk, J., & Reid, J. (1985). Informant variance: The issue of parent–child disagreement. *Journal of the American Academy of Child Psychiatry, 24,* 437–441.

Kaufman, J., Birmaher, B., Brent, D., Rao, U., Flynn, C., Moreci, P., Williamson, D., & Ryan, N. (1997). The Schedule for Affective Disorders and Schizophrenia for School-aged Children—Present and Lifetime Version (K-SADS-PL): Initial reliability and validity data. *Journal of the American Academy of Child and Adolescent Psychiatry, 36,* 980–988.

Kendall, P. C., & Flannery-Schroeder, E. C. (1998). Methodological issues in treatment research for anxiety disorders in youth. *Journal of Abnormal Child Psychology, 26,* 27–38.

Kendall, P. C., Flannery-Schroeder, E. C., Panichelli-Mindel, S. M., Southam-Gerow, M., Henin, A., & Warman, M. (1997). Therapy for youths with anxiety disorders: A second randomized clinical trial. *Journal of Consulting and Clinical Psychology, 65*, 366–380.

Kovacs, M., & Devlin, B. (1998). Internalizing disorders. *Journal of Child Psychology, Psychiatry, and Allied Disciplines, 39*, 47–63.

Krohne, H. W., & Hock, M. (1991). Relationships between restrictive mother–child interactions and anxiety of the child. *Anxiety Research, 4*, 109–124.

La Greca, A. M. (1998). *Social anxiety scales for children and adolescents: Manual and instructions for the SASC, SASC-R, SAS-A*. Miami, FL: University of Miami, Department of Psychology.

La Greca, A. M., Dandes, S. K., Wick, P., Shaw, K., & Stone, W. L. (1988). Development of the Social Anxiety Scale for Children: Reliability and concurrent validity. *Journal of Clinical Child Psychology, 17*, 84–91.

La Greca, A. M., & Lopez, N. (1998). Social anxiety among adolescents: Linkages with peer relations and friendships. *Journal of Abnormal Child Psychology, 26*, 83–94.

La Greca, A., & Stone, W. L. (1993). Social Anxiety Scale for Children—Revised: Factor structure and concurrent validity. *Journal of Clinical Child Psychology, 22*, 17–27.

Langley, A. K., Bergman, L. R., & Piacentini, J. C. (2002). Assessment of childhood anxiety. *International Review of Psychiatry, 14*, 102–113.

Lau, J. J., Calamari, J. E., & Waraczynski, M. (1996). Panic attack symptomatology and anxiety sensitivity in adolescents. *Journal of Anxiety Disorders, 10*, 355–364.

Leary, M. R. (1983). *Understanding social anxiety: Social, personality, and clinical perspectives*. Beverly Hills, CA: Sage.

Levi, R., & Drotar, D. (1998). Critical issues and needs in health-related quality of life assessment of children and adolescents with chronic health conditions. In D. Drotar (Ed.), *Measuring health-related quality of life in children and adolescents: Implications for research and practice* (pp. 3–23). Mahwah, NJ: Erlbaum.

Lilienfeld, S. O., Jacob, R. G., & Turner, S. M. (1989). Comment on Holloway and McNally's (1987) "Effects of anxiety sensitivity on the response to hyperventilation." *Journal of Abnormal Psychology, 98*, 100–102.

Manassis, K. (2000). Childhood anxiety disorders: Lessons from the literature. *Canadian Journal of Psychiatry, 45*, 724–730.

March, J. (1998). *Manual for the Multidimensional Anxiety Scale for Children (MASC)*. Toronto: Multi-Health Systems.

March, J., Parker, J., Sullivan, K., Stallings, P., & Conners, C. K. (1997). The Multidimensional Anxiety Scale for Children (MASC): Factor structure, reliability, and validity. *Journal of the American Academy of Child and Adolescent Psychiatry, 36*, 554–565.

Masia, C. L., & Morris, T. L. (1998). Parental factors associated with social anxiety: Methodological limitations and suggestions for integrated behavioral research. *Clinical Psychology: Science and Practice, 5*, 211–228.

Mattis, S. G., & Ollendick, T. H. (1997). Children's cognitive responses to the somatic symptoms of panic. *Journal of Abnormal Child Psychology, 25*, 47–57.

Morris, R. J., & Kratochwill, T. R. (1983). *Treating children's fears and phobias: A behavioral approach.* Elmsford, NY: Pergamon.

Morris, T. L., & Masia, C. L. (1998). Psychometric evaluation of the Social Phobia and Anxiety Inventory for Children: Concurrent validity and normative data. *Journal of Clinical Child Psychology, 27,* 452–458.

Morris, T. L., Messer, S. C., & Gross, A. M. (1995). Enhancement of the social interaction and status of neglected children: A peer-pairing approach. *Journal of Clinical Child Psychology, 25,* 11–20.

Muris, P., Mayer, B., Bartelds, E., Tierney, S., & Bogie, N. (2001). The revised version of the Screen for Child Anxiety Related Emotional Disorders (SCARED-R): Treatment sensitivity in an early intervention trial for childhood anxiety disorders. *British Journal of Clinical Psychology, 40,* 323–336.

Muris, P., Merckelbach, H., & Damsma, E. (2000). Threat perception bias in nonreferred socially anxious children. *Journal of Clinical Child Psychology, 29,* 348–359.

Muris, P., Merckelbach, H., Koerver, P., & Meesters, C. (2000). Screening for trauma in children and adolescents: The validity of the Traumatic Stress Disorder scale of the Screen for Child Anxiety Related Emotional Disorders. *Journal of Clinical Child Psychology, 29,* 406–413.

Muris, P., Merckelbach, H., Van Brakel, A., & Mayer, B. (1999). The Screen for Child Anxiety Related Emotional Disorders (SCARED): Further evidence for its reliability and validity. *Anxiety, Stress, and Coping, 12,* 411–425.

Muris, P., Schmidt, H., & Merckelbach, H. (2000). Correlations among two self-report questionnaires for measuring DSM-defined anxiety disorder symptoms in children: The Screen for Child Anxiety Related Emotional Disorders and the Spence Children's Anxiety Scale. *Personality and Individual Differences, 28,* 333–346.

Nader, K. O. (1997). Assessing traumatic experiences in children. In J. P. Wilson & T. M. Keane (Eds.), *Assessing psychological trauma and PTSD* (pp. 291–348). New York: Guilford Press.

Newcomb, A. F., Bukowski, W. M., & Pattee, L. (1993). Children's peer relations: A meta-analytic review of popular, rejected, neglected, controversial, and average sociometric status. *Psychological Bulletin, 113,* 99–128.

Ollendick, T. H. (1981). Assessment of social interaction skills in school children. *Behavioral Counseling Quarterly, 1,* 227–243.

Ollendick, T. H. (1983). Reliability and validity of the Revised Fear Survey Schedule for Children (FSSC-R). *Behaviour Research and Therapy, 23,* 465–467.

Ollendick, T. H., Meader, A. E., & Villanis, C. (1986). Relationship between the Children's Assertiveness Inventory (CAI) and the Revised Behavioural Assertiveness Test for Children (BAT-CR). *Child and Family Behavior Therapy, 8,* 27–36.

Ollendick, T. H., Weist, M. D., Borden, C. M., & Greene, R. W. (1992). Sociometric status and academic, behavioral, and psychological adjustment: A five-year longitudinal study. *Journal of Consulting and Clinical Psychology, 60,* 80–87.

Perrin, S., & Last, C. G. (1992). Do childhood anxiety measures measure anxiety? *Journal of Abnormal Child Psychology, 20,* 567–578.

Peterson, R. A., & Reiss, S. (1987). *Anxiety Sensitivity Index manual.* Orland Park, IL: International Diagnostic Systems.

Pynoos, R. S., & Nader, K. O. (1989). Children's memory and proximity to violence. *Journal of the American Academy of Child and Adolescent Psychiatry, 28*, 236–241.

Quay, H. C., & La Greca, A. M. (1986). Disorders of anxiety, withdrawal, and dysphoria. In H. C. Quay & J. S. Weny (Eds.), *Psychopathological disorders of childhood* (3rd ed., pp. 71–110). New York: Wiley.

Rapee, R. M. (1997). Potential role of childrearing practices in the development of anxiety and depression. *Clinical Psychology Review, 17*, 47–67.

Rapee, R. M., Barrett, P.M., Dadds, M. R., & Evans, L. (1994). Reliability of the DSM-III-R childhood anxiety disorders using structured interview: Interrater and parent–child agreement. *Journal of the American Academy of Child and Adolescent Psychiatry, 33*, 984–992.

Reiss, S. (1991). Expectancy model of fear, anxiety, and panic. *Clinical Psychology Review, 11*, 141–153.

Reiss, S., Silverman, W. K., & Weems, C. F. (2001). Anxiety sensitivity. In M. W. Vasey & M. R. Dadds (Eds.), *The developmental psychopathology of anxiety* (pp. 45–59). New York: Oxford University Press.

Reynolds, C. R., & Richmond, B. O. (1978). What I think and feel: A revised measure of children's manifest anxiety. *Journal of Abnormal Child Psychology, 6*, 271–280.

Scahill, L., Riddle, M. A., McSwiggen-Hardin, M., & Ort, S. I. (1997). Children's Yale–Brown Obsessive Compulsive Scale. *Journal of the American Academy of Child and Adolescent Psychiatry, 36*, 844–852.

Schniering, C. A., Hudson, J. L., & Rapee, R. M. (2000). Issues in the diagnosis and assessment of anxiety disorders in children and adolescents. *Clinical Psychology Review, 20*, 453–478.

Shaffer, D., Fisher, P., Lucas, C., Dulcan, M. K., & Schwab-Stone, M. E. (2000). NIMH Diagnostic Interview Schedule for Children—Version IV (NIMH DISC-IV): Description, differences from previous versions, and reliability of some common diagnoses. *Journal of the American Academy of Child and Adolescent Psychiatry, 39*, 28–38.

Sheslow, D. V., Bondy, A. S., & Nelson, R. O. (1982). A comparison of graduated exposure, verbal coping skills, and their combination in the treatment of children's fear of the dark. *Child and Family Behavior Therapy, 4*, 33–45.

Silverman, W. K., & Albano, A. M. (1996). *The Anxiety Disorders Interview Schedule for Children for DSM-IV: Child and parent versions.* San Antonio, TX: Psychological Corporation.

Silverman, W. K., Fleisig, W., Rabian, B., & Peterson, R. A. (1991). Childhood Anxiety Sensitivity Index. *Journal of Clinical Child Psychology, 20*, 162–168.

Silverman, W. K., Ginsburg, G. S., & Goedhart, A. W. (1999). Factor structure of the Childhood Anxiety Sensitivity Index. *Behaviour Research and Therapy, 37*, 903–917.

Silverman, W. K., Saavedra, L. M., & Pina, A. A. (2001). Test–retest reliability of anxiety symptoms and diagnoses with Anxiety Disorders Interview Schedule for DSM-IV: Child and parent versions. *Journal of the American Academy of Child and Adolescent Psychiatry, 40*, 937–944.

Silverman, W. K., & Weems, C. F. (1999). Anxiety sensitivity in children. In S. Taylor

(Ed.), *Anxiety sensitivity: Theory research and treatment of the fear of anxiety* (pp. 239–268). Mahwah, NJ: Erlbaum.

Spence, S. H. (1997). Structure of anxiety symptoms among children: A confirmatory factor-analytic study. *Journal of Abnormal Psychology, 106,* 280–297.

Spence, S. H. (1998). A measure of anxiety symptoms among children. *Behaviour Research and Therapy, 36,* 545–566.

Spence, S. H., Donovan, C., & Brechman-Toussaint, M. (1999). Social skills, social outcomes, and cognitive features of childhood social phobia. *Journal of Abnormal Psychology, 108,* 211–221.

Spielberger, C. D. (1973). *Manual for the State–Trait Anxiety Inventory for Children.* Palo Alto, CA: Consulting Psychologists Press.

Sprafkin, J., Gadow, K. D., Salisbury, H., Schneider, J., & Loney, J. (2002). Further evidence of reliability and validity of the Child Symptom Inventory–4: Parent Checklist in clinically referred boys. *Journal of Clinical Child and Adolescent Psychology, 31,* 513–524.

Stallings, P., & March, J. S. (1995). Assessment. In J. S. March (Ed.), *Anxiety disorders in children and adolescents* (pp. 125–147). New York: Guilford Press.

Stark, D., Kaslow, N. J., & Laurent, J. (1993). The assessment of depression in children: Are we assessing depression or the broad-band construct of negative affectivity? *Journal of Emotional and Behavioral Disorders, 1,* 149–159.

Stone, W. L., & Lemanek, K. L. (1990). Developmental issues in children's self-reports. In A. M. La Greca (Ed.), *Through the eyes of the child: Obtaining self-reports from children and adolescents* (pp. 18–56). Boston: Allyn & Bacon.

Strauss, C. C., Frame, C. L., & Forehand, R. (1987). Psychosocial impairment associated with anxiety in children. *Journal of Clinical Child Psychology, 16,* 235–239.

Strauss, C. C., & Last, C. G. (1993). Social and simple phobias in children. *Journal of Anxiety Disorders, 7,* 141–152.

Vasey, M. W., & Lonigan, C. J. (2000). Considering the clinical utility of performance-based measures of childhood anxiety. *Journal of Clinical Child Psychology, 29,* 493–508.

Vernberg, E. M., Abwender, D. A., Ewell, K. K., & Beery, S. H. (1992). Social anxiety and peer relationships in early adolescence: A prospective analysis. *Journal of Clinical Child Psychology, 21,* 189–196.

Watson, D., & Friend, R. (1969). Measurement of social-evaluative anxiety. *Journal of Consulting and Clinical Psychology, 33,* 448–457.

Weems, C. F., Hammond-Laurence, K., Silverman, W. K., & Ginsburg, G. S. (1998). Testing the utility of the anxiety sensitivity construct in children and adolescents referred for anxiety disorders. *Journal of Clinical Child Psychology, 27,* 69–77.

Wood, J. J., Piacentini, J. C., Bergman, R. L., McCracken, J., & Barrios, V. (2002). Concurrent validity of the anxiety disorders section of the Anxiety Disorders Interview Schedule for DSM-IV: Child and parent versions. *Journal of Clinical Child and Adolescent Psychology, 31,* 335–342.

World Health Organization. (1948). *World Health Organization constitution.* Geneva: Author.

Part II

DISORDERS

Chapter 6

Generalized
Anxiety Disorder

ELLEN C. FLANNERY-SCHROEDER

Worry is perhaps one of the most characteristic features of anxiety. Whereas worry in adults has been a focus of much attention and clinical concern, worry in children has not received parallel attention. Given the paucity of research on childhood worry, the current state of knowledge should be considered formative and incomplete. Because of this, researchers on child anxiety have begun a strong and methodologically rigorous journey toward a thorough understanding of childhood worry and anxiety disorders more generally.

Worry is considered by some to be the defining feature of generalized anxiety disorder (GAD). Although worry is undoubtedly a normative human experience, worry in GAD tends to be more intense, prolonged, and uncontrollable. This chapter traces the historical origins of GAD, describes its characteristic and associated features and course, and examines the empirical findings regarding epidemiology and developmental factors. Treatment approaches and future directions are also examined.

HISTORICAL PERSPECTIVE

The childhood experience of excessive or unfounded worry was first referred to as overanxious reaction in DSM-II (American Psychiatric Association [APA], 1968). The syndrome underwent revisions through DSM-III (APA, 1980) and DSM-III-R (APA, 1997), when the disorder became known as "overanxious disorder" (OAD). However, despite the diagnostic revisions, the category of overanxious disorder was criticized. Researchers and clinicians alike complained that OAD criteria were vague, that symptom overlap with other disorders was problematic, and that the disorder was prone to overdiagnosis (e.g., Beidel, 1991; Klein & Last, 1989; Silverman, 1992; Werry, 1991). Lower interrater reliability was found for OAD than for other childhood anxiety disorders (Silverman & Eisen, 1992; Silverman & Nelles, 1988). Additional concerns included the large number of nondisordered children experiencing OAD symptoms (Bell-Dolan, Last, & Strauss, 1990), as well as the question of child-reported impairment caused by OAD (Beidel, Silverman, & Hammond-Laurence, 1996). DSM-IV (APA, 1994) responded to these problems by eliminating the diagnosis of OAD. The disorder was subsumed by generalized anxiety disorder—previously the "adult" version of OAD. Much of the research reported herein involved DSM diagnoses of OAD; recent research on GAD in children is reported whenever possible. Diagnoses of OAD using DSM-III-R and of GAD using DSM-IV are believed to be quite similar. In fact, in a comparative study of these disorders, Kendall and Warman (1996) found tremendous overlap (i.e., nonsignificant differences) between diagnoses of the disorders. In a similar vein, the DSM-IV diagnosis of GAD in children has been empirically evaluated by Tracey, Chorpita, Douban, and Barlow (1997). Tracey and colleagues found the DSM-IV GAD criteria to reliably distinguish children with GAD from those with other anxiety disorders and to demonstrate good agreement between child and parent reports and clinician ratings of GAD severity. Developmental differences (e.g., older children reporting more symptoms) did not appear to necessitate separate criteria for childhood and adulthood GAD. Overall, results supported the utility of the criteria for children and adolescents.

PHENOMENOLOGY

The *Diagnostic and Statistical Manual of Mental Disorders, Fourth Edition, Text Revision* (DSM-IV-TR; APA, 2000) diagnosis of GAD is characterized by persistent worry regarding multiple life domains, events, or activities. Children with GAD are not merely worrying about an upcoming test, for example, but about their personal future, health, performance, and safety *and* the future, health, performance, and safety of others. A recent study of children referred for treatment to an anxiety clinic demonstrated health, school, disasters, and personal harm to be the main domains of worry (Weems, Silverman, & La Greca, 2000). Although worry is not a symptom limited to GAD, these areas of worry are likely to be reflective of or similar to the main areas of worry in GAD. The worry is present more days than not, is difficult to control, and is enduring (i.e., it lasts more than 6 months). Additionally, physiological symptoms (e.g., restlessness, fatigue, muscle tension, sleep disturbance) and cognitive symptoms (e.g., irritability and concentration difficulties) may accompany the worry. Somatic complaints such as muscle tension, stomachaches, and headaches are common.

Children with GAD are frequently perfectionistic. They show cognitive distortions in which they believe a small error to be a sign of complete failure. If the task cannot be completed perfectly, it will not be completed at all. It is not uncommon for children with GAD to abandon or avoid activities if they perceive that their performance may fall shy of perfection. In this vein, children with GAD can be excessively self-critical. Additionally, children with GAD may require frequent and excessive reassurances and frequently have marked self-consciousness. They may be unable to progress in tasks without constant reassurances that they are "on the right track" or "doing fine." Self-consciousness may manifest as rigid adherence to social and peer norms (e.g., overconformity in dress, mannerism, and behavior) or an unwillingness to perform behaviors that might be "evaluated" by others (e.g., refusal to read or sing aloud). Children with GAD have been labeled "hypermature" and like "little adults" (Kendall, Krain, & Treadwell, 1999; Strauss, 1990). In the words of Kendall and colleagues, children's "anxieties about needing to meet deadlines, keeping appointments, and adhering to rules, and their inquiries about the dangers of situations, often create this illusion of maturity" (Kendall et al., 1999, p. 155). This "illusion of maturity" makes problem identification difficult—adults perceive these perfectionistic, eager-to-please, rule-abiding behaviors as both desirable and valuable.

Some researchers (e.g., Rapee, 1991) have suggested that GAD may be nothing more than high levels of trait anxiety. Differences between the personality or temperamental characteristic of high trait anxiety and clinically significant generalized anxiety are often difficult to discern. In some respects, GAD may be regarded as a maladaptive personality style.

Anxiety disorders in general, and GAD specifically, appear to be related to abnormalities in threat perception (e.g., Butler & Mathews, 1983; Muris et al., 2000). Several researchers have suggested that individuals with anxiety disorders tend to overestimate the likelihood and catastrophize the outcomes of dangerous events. Rapee (1991) has suggested that GAD involves not only a biased perception of threat but also a low perception of control over one's situation and/or environment. Others (Woody & Rachman, 1994) have proposed that individuals with GAD fail to perceive indices of safety. Woody and Rachman theorize that increased perception of threat results in an inability to identify safety signals, which, in turn, results in the continued experience or maintenance of anxiety.

NATURAL HISTORY

Community prevalence rates for OAD/GAD range between 2 and 19% (e.g., Cohen et al., 1993; McGee et al., 1990; Werry, 1991). Some have noted, however, that the available epidemiological data for child anxiety disorders are based on prevalence of anxiety symptoms rather than on the full disorder (e.g., Orvaschel & Weissman, 1986). Prevalence rates utilizing strict diagnostic criteria range from 2 to 4% (e.g., Anderson, Williams, McGee, & Silva, 1987; Bowen, Offord, & Boyle, 1990). GAD prevalence rates in child psychiatry clinics have been reported to be around 10–14% (Beitchman, Wekerle, & Hood, 1987; Silverman & Nelles, 1988), whereas referrals to specialized anxiety clinics have ranged from 15% (Last, Strauss, & Francis, 1987) to 58% (Kendall et al., 1997).

GAD is characterized by an early but slow and insidious onset (Brown, Barlow, & Liebowitz, 1994; Rapee, 1985, 1991). Many adults with GAD report having been anxious for as long as they can remember (Rapee, 1985). GAD does not appear to be differentially diagnosed by gender at least until early adolescence (Kendall, 1994; Last, Strauss, & Francis, 1987). Gender patterns then begin to parallel those in the adult literature— more girls than boys are diagnosed with GAD (Bowen et al., 1990; McGee et al., 1990; Rapee, 1991). This difference appears to be the result of fewer males (rather than more females) being diagnosed (Velez, Johnson, & Cohen, 1989). However, some developmental differences have been noted. Children under 12 years have been found to experience fewer GAD symptoms than older children, or inversely, older children report more symptoms of GAD than do younger children (Strauss, Lease, Last, & Francis, 1988; Tracey et al., 1997).

Several studies have demonstrated OAD to be associated with problems such as major depression (Last, Hersen, Kazdin, Finkelstein, & Strauss, 1987), suicide attempts and ideation (Brent et al., 1986), and low self-esteem (Strauss, Last, & Francis, 1988, cited in Strauss, 1988). These correlates are more often seen in older preadolescents and adolescent youths and are likely to have significant impact on children's adjustment. OAD/GAD in childhood has been speculated to be a precursor to GAD in adulthood (Gittelman, 1984). Beidel (1991), however, hypothesizes that childhood OAD/GAD may merely represent a vulnerability to not only GAD but also other anxiety disorders in adulthood. Left untreated, GAD can result in significant impairment in life tasks and major costs to the community (Massion, Warshaw, & Keller, 1993; Roy-Burne & Katon, 1997).

ETIOLOGY

Research has identified several risk factors for anxiety disorder, including attachment style, child temperament, parental anxiety, and certain parenting characteristics. Little research has focused on the etiology of GAD specifically; thus this review is applicable to anxiety disorders in general and to GAD where possible.

Attachment style has been identified as a potential risk factor for childhood anxiety (e.g., Erickson, Sroufe, & Egeland, 1985; Lewis, Feiring, McGafey, & Jaskir, 1984; Sroufe, Egeland, & Kreutzer, 1990). Bowlby (1982) suggested that anxiety in adulthood may be related to an insecure attachment in childhood. According to Bowlby, attachment is the child's attempt to ensure safety and security in his or her world. If the attachment figure is perceived as unavailable, the child may come to experience the world as dangerous and threatening. This perception parallels the aforementioned research suggesting that individuals with GAD overestimate the likelihood and consequences of dangerous events while underestimating their ability to cope with the events. Warren and colleagues found anxious-resistant attachment style at 12 months to be associated with greater incidence of anxiety disorder at 17½ years of age (Warren, Huston, Egeland, & Sroufe, 1997). Cassidy (1995), on the other hand, has examined the role of childhood attachment as a precursor of GAD, specifically. In both analogue and clinical samples, investigators examined the relationship between attachment (as measured by the Inventory of Adult Attachment [INVAA]; Lichtenstein & Cassidy, 1991) and GAD diagnosis. In the analogue sample, participants with GAD symptoms reported experiencing significantly higher rejection, role reversal, and enmeshment in childhood and greater anger and vulnerability related to their mothers in adulthood than did the nonanxious participants. In the clinical sample, participants with GAD reported greater role reversal and enmeshment in childhood, more anger and vulnerability related to their mothers in adulthood, and fewer childhood memories than did control participants. Although the attachment measure (i.e., INVAA) used by Cassidy and colleagues does not measure secure versus insecure attachment, it is suggestive of a connection between attachment and GAD and provides an impetus and direction for future studies.

Additionally, children who possess certain temperamental characteristics appear to be at increased risk for the development of a childhood anxiety disorder. Child temperament has been the focus of both retrospective and prospective studies of etiology of anxiety. Rapee and Szollos (1997) conducted a retrospective study of mothers of anxious and nonanxious children ages 7–16. Mothers of anxious children reported that their children had experienced significantly more bouts of crying, sleep difficulties, pain, and gas in the first year of life than mothers of nonanxious children. In addition, these mothers, compared with mothers of nonanxious children, reported that their children were more fearful from birth to age 2 and had greater difficulties calming themselves after distress. No differences among anxiety disorder diagnosis (separation anxiety, social phobia, generalized anxiety) were found for these temperamental characteristics (i.e., difficult/colicky and fearful disposition).

Behavioral inhibition, a temperamental feature characterized by irritability in infancy, fearfulness in toddlerhood, and shyness, wariness, and withdrawal in childhood, has been associated with an increased vulnerability to anxiety disorder(s) (e.g., Biederman et al., 1993; Kagan, 1997; Rosenbaum et al., 1993). Kagan (1997) found 15–20% of European American children to be predisposed to this temperamental trait. Biederman and colleagues found that rates of anxiety disorders were highest among children who had been identified as behaviorally inhibited throughout childhood (Biederman, Rosenbaum, Chaloff, & Kagan, 1995). Prospective studies have demonstrated that children identified as behaviorally inhibited at 21 months were more likely than uninhibited children to develop anxiety disorders over the next 5–10 years (Biederman et al., 1993; Hirshfeld et al., 1992). Additionally, inhibited children have a greater likelihood of having a parent with an anxiety disorder (Biederman et al., 1995; Rosenbaum et al., 1993). Collectively, the research is strongly suggestive of a relationship between behavioral inhibition and increased risk for anxiety disorder.

Parental anxiety has been demonstrated to be predictive of anxiety disorders in children. Anxious children are more likely than nonanxious peers to have an anxious parent (Last, Hersen, Kazdin, Francis, & Grubb, 1987; Turner, Beidel, & Costello, 1987; Weissman, Leckman, Merikangas, Gammon, & Prusoff, 1984). Also, parents with anxiety disorders are more likely to have a child at increased risk for anxiety (Rosenbaum et al., 1993). However, parental anxiety is likely to be a factor that is not directly, but indirectly, linked to child anxiety via genetics (e.g., temperament) and/or environmental factors (e.g., parenting style; Donovan & Spence, 2000).

Last, several parenting characteristics and/or styles have been associated with child anxiety. Parenting variables such as reinforcement of avoidant behaviors, modeling of social interaction, and parental overprotection have been subjects of study. Barrett, Dadds, Rapee, and Ryan (1996) found parents of anxious children to be more likely to reinforce avoidant strategies than other parents. In the Barrett et al. study, children were presented with hypothetical scenerios and asked about the likelihood of their behavior. The children were again asked about their likely response(s) after a 5-minute family discussion of the scenerio. After the discussion, anxious children were significantly more likely to provide an avoidant response. Thus it appears that parents of anxious children may reinforce and/or agree with avoidant behaviors (Dadds, Barrett, Rapee, & Ryan, 1996).

Some research evidence suggests that adults with social phobia selectively recall their parents to have exhibited less social interaction than nonanxious control participants (Rapee & Melville, 1997). Additionally, parental characteristics, including overcontrol and overprotection, appear to be associated with low self-efficacy in children, a factor that may directly or indirectly be linked to childhood anxiety (Hudson & Rapee, 2001; Khrone, 1990; Khrone & Hock, 1991). Similarly, in an investigation of parental rearing behaviors and anxiety symptoms in nonclinical children, Muris and Merckelbach (1998) found children's perceptions of parental control and anxious rearing to be correlated with increases in anxious symptomatology, especially symptoms of GAD.

TREATMENT

Cognitive-Behavioral Treatment

In response to increasing recognition of the debilitating nature of childhood anxiety disorders, treatment research has flourished, and cognitive-behavioral interventions have shown real promise in helping children with clinical levels of disorder (e.g., Barrett, Dadds, & Rapee, 1996; Cobham, Dadds, & Spence, 1998; Kendall, 1994; Kendall et al., 1997). In fact, cognitive-behavioral treatments for anxiety disorders (e.g., Kendall, 1994; Kendall et al., 1997) have been deemed "probably efficacious" as determined by proposed criteria (Chambless & Hollon, 1998). Although the majority of treatments aimed at child anxiety are not specific to anxiety disorder, most are targeted at such disorders as GAD, social phobia, and separation anxiety. Three studies, however, have been interventions aimed at treating OAD/GAD. This section reviews the treatment research specifically targeting OAD/GAD, followed by a review of treatment research targeting child anxiety more generally (i.e., targeting any of the three aforementioned disorders).

Kane and Kendall (1989) utilized a multiple-baseline evaluation of a cognitive-behavioral treatment for OAD. Participants included four children (ages 9–13) diagnosed with OAD via a structured diagnostic interview. Dependent measures included child self-report, parent report, teacher report, and clinician report of anxiety and associated symptomatology. Children attended 16–20 sessions biweekly; assessments were conducted pre-, mid-, and posttreatment, as well as 3–6 months following treatment. The treatment consisted of four major components: (1) recognizing anxious feelings and physical reactions to anxiety; (2) identifying and modifying negative self-statements; (3) generating strategies to cope effectively in anxiety-provoking situations; and (4) rating and rewarding attempts at coping. The treatment was conducted in two parts: instruction in coping skills and practice in use of skills in increasingly anxiety-provoking situations. Posttreatment results indicated improvement on child self-report, parent report, and clinician report, with many indices of anxious behavior falling into the normative range. Follow-up results were somewhat varied. Two children clearly maintained gains; the other two children maintained gains according to self-reports, yet parent reports indicated the reemergence of some anxious behavior.

In another study of OAD, Eisen and Silverman (1993) evaluated the effectiveness of cognitive therapy, relaxation training, and their combination with four children (ages 6–15). The order of presentation of the cognitive therapy and relaxation training was counterbalanced; the combination component was always added last. The children were diagnosed via structured interview and completed assessments pre- and posttreatment and at a 6-month follow-up. Dependent measures included child, parent, and clinician reports of anxiety and associated symptomatology. Results indicated that all children improved on self-, parent, and clinician report. Most indices of anxiety fell from clinical to normative levels posttreatment. Two of the four children no longer met criteria for OAD. Follow-up results demonstrated maintenance of treatment gains; however, two of the children were still experiencing some problems in limited areas. The relative efficacy of cognitive therapy versus relaxation training was unclear; however, the combined treatment appeared to be associated with the greatest decreases in anxiety. In addition, the authors found comorbidity to be related to a poorer prognostic outcome.

In a more recent evaluation of cognitive-behavioral treatment for OAD/GAD, Eisen and Silverman (1998) used a multiple-baseline design with four children with OAD/GAD. Experimental participants were differentially prescribed treatments (cognitive therapy and exposure or relaxation training and exposure), depending on problematic response classes (cognitive or somatic, respectively). Control participants received nonprescriptive treatments (i.e., cognitive-response-class treatment for somatic symptoms or somatic-response-class treatment for somatic symptoms). Each treatment lasted 5 weeks (10 sessions). Dependent measures included child, parent, and clinical reports of anxiety and associated symptoms. Additionally, measurements of heart rate in anxiety-eliciting situations were collected. Results demonstrated that, although both prescriptive and nonprescriptive treatments effected change, the prescriptive treatments led to positive end-state functioning, whereas the nonprescriptive treatments did not. Positive end-state functioning was defined as return to within one standard deviation of normative scores and/or clinical cutoff scores on two specific response-class measures and receipt of a clinician-rated subclinical severity score for the OAD/GAD diagnosis.

In the first of several randomized clinical trials investigating the effectiveness of cognitive-behavioral treatments for childhood anxiety (e.g., GAD, social phobia, and/or separation anxiety), Kendall (1994) randomly assigned 47 children with anxiety disorders to either a cognitive-behavioral treatment or a wait-list control condition. Dependent measures included child self-report, parent report, teacher report, and diagnosis via structured diagnostic interview. Results indicated that 64% of treated children no longer exhibited primary anxiety disorder symptoms at posttreatment. In addition, improvements were noted on self-report measures of coping and symptomatology and on parent-report measures of child behavior. Teacher reports demonstrated that 60% of treated children were returned to nondeviant levels at posttreatment. A 1-year follow-up (Kendall, 1994) and a 3-year follow-up (Kendall & Southam-Gerow, 1996) demonstrated maintenance of treatment gains. An examination of differential outcome and differential maintenance of treatment gains among the three anxiety disorders found no significant differences.

Kendall and colleagues (1997) completed a second randomized clinical trial in which 94 children with anxiety disorders were randomly assigned to a cognitive-behavioral treatment or a wait list. Seventy-one percent of treated children no longer had their primary diagnoses at posttreatment and treated children evidenced significantly greater gains on self- and parent-reported ratings of anxiety. Maintenance of treatment gains was evident at a 1-year follow-up. Again, no significant differences were found in outcome or maintenance among the three anxiety disorders studied. Kendall and colleagues are currently examining the results of a 7-year follow-up conducted with these 94 children, and preliminary results suggest excellent maintenance of treatment gains.

Barrett and colleagues (1996), using a modification of Kendall's (2000) Coping Cat program with Australian youth, added a family-management component to the cognitive-behavioral treatment with good effects. Seventy-nine children with anxiety disorders were randomly assigned to one of three conditions: cognitive-behavioral treatment (CBT), cognitive-behavioral treatment plus family management (FAM), and a wait-list control group. Approximately 70% of treated children versus 26% of wait-list children did not meet criteria for an anxiety disorder at posttreatment. Results suggested that younger children had better outcomes in the CBT versus FAM condition, whereas no differential effects were found between the two active treatments for older children. One-year and 6-year follow-ups demonstrated maintenance of treatment effects (Barrett et al., 1996; Barrett, Duffy, Dadds, & Rapee, 2001). Several other researchers have documented the efficacy of cognitive-behavioral interventions for childhood anxiety (e.g., Silverman et al., 1999; Spence, Donovan, & Brechman-Toussaint, 2000).

Several researchers have adapted Kendall's protocol for use in treating groups of children with anxiety disorders (e.g., Barrett, 1998; Flannery-Schroeder & Kendall, 2000; Mendlowitz, et al., 1999; Silverman, et al., 1999). Silverman and colleagues (1999) and Barrett (1998) compared a cognitive-behavioral treatment with a wait-list control condition. Results demonstrated that 64% and 75%, respectively, of participants no longer met criteria for their primary anxiety disorder. Self-report measures also demonstrated differential gains for treatment versus control conditions, and results were maintained at 1-year follow-ups. Flannery-Schroeder and Kendall (2000) compared individual and group formats to a wait-list control condition. Analyses revealed that 73% of individual and 50% of group (versus 8% of wait list) participants failed to meet diagnostic criteria for their primary anxiety disorder at posttreatment. Self-report measures of adaptive functioning also demonstrated the superiority of the treatment conditions. Treatment gains were maintained at a 3-month follow-up. Similarly, Mendlowitz and colleagues (1999) found cognitive-behavioral group interventions to reduce symptoms of anxiety and depression in a sample of children with anxiety disorders.

In sum, cognitive-behavioral treatments aimed at childhood anxiety disorders have shown both good efficacy and effectiveness. However, additional research is necessary to begin to examine which therapeutic factors, techniques, or both are best suited for specific anxiety disorders.

Pharmacological Interventions

Numerous pharmacological agents—including benzodiazepines, tricyclic antidepressants, serotonin reuptake inhibitors, monoamine oxidase inhibitors, and beta-adrenergic blockers—have been used to treat child anxiety. Benzodiazepines have been used most frequently.

In a review of systematic pharmacological trials for childhood anxiety disorders, Allen, Leonard, and Swedo (1995) found only 13 controlled studies; only one of these studies involved OAD/GAD. Simeon and colleagues (1992) conducted a controlled trial with 30 children and adolescents diagnosed with overanxious or avoidant disorders. Results found no significant difference between alprazolam and placebo, and there was an indication that participants with OAD may have been less responsive to alprazolam than the sample as a whole. Several open trials have demonstrated improvements in anxious symptomatology with both fluoxetine

(Birmaher, et al., 1994) and buspirone (Kutcher, Reiter, Gardner, & Klein, 1992). Additional studies using controlled, double-blind designs with well-defined patient populations are necessary before researchers will possess adequate knowledge regarding the costs, risks, and benefits of pharmacological interventions for childhood anxiety.

CONCLUSIONS

Generalized anxiety disorder is characterized by persistent and excessive worry about two or more life domains. Children with GAD tend to be perfectionistic, self-critical, self-conscious, and "hypermature." Due to changing diagnostic criteria, relatively few studies have investigated GAD in childhood. This dearth of research should stand as an impetus for methodologically rigorous examinations of risk and protective factors, prevention and intervention efforts, family factors, and additional study of psychotherapeutic and pharmacological interventions. Child anxiety researchers have only just begun the journey toward a thorough understanding of childhood GAD and anxiety disorders more generally.

REFERENCES

Allen, A. J., Leonard, H., & Swedo, S. E. (1995). Current knowledge of medications for the treatment of childhood anxiety disorders. *Journal of the American Academy of Child and Adolescent Psychiatry, 34,* 976–986.

American Psychiatric Association. (1968). *Diagnostic and statistical manual of mental disorders* (2nd ed.). Washington, DC: Author.

American Psychiatric Association. (1980). *Diagnostic and statistical manual of mental disorders* (3rd ed.). Washington, DC: Author.

American Psychiatric Association. (1987). *Diagnostic and statistical manual of mental disorders* (3rd ed., rev.). Washington, DC: Author.

American Psychiatric Association. (1994). *Diagnostic and statistical manual of mental disorders* (4th ed.). Washington, DC: Author.

American Psychiatric Association. (2000). *Diagnostic and statistical manual of mental disorders* (4th ed., text rev.). Washington, DC: Author.

Anderson, J. C., Williams, S., McGee, R., & Silva, P. A. (1987). DSM-III disorders in preadolescent children. *Archives of General Psychiatry, 44,* 69–76.

Barrett, P., Dadds, M., & Rapee, R. (1996). Family treatment of child anxiety: A controlled trial. *Journal of Consulting and Clinical Psychology, 64,* 333–342.

Barrett, P. M. (1998). Evaluation of cognitive-behavioral group treatments for childhood anxiety disorders. *Journal of Clinical Child Psychology, 27,* 459–468.

Barrett, P. M., Dadds, M. R., Rapee, R. M., & Ryan, S. M. (1996). Family enhancement of cognitive style in anxious and aggressive children. *Journal of Abnormal Child Psychology, 24,* 187–203.

Barrett, P. M., Duffy, A. L., Dadds, M. R., & Rapee, R. M. (2001). Cognitive-behavioral treatment of anxiety disorders in children: Long-term (6-year) follow-up. *Journal of Consulting and Clinical Psychology, 69,* 135–141.

Beidel, D. C. (1991). Social phobia and overanxious disorder in school-age children. *Journal of the American Academy of Child and Adolescent Psychiatry, 30,* 545–552.

Beidel, D. C., Silverman, W., & Hammond-Laurence, K. (1996). Overanxious disorder: Subsyndromal state or specific disorder? A comparison of clinic and community samples. *Journal of Clinical Child Psychology, 25,* 25–32.

Beitchman, J. H., Wekerle, C., & Hood, J. (1987). Diagnostic continuity from preschool to middle childhood. *Journal of the American Academy of Child and Adolescent Psychiatry, 26,* 694–699.

Bell-Dolan, D. J., Last, C. G., & Strauss, C. C. (1990). Symptoms of anxiety disorders in normal children. *Journal of the American Academy of Child and Adolescent Psychiatry, 29,* 759–765.

Biederman, J., Rosenbaum, J. F., Bolduc-Murphy, E. A., Faraone, S. V., Chaloff, J., Hirshfeld, D. R., & Kagan, J. (1993). A 3-year follow-up of children with and without behavioral inhibition. *Journal of the American Academy of Child and Adolescent Psychiatry, 32,* 814–821.

Biederman, J., Rosenbaum, J. F., Chaloff, J., & Kagan, J. (1995). Behavioral inhibition as a risk factor for anxiety disorders. In J. S. March (Ed.), *Anxiety disorders in children and adolescents* (pp. 61–81). New York: Guilford Press.

Birmaher, B., Waterman, G. S., Ryan, N., Cully, M., Balach, L., Ingram, J., & Brodsky, M. (1994). Fluoxetine for childhood anxiety disorders. *Journal of the American Academy of Child and Adolescent Psychiatry, 33,* 993–999.

Bowen, R. C., Offord, D. R., & Boyle, M. H. (1990). The prevalence of overanxious disorder and separation disorder in the community: Results from the Ontario Mental Health Study. *Journal of the American Academy of Child and Adolescent Psychiatry, 29,* 753–758.

Bowlby, J. (1982). *Attachment and loss.* New York: Basic Books.

Brent, D. A., Kalas, R., Edelbrock, C., Costello, A. J., Dulcan, M. K., & Conover, N. (1986). Psychopathology and its relationship to suicidal ideation in childhood and adolescence. *Journal of the American Academy of Child Psychiatry, 25,* 666–673.

Brown, T. A., Barlow, D. H., & Liebowitz, M. R. (1994). The empirical basis of generalized anxiety disorder. *American Journal of Psychiatry, 151,* 1272–1280.

Butler, G., & Mathews, A. (1983). Cognitive process in anxiety. *Advances in Behavior Research and Therapy, 5,* 51–62.

Cassidy, J. (1995). Attachment and generalized anxiety disorder. In D. Cicchetti & S. L. Toth (Eds.), *Emotion, cognition, and representation* (pp. 343–370). Rochester, NY: University of Rochester Press.

Chambless, D. L., & Hollon, S. D. (1998). Defining empirically supported therapies. *Journal of Consulting and Clinical Psychology, 66,* 7–18.

Cobham, V. E., Dadds, M. R., & Spence, S. H. (1998). The role of parental anxiety in the treatment of childhood anxiety. *Journal of Consulting and Clinical Psychology, 66,* 893–905.

Cohen, P., Cohen, J., Kasen, S., Velez, C. N., Hartmark, C., Johnson, J., Rojas, M.,

Brook, J., & Streuning, E. L. (1993). An epidemiological study of disorders in late childhood and adolescence: Age and gender specific prevalence. *Journal of Child Psychology and Psychiatry, 34,* 851–867.

Dadds, M. R., Barrett, P. M., Rapee, R. M., & Ryan, S. M. (1996). Family process and child anxiety and aggression: An observational analysis of the FEAR effect. *Journal of Abnormal Child Psychology, 24,* 715–734.

Donovan, C. L., & Spence, S. H. (2000). Prevention of childhood anxiety disorders. *Clinical Psychology Review, 20,* 509–531.

Eisen, A R., & Silverman, W. K. (1993). Should I relax or change my thoughts? A preliminary examination of cognitive therapy, relaxation training, and their combination with overanxious children. *Journal of Cognitive Psychotherapy, 7,* 265–279.

Eisen, A. R., & Silverman, W. K. (1998). Prescriptive treatment for generalized anxiety disorder in children. *Behavior Therapy, 29,* 105–121.

Erickson, M. F., Sroufe, L. A., & Egeland, B. (1985). The relationship between quality of attachment and behavior problems in preschool and a high-risk sample. *Monographs of the Society for Research in Child Development, 50,* 147–166.

Flannery-Schroeder, E. C., & Kendall, P. C. (2000). Group and individual cognitive-behavioral treatments for youth with anxiety disorders: A randomized clinical trial. *Cognitive Therapy and Research, 24,* 251–278.

Gittelman, R. (1984). Anxiety disorders in children. In L. Grinspoon (Ed.), *Psychiatry update* (Vol. 3, pp. 410–418). Washington, DC: American Psychiatric Association.

Hirshfeld, D. R., Rosenbaum, J. F., Biederman, J., Bolduc, E. A., Faraone, S. V., Snidman, N., Reznick, J. S., & Kagan, J. (1992). Stable behavioral inhibition and its association with anxiety disorder. *Journal of the American Academy of Child and Adolescent Psychiatry, 31,* 103–111.

Hudson, J. L., & Rapee, R. M. (2001). Parent–child interactions and the anxiety disorders: An observational analysis. *Behaviour Research and Therapy, 39,* 31–47.

Kagan, J. (1997). Temperament and the reactions to unfamiliarity. *Child Development, 68,* 139–143.

Kane, M. T., & Kendall, P. C. (1989). Anxiety disorders in children: A multiple baseline evaluation of a cognitive-behavioral treatment. *Behavior Therapy, 20,* 499–508.

Kendall, P. C. (1994). Treating anxiety disorders in children: Results of a randomized clinical trial. *Journal of Consulting and Clinical Psychology, 62,* 100–110.

Kendall, P. C. (2000). *Cognitive-behavioral therapy for anxious children: Therapist manual* (2nd ed.). Ardmore, PA: Workbook Publishing.

Kendall, P. C., Flannery-Schroeder, E., Panichelli-Mindel, S. M., Southam-Gerow, M., Henin, A., & Warman, M. (1997). Therapy for youths with anxiety disorders: A second randomized clinical trial. *Journal of Consulting and Clinical Psychology, 65,* 366–380.

Kendall, P. C., Krain, A., & Treadwell, K. (1999). Generalized anxiety disorders. In R. T. Ammerman, M. Hersen, & C. G. Last (Eds.), *Handbook of prescriptive treatments for children and adolescents* (2nd ed., pp. 155–171). Needham Heights, MA: Allyn & Bacon.

Kendall, P. C., & Southam-Gerow, M. (1996). Long-term follow-up of a cognitive-behavioral therapy for anxiety-disordered youth. *Journal of Consulting and Clinical Psychology, 64,* 724–730.

Kendall, P. C., & Warman, M. J. (1996). Anxiety disorders in youth: Diagnostic consistency across DSM-III-R and DSM-IV. *Journal of Anxiety Disorders, 10,* 453–463.

Khrone, H. W. (1990). Parental childrearing and anxiety development. In K. Hurrelmann & F. Losel (Eds.), *Health hazards in adolescence* (pp. 115–130). New York: de Gruyter.

Khrone, H. W., & Hock, M. (1991). Relationships between restrictive mother–child interactions and anxiety of the child. *Anxiety Research, 4,* 109–124.

Klein, R. G., & Last, C. G. (1989). Anxiety disorder in children. *Developmental Clinical Psychology and Psychiatry, 20,* 76–83.

Kutcher, S. P., Reiter, S., Gardner, D. M., & Klein, R. G. (1992). The pharmacotherapy of anxiety disorders in children and adolescents. *Psychiatric Clinics of North America, 15,* 41–67.

Last, C. G., Hersen, M., Kazdin, A. E., Finkelstein, R., & Strauss, C. C. (1987). Comparison of DSM-III separation anxiety and overanxious disorders: Demographic characteristics and patterns of comorbidity. *Journal of the American Academy of Child and Adolescent Psychiatry, 26,* 527–531.

Last, C. G., Hersen, M., Kazdin, A. E., Francis, G., & Grubb, H. J. (1987). Psychiatric illness in the mothers of anxious children. *American Journal of Psychiatry, 144,* 1580–1583.

Last, C. G., Strauss, C. C., & Francis, G. (1987). Comorbidity among childhood anxiety disorders. *Journal of Nervous and Mental Disease, 175,* 726–730.

Lewis, M., Feiring, C., McGafey, C., & Jaskir, J. (1984). Predicting psychopathology in six-year-olds from early social relations. *Child Development, 55,* 123–136.

Lichtenstein, J., & Cassidy, J. (1991, April). *The Inventory of Adult Attachment: Validation of a new measure.* Paper presented at the annual meeting of the Society for Research in Child Development, Seattle, WA.

Massion, A. O., Warshaw, M. G., & Keller, M. B. (1993). Quality of life and psychiatric morbidity in panic disorder and generalized anxiety disorder. *American Journal of Psychiatry, 150,* 600–607.

McGee, R., Feehan, M., Williams, S., Partridge, F., Silva, P., & Kelly, J. (1990). DSM-III disorders in a large sample of adolescents. *Journal of the American Academy of Child and Adolescent Psychiatry, 26,* 611–619.

Mendlowitz, S. L., Manassis, K., Bradley, S., Scapillato, D., Miezitis, S., & Shaw, B. F. (1999). Cognitive-behavioral group treatments in childhood anxiety disorders: The role of parental involvement. *Journal of the American Academy of Child and Adolescent Psychiatry, 38,* 1223–1229.

Muris, P., Kindt, M., Bögels, S., Merckelbach, H., Gadet, B., & Moulaert, V. (2000). Anxiety and threat perception abnormalities in normal children. *Journal of Psychopathology and Behavioral Assessment, 22,* 183–199.

Muris, P., & Merckelbach, H. (1998). Perceived parental rearing behavior and anxiety disorder symptoms in normal children. *Personality and Individual Differences, 25,* 1199–1206.

Orvaschel, H., & Weissman, M. M. (1986). Epidemiology of anxiety disorders in children: A review. In R. Gittelman (Ed.), *Anxiety disorders of childhood* (pp. 58–72). New York: Guilford Press.

Rapee, R. M. (1985). Distinctions between panic disorder and generalized anxiety disorder: Clinical presentation. *Australian and New Zealand Journal of Psychiatry, 19,* 227–232.

Rapee, R. M. (1991). Generalized anxiety disorder: A review of clinical features and theoretical concepts. *Clinical Psychology Review, 11,* 419–440.

Rapee, R. M., & Melville, L. F. (1997). Retrospective recall of family factors in social phobia and panic disorder. *Depression and Anxiety, 5,* 7–11.

Rapee, R. M., & Szollos, A. (1997, November). Early life events in anxious children. Paper presented at the annual Association for the Advancement of Behavior Therapy Convention, Miami, FL.

Rosenbaum, J. F., Biederman, J., Bolduc-Murphy, E. A., Faraone, S. V., Chaloff, J., Hirshfeld, D. R., & Kagan, J. (1993). Behavioral inhibition in childhood: A risk factor for anxiety disorders. *Harvard Review of Psychiatry, 1,* 2–16.

Roy-Burne, P. P., & Katon, W. (1997). Generalized anxiety disorder in primary care: The precursor/modifier pathway to increased health care utilization. *Journal of Clinical Psychiatry, 58*(Suppl. 3), 34–38.

Silverman, W. K. (1992). Taxonomy of anxiety disorders in children. In G. D. Burrows, R. Noyes, & S. M. Roth (Eds.), *Handbook of anxiety* (Vol. 5, pp. 281–308). Amsterdam: Elsevier.

Silverman, W. K., & Eisen, A. R. (1992). Age differences in the reliability of parent and child reports of child anxious symptomatology using a structured interview. *Journal of the American Academy of Child and Adolescent Psychiatry, 31,* 117–124.

Silverman, W. K., Kurtines, W. M., Ginsburg, G. S., Weems, C. F., Lumpkin, P. W., & Carmichael, D. H. (1999). Treating anxiety disorders in children with group cognitive-behavioral therapy: A randomized clinical trial. *Journal of Consulting and Clinical Psychology, 67,* 995–1003.

Silverman, W. K., & Nelles, W. B. (1988). The Anxiety Disorders Interview Schedule for Children. *Journal of the American Academy of Child and Adolescent Psychiatry, 27,* 772–778.

Simeon, J. G., Ferguson, H. B., Knott, V., Roberts, N., Gauthier, B., Dubois, C., & Wiggins, D. (1992). Clinical, cognitive, and neurophysiological effects of alprazolam in children and adolescents with overanxious and avoidant disorders. *Journal of the American Academy of Child and Adolescent Psychiatry, 31,* 29–33.

Spence, S. H., Donovan, C., & Brechman-Toussaint, M. (2000). The treatment of childhood social phobia: The effectiveness of a social skills training-based, cognitive-behavioral intervention with and without parental involvement. *Journal of Child Psychology and Psychiatry, 41,* 713–726.

Sroufe, L. A., Egeland, B., & Kreutzer, T. (1990). The fate of early experience following developmental change: Longitudinal approaches to individual adaptation in childhood. *Child Development, 61,* 1363–1373.

Strauss, C. C. (1988). Social deficits of children with internalizing disorders. In B. B. Lahey & A. E. Kazdin (Eds.), *Advances in clinical child psychology* (Vol. 11, pp. 159–191). New York: Plenum Press.

Strauss, C. C. (1990). Overanxious disorder in childhood. In M. Hersen & C. G. Last (Eds.), *Handbook of child and adult psychopathology: A longitudinal perspective* (pp. 237–246). New York: Pergamon Press.

Strauss, C. C., Lease, C. A., Last, C. G., & Francis, G. (1988). Overanxious disorder: An examination of developmental differences. *Journal of Abnormal Child Psychology, 16*, 433–443.

Tracey, S. A., Chorpita, B. F., Douban, J., & Barlow, D. H. (1997). Empirical evaluation of DSM-IV generalized anxiety disorder criteria in children and adolescents. *Journal of Clinical Child Psychology, 26*, 404–414.

Turner, S. M., Beidel, D. C., & Costello, A. (1987). Psychopathology in the offspring of anxiety disordered patients. *Journal of Consulting and Clinical Psychology, 55*, 229–235.

Velez, C. N., Johnson, J., & Cohen, P. (1989). A longitudinal analysis of selected risk factors of childhood psychopathology. *Journal of the American Academy of Child and Adolescent Psychiatry, 28*, 861–864.

Warren, S. L., Huston, L., Egeland, B., & Sroufe, L. A. (1997). Child and adolescent anxiety disorders and early attachment. *Journal of the American Academy of Child and Adolescent Psychiatry, 36*, 637–644.

Weems, C. F., Silverman, W. K., & La Greca, A. M. (2000). What do youth referred for anxiety problems worry about? Worry and its relation to anxiety and anxiety disorders in children and adolescents. *Journal of Abnormal Child Psychology, 28*, 63–72.

Weissman, M. M., Leckman, J. F., Merikangas, K. R., Gammon, G. D., & Prusoff, B. A. (1984). Depression and anxiety disorders in parents and children: Results from the Yale Family Study. *Archives of General Psychiatry, 41*, 845–852.

Werry, J. S. (1991). Overanxious disorder: A review of its taxonomic properties. *Journal of the American Academy of Child and Adolescent Psychiatry, 30*, 533–544.

Woody, S., & Rachman, S. (1994). Generalized anxiety disorder (GAD) as an unsuccessful search for safety. *Clinical Psychology Review, 14*, 743–753.

Chapter 7

Social Phobia

DEBORAH C. BEIDEL
TRACY L. MORRIS
MARQUETTE W. TURNER

Sociability, a preference for affiliation and the companionship of others rather than solitude, appears to be a basic and consistently identified dimension of personality (Buss & Plomin, 1984; Thomas & Chess, 1977). Shyness, another commonly identified behavior, is a form of social withdrawal that is characterized by social evaluative concerns, particularly in novel settings (Rubin & Asendorpf, 1993). Thus sociability refers to the desire for social affiliation, whereas shyness refers to distress and inhibited behaviors in social interactions. Empirically, sociability and social withdrawal represent distinct traits (Cheek & Buss, 1981), are detected at a very early age, and are stable across periods of developmental change (Broberg, Lamb, & Hwang, 1990; Kagan, Reznick, Clarke, Snidman, & Garcia-Coll, 1984). Any individual's social behavior may be characterized according to these two dimensions. For example, those who are low on sociability may have little desire for and receive very little satisfaction from social interactions with others. When in social encounters, they may not interact but nonetheless show (or feel) very little emotional distress. Others may have a strong desire for social encounters but become so distressed when in the company of others that they are unable to engage in rewarding interpersonal interactions. These children, who profess a desire for social encounters but who become significantly distressed when doing so, may meet diagnostic criteria for social phobia.

The recognition of individual differences in sociability and the labeling of individuals as shy is not a new concept. Case descriptions of those who would meet criteria for social phobia have been documented since the time of Hippocrates (Marks, 1985). In 1970, Marks described the phenomenology of socially phobic adults, and in 1980 this diagnostic condition was codified in the American psychiatric nomenclature with the publication of the third edition of the *Diagnostic and Statistical Manual of Mental Disorders* (DSM-III; American Psychiatric Association, 1980). However, despite this recognition, social phobia initially received very little attention from child researchers, possibly because fears in children are considered to be common (Barrios & O'Dell, 1989) and because of the belief that shy children subsequently "outgrow" this condition (e.g., Bruch, Giordano, & Pearl, 1986). Another possibility is that, although children who were fearful of social encounters could have been given the diagnosis of social phobia, other diagnostic conditions (listed in the section on children and adolescents in DSM-III-R; American Psychiatric Association, 1987) also contained criteria that tapped social-evaluative fears. Thus, until the past decade (Beidel, 1991; Beidel & Turner, 1988, Francis, Last & Strauss, 1992; Strauss & Last, 1993), social phobia in children as a distinct diagnostic entity was virtually ignored in the scientific literature.

SYMPTOM PICTURE

Social phobia is a marked and persistent fear of social situations characterized by pervasive social inhibition and timidity. Based on adult retrospective reports, the average age of onset is early to middle adolescence (Liebowitz, Gorman, Fyer, & Klein,1985; Turner, Beidel, Dancu, & Keys, 1986), but cases of social phobia have been documented in children as young as age 8 (Beidel & Turner, 1988; Schneier, Johnson, Hornig, Liebowitz, & Weissman, 1992). Last and her colleagues (Last, Perrin, Hersen, & Kazdin, 1992; Strauss & Last, 1993) reported an average age of onset ranging from 11.3 to 12.3 years, based on child and adolescent clinic-referred samples. Similarly, among a Canadian epidemiological sample, 12.7 years was reported as the median age of onset (DeWit, Ogborne, Offord, & MacDonald, 1999). Prior to DSM-IV (American Psychiatric Association, 1994), it was estimated that about 1% of the general child population suffered from social phobia (Anderson, Williams, McGee, & Silva, 1987; Kashani & Orvaschel, 1990). However, these early figures likely underestimate the prevalence of this disorder. As noted, the diagnostic schema of DSM-III-R allowed for children with social fears to be assigned this diagnosis. However, other disorders, such as avoidant disorder of childhood or overanxious disorder, also contained criteria addressing social fears. In light of the changes in DSM-IV (elimination of avoidant disorder of childhood and of social fears from the criteria for overanxious disorder, now included under generalized anxiety disorder), the prevalence rate of social phobia is no doubt higher. As one example, Kendall and Warman (1996) reported that, using DSM-III-R criteria, 18% of a clinic sample were diagnosed with social phobia, whereas using DSM-IV criteria, 40% of the sample were diagnosed with social phobia. Using a sample of German adolescents, the prevalence of social phobia was reported to be 1.6% of adolescents (ages 12–17; Essau, Conradt, & Petermann, 1999). It also is important to note that the prevalence of social phobia increases as children age (Essau et al., 1999; Kashani & Orvaschel, 1990); therefore, more adolescents than preadolescent children suffer from this disorder. The gender distribution for social phobia is approximately equal, and both European American and African American children show a similar clinical presentation (Beidel, Turner, & Morris, 1999).

Children with social phobia report distress in a broad range of interpersonal encounters. In a recent study of the psychopathology of childhood social phobia, Beidel and colleagues (1999) examined the range of situations reported as distressful for preadolescent children with this disorder. As depicted in Table 7.1, children endorse moderate to severe distress across a variety of social and performance settings. Strauss and Last (1993) reported a similar range of distressing situations plus a category called "school," referring to social distress in the school setting. In both studies, many of the situations describe specific behaviors performed in front of others (writing, eating, speaking) and more general conversational interactions. Currently, in DSM-IV, the generalized subtype is used for individuals who experience distress across a range of social settings. Among adults, about 70% of those with social phobia are of the generalized subtype (Turner, Beidel, & Jacob, 1994). Among preadolescent children, 89% of one sample had the generalized subtype (Beidel et al., 1999). Among an adolescent sample (Hofmann et al., 1999), 45.5% were judged as the generalized subtype, although this study used a numerical count of situations, which is not the usual practice for making this type of determination.

Children with social phobia have reported that distressful events occur approximately every other day, significantly more often than for normal controls (Beidel, 1991). Consistent with Strauss and Last's (1993) observation that school is a fearful setting, 60% of the distressing events occurred at school. Within this setting, the most common distressing event was an unstructured peer encounter (e.g., having to talk to another child), followed by taking tests, performing in front of others, and reading aloud. Hofmann and colleagues (1999) reported that adolescents most often endorsed the informal speaking/interaction tasks as their most fear-provoking situations. When these events occurred, the children with social phobia were signifi-

TABLE 7.1. Types of Social Situations Feared by Children
with Social Phobia

Situation	% Endorsing at least moderate distress
Reading aloud in front of the class	71
Musical or athletic performances	61
Joining in on a conversation	59
Speaking to adults	59
Starting a conversation	58
Writing on the blackboard	51
Ordering food in a restaurant	50
Attending dances or activity nights	50
Taking tests	48
Parties	47
Answering a question in class	46
Working or playing with other children	45
Asking the teacher for help	44
Physical education class	37
Group or team meetings	36
Having a picture taken	32
Using school or public bathrooms	24
Inviting a friend to get together	24
Eating in the school cafeteria	23
Walking in the hallway/hanging out at lockers	16
Answering or talking on the telephone	13
Eating in front of others	10

cantly more likely to respond negatively and to report higher levels of subjective distress. Furthermore, a number of these negative coping responses (8%) involved behavioral avoidance (Beidel, 1991). Interestingly, avoidance behaviors also may increase with increasing age, as Essau and her colleagues noted that 65.4% of their adolescent sample with significant social fears reported at least occasional social avoidance. As noted, although formal speaking situations are the most universally feared, the most frequent distressful encounter is interpersonal conversation. Thus, in addition to performance situations, clinicians need to be attuned to the potentially anxiety-producing consequences of interpersonal encounters.

Although social phobia can be diagnosed in children, adolescents, and adults, the disorder does not manifest itself identically across different developmental stages. In a comparison of the epidemiological and clinical presentations of social phobia in adults and children, Beidel and Turner (1993) reported similar prevalence rates. In addition, similar coexisting diagnoses (generalized anxiety disorder in adults, overanxious disorder in children, and specific phobia in both adults and children) also were common among individuals with social phobia (Beidel & Turner, 1993; Last,

Strauss, & Francis, 1987; Turner, Beidel, Borden, Stanley, & Jacob, 1991). Both adults and children endorsed distress across a broad range of potentially fearful situations. Formal speaking was the most commonly endorsed event, and the physical complaints characteristic of socially phobic adults also were common for children with this disorder. However, when in anxiety-producing situations, children did not report the occurrence of negative cognitions with the same frequency as adults.

When in socially distressful situations, children with social phobia endorse a range of physical symptoms that include heart palpitations (70.8%), shakiness (66.7%), flushes and chills (62.5%), sweating (54.2%), and nausea (54.2%; Beidel, Christ, & Long, 1991). With respect to other clinical correlates, children with social phobia endorse high trait anxiety, dysphoria or depression, a restricted range of social situations, and loneliness (Beidel et al., 1999). Additionally, several studies have documented the existence of poor social skills among this population (Beidel et al., 1999; Spence, Donovan, & Brechman-Toussaint, 1999). Furthermore, a substantial percentage of children and adolescents with social phobia present with additional comorbid conditions. Among preadolescent children, 60% of one sample had a comorbid disorder, including generalized anxiety disorder (10% of the sample), attention-deficit/hyperactivity disorder (10%), specific phobia (10%), selective mutism (8%), separation anxiety disorder (6%), obsessive–compulsive disorder (6%), depression (6%), panic disorder (2%), and adjustment disorder with anxious and depressed mood (2%; Beidel et al., 1999) . Among adolescents with this disorder, 41.2% were reported to have a somatoform disorder, 29.4% had a depressive disorder, and 23.5% had a substance abuse disorder (Essau et al., 1999).

Although functional interference is not necessary in order to assign a diagnosis of social phobia, the disorder often results in significant immediate and long-term sequelae. Functional impairment includes depression (Last & Perrin, 1993), social isolation and loneliness (Beidel et al., 1999), and school refusal (Last, Hersen, Kazdin, & Orvaschel, 1991). Additionally, Last and Perrin (1993) noted that among anxious children, social phobia was much more likely to precede the onset of depression than vice versa. Among adolescents with this disorder, Essau and colleagues (1999) reported that 60% reported impairment at school, 26.7% endorsed impairment in leisure activity, and 53.3% reported impairment in social contacts. Conduct problems and oppositional behaviors have been reported among adolescents with social phobia (Clark, 1993), as has substance abuse and dependence (Clark, 1993; DeWit, MacDonald, & Offord, 1999; Essau et al., 1999).

Those with social phobia exhibit deficient social skills. Among preadolescent children, those with social phobia were judged by independent observers to have significantly poorer social skills both in social interactions and when reading in front of a small audience than do age-matched, nonanxious peers (Beidel et al., 1999). These children also were judged to be significantly more anxious when engaged in those situations. Similar findings were reported by Spence and colleagues (1999). In that study, children with social phobia showed significant social skill deficits (when compared with children without a disorder). Results were consistent across self-report and parental report of social skills and assertiveness, as well as by direct observation in a role-play situation. Furthermore, some preliminary data from our clinic reveal that socially anxious children are less likely than nonanxious peers to engage in social activities such as conversing with others, attending social events, and participating in class (Ferrell, Beidel, & Turner, 2001) and that these differences become more pronounced between the ages of 10 and 11–12. As noted in the upcoming section on Etiology, social reticence and anxiety may prevent engagement in social interactions (Rubin, LeMare, & Lollis, 1990), which in turn prevents the acquisition of social skills. This, in turn, can lead to further avoidance and distress. Such a developmental pathway would suggest that interventions would have to include attention to the acquisition of social skills, as well as the elimination of social distress.

NATURAL HISTORY

No studies of the long-term outcome of social phobia currently exist, perhaps because until recently shyness in children was considered a temporary condition. Retrospective studies of college students note that the majority of those who reported being shy as children had outgrown their shyness by the time they reached adulthood. Similarly, and more recently, a retrospective study found that half of those with a history of social phobia recovered from the disorder (DeWit, Ogborne, et al., 1999). In this study, the strongest predictor was a later age of onset of social fears. In fact, those who reported an onset of social phobia after the age of 13 were 8.59 times more likely to recover from the disorder than those who reported the onset prior to the age of 7. These results are consistent with earlier retrospective findings of Davidson (1993), who reported that age of onset prior to age 11 predicted nonrecovery in adulthood.

As noted, these studies are based on retrospective reports of adults with this disorder. To date, there are no longitudinal studies beginning with children who are diagnosed with social phobia. However, 25–30-year longitudinal studies of shy children (Caspi, Edler, & Bem, 1988; Kerr, Lambert, & Bem, 1996) suggest that shy boys marry later and become parents later than nonshy boys, whereas shy girls had a lower likelihood of attending college than nonshy girls. Furthermore, 42% of children consistently rated as shy had anxiety problems in adolescence, as rated by behavior-problem checklists, in comparison with only 11% of children never rated as shy (Prior, Smart, Sanson, & Oberklaid, 2000). Similarly, long-term follow-up studies of behaviorally inhibited infants and toddlers found that (1) social phobia was more frequent among inhibited children than among uninhibited children (Kagan, 1997) and (2) inhibited children were more likely to have a less positive and active social life as adults, a later move away from the family of origin, and, for males, higher negative emotionality (Gest, 1997). In summary, retrospective studies suggest that some individuals with social phobia may overcome their condition, but this is not likely to occur if there is an early age of onset. Although no prospective studies of children with social phobia exist, prospective studies of children characterized as shy or behaviorally inhibited suggest that a proportion of them will develop anxiety during adolescence. However, to date it is unclear how to determine which children are likely to develop more severe disorders.

ETIOLOGY

Etiological factors are usually divided into one of two groups: psychological factors and biological factors. Within the psychological dimension, three pathways are considered: direct conditioning, social learning (modeling), and information transfer. In one of the first studies to look at the onset of social phobia, Ost (1985) reported that 58% of those with the diagnosis attributed its onset to a direct traumatic conditioning event. More recently, among a sample of adults with social phobia, 44% reported a conditioning experience that marked the onset or exacerbation of social phobia (Stemberger, Turner, Beidel, & Calhoun, 1995). Interestingly, 20% of adults without a history of social phobia also reported a history of traumatic conditioning events, yet they did not develop social phobia. When examined by social-phobia subtype, 40% of those with the generalized subtype and 56% of those with the nongeneralized (specific) subtype reported traumatic conditioning events, but only the rate for the specific subtype was significantly higher than the rate for the normal control group. These data illustrate an important point. First, a sizeable number of individuals with social phobia cannot recall a specific event that precipitated the onset of their disorder. Second, 1 out of 5 normal controls reported experiencing a traumatic social event, yet never developed social phobia. Thus, although conditioning experiences may play a role, they do not appear necessary or sufficient for the onset of the disorder.

Direct conditioning experiences are only one of the hypothesized psychological pathways to the onset of the disorder. Several retrospective reports of adults with social phobia suggest that they had at least one parent who was shy, reticent, or avoidant of social interactions (Brown & Lloyd, 1975). It is important to note that, usually, data from family studies are used to argue for a biological etiology. However, Mineka and her colleagues (e.g., Mineka & Cook, 1988) have clearly demonstrated that emotion, as well as avoidant behavior, can be acquired through behavioral observation. Thus it is equally as likely that children might acquire these shy and reticent behaviors through modeling (social learning) as it is that they are simply a result of direct genetic transmission (see Masia & Morris, 1998).

The least studied form of learning with respect to social fears (and fears in general) is information transfer (Beidel & Turner, 1998). Ost (1985) reported that 3% of adults with social phobia reported that their fears were acquired through information transfer. Based on retrospective data supplied by adults with social phobia, childhood histories suggest a pattern of familial communication characterized by concern about the opinions of others, isolation of the child, and emphasis on shame (Bruch & Heimberg, 1994; Bruch, Heimberg, Berger, & Collins, 1989). However, because of their retrospective nature and the fact that these individuals were suffering from a disorder, the veracity of these data may be affected by time or the perception of an individual with a disorder. More recently, observational studies of parent–child interaction suggest that parents may play a role in fostering fear and avoidance behavior in children (Greco & Morris, 2002; Turner, Beidel, Roberson-Nay, & Tervo, 2003). Continued observational investigation is needed to further elucidate patterns of interaction involved in the development of specific forms of anxiety.

In addition to hypothesized psychological etiologies, biological factors also may play a role in the onset of social phobia. Torgersen (1983) reported that the proband-wise concordance rate for any anxiety disorders category (except GAD) was higher for monozygotic (MZ) than dizygotic (DZ) twins (34% vs. 17%, respectively) but that no co-twin had the same anxiety disorder as the proband. Andrews, Stewart, Allen, and Henderson (1990) reached similar conclusions. Kendler and his colleagues (Kendler et al., 1992) reported that the familial aggregation of agoraphobia, social phobia, situational phobia, and specific phobia was consistent with "phobia proneness," with heritability estimates indicating that "genetic factors play a significant but by no means overwhelming role in the etiology of phobias" (Kendler et al.,1992, p. 279). Thus the data did not support a one-to-one genetic transmission.

In a study of the family history of children with anxiety disorders (Last et al., 1991), social phobia and avoidant disorder were significantly more prevalent among the first-degree relatives of anxious children than among the relatives of the normal controls, but there was no difference in prevalence rates for these disorders between groups with anxiety and with attention-deficit/hyperactivity disorder (ADHD). A recently published study (Fyer, Mannuzza, Chapman, Liebowitz, & Klein, 1993) indicated a significantly increased risk for social phobia in the adult relatives of adult patients with social phobia compared with adult relatives of normal controls (16% vs. 5%). More recently, rates of psychopathology in the offspring of parents with social phobia have been examined (Mancini, Van Ameringen, Szatmari, Fugere, & Boyle, 1996). Results indicated that 49% of the offspring had at least one DSM-III-R anxiety disorder, most commonly overanxious disorder (30%), social phobia (23%), and separation anxiety disorder (19%). However, this was an uncontrolled family study, and those who conducted assessments on the children were not blind to parental diagnosis. Thus these data must be interpreted cautiously.

TREATMENT

The extant treatment literature for youth with social anxiety disorder is quite sparse. That is, few studies have focused specifically on the psychosocial or pharmacological treatment of social phobia in childhood. Several studies have included children with social phobia as part of a larger sample of children with various anxiety disorders. Additionally, several investigations have included children meeting DSM-III-R diagnostic criteria for avoidant disorder, since subsumed under social phobia in DSM-IV. Because so few studies have included samples of children with only social phobia, all of the studies noted previously are included as part of this review.

Cognitive-Behavioral Treatment

Initially, most studies focused on samples of children who had one of several different anxiety disorders. These treatments were broadly based and, as noted, were used to address generalized anxiety disorder (overanxious disorder), avoidant disorder (social phobia), or separation anxiety disorder. In a series of studies, Kendall and his colleagues (Flannery-Schroeder & Kendall, 2000; Kendall, 1994; Kendall et al., 1997) reported that children treated with cognitive-behavioral treatment (CBT), either individually or in groups, had significantly lower general anxiety and enhanced coping abilities and improved on parents' ratings of anxiety, depression, and social competence compared with controls. Treatment gains were maintained at 3.35-year follow-up (Kendall & Southam-Gerow, 1996). However, the percentage of children in the sample with social phobia was quite small, and, in some cases, children's social functioning did not improve (e.g., social anxiety, friendships, and social activities; Flannery-Schroeder & Kendall,

2000), suggesting that this intervention, although effective for anxiety, may not address unique aspects of social phobia.

Similar to the research of Kendall and his colleagues, Silverman and her colleagues examined the effectiveness of group and individual CBT for children with various anxiety disorders (Silverman, Kurtines, Ginsburg, Weems, Lumpkin, & Carmichael, 1999); 27% of the sample had a primary diagnosis of social phobia. Results indicated that 64% of children in group cognitive-behavioral treatment (GCBT) no longer met criteria for their primary diagnosis at posttreatment compared with 13% of wait-list controls. Silverman's individual exposure-based CBT (Silverman, Kurtines, Ginsberg, Weems, Rabian, & Serafini, 1999) also was compared with an active control condition. Ten percent of the sample had a primary diagnosis of social phobia. Based on the small proportion of children with social phobia in this sample, outcome analyses were conducted for the total sample and for children with simple phobia only. Findings revealed that although the active treatment was effective, even the active control group produced meaningful changes in phobic symptoms at posttreatment and at follow-up. Although the studies of Kendall and colleagues and Silverman and colleagues have some implications for the treatment of childhood social phobia, the results must be interpreted cautiously. The samples included only a few children with social phobia or DSM-III-R avoidant disorder, thus it is difficult to determine the utility of these treatments for children and adolescents with social phobia.

The first treatment program designed specifically for socially phobic youths (in this case, adolescents) is termed Group Cognitive-Behavioral Treatment for Adolescents (GCBT-A). The initial publication was a series of 5 case studies (Albano, Marten, Holt, Heimberg, & Barlow, 1995). GCBT-A consists of psychoeducation, skill building (such as social skills, problem solving, and assertiveness training), cognitive restructuring, and behavioral exposure to socially distressing or fearful situations. At posttreatment, 4 of the 5 adolescents were judged to have only subclinical levels of social phobia, and 1 year later, 4 did not meet DSM-III-R diagnostic criteria for social phobia. More recently, Hayward and colleagues (2000) compared GCBT-A to a no-treatment control group. At posttreatment, 45% of those treated with GCBT-A did not meet criteria for social phobia, compared with 4% in the no-treatment control group. However, considerable residual social-phobia symptoms remained at posttreatment, and 1 year later, there were no significant group differences in the frequency of social phobia diagnosis or in mean scores on a self-report social phobia inventory.

Spence, Donovan, and Brechman-Toussaint (2000) examined the effectiveness of including a social-skills-training component in their CBT for children with social phobia. This study also examined the role of parental involvement and, thus, is discussed in a later section. In the only other controlled trial of behavioral treatment for preadolescent children with social phobia, Beidel, Turner, and Morris (2000) compared a multi-component behavioral treatment for childhood social phobia with an active, nonspecific intervention. Sixty-seven children were randomly assigned to either the active treatment Social Effectiveness Therapy for Children (SET-C), or to an active nonspecific control, called Testbusters. SET-C is a multifaceted behavioral treatment that includes group social skills training, peer-generalization experiences, and individual *in vivo* exposure. At posttreatment, 67% of those treated with SET-C no longer met criteria for social phobia, compared with 5% for the Testbusters group. Furthermore, in terms of clinical significance, children in the SET-C group were less anxious, less avoidant of social situations, more skillful in their social interactions, and engaged in more social discourse, as reported by children, parents, and independent evaluators. At 3-year follow-up, children treated with SET-C maintained their improved status. The results of this investigation are notably encouraging because, unlike in previous investigations, SET-C was compared with an active, nonspecific control.

Finally, Masia, Klein, Storch, and Corda (2001) investigated a 14-session group treatment program for 6 adolescents with social anxiety disorder. Conducted in the school setting, the treatment program included social skills training and *in vivo* exposure sessions. The results showed significant improvement on clinician severity ratings of social anxiety disorder but no significant change in the adolescents' self-reports of social fears. The pilot nature of this study means that the results must be considered preliminary. However, if replicated, accessibility of the intervention may be maximized by conducting it in a group setting.

Pharmacological Treatment

Although several classes of medication have been studied for their effectiveness in children with social phobia or related conditions such as selective mutism, selective serotonin reuptake inhibitors (SSRIs) are usually considered the first-line pharmacological agent. Three advantages of SSRIs include their high tolerance levels, minimal side effects, and lack of need for blood-level monitoring (Kratochvil, Kutcher, Reiter, & March, 1999; Pine & Grun, 1998; Velosa & Riddle, 2000). The most common SSRIs include fluvoxamine (Luvox), fluoxetine (Prozac), sertraline (Zoloft), and paroxetine (Paxil). Among the eight published trials, six have evaluated SSRIs (Birmaher et al., 1994; Black & Uhde, 1994; Compton et al., 2001; Dummit, Klein, Tancer, Asche, & Martin, 1996; Fairbanks et al., 1997; Research Units of Pediatric Psychopharmacology [RUPP] Anxiety Study Group, 2001). In general, only minimal, if any, side effects (headaches, nausea, drowsiness, insomnia, jitteriness, and stomachaches) have been reported (Velosa & Riddle, 2000). A more severe side effect, disinhibition, which required the discontinuation of fluoxetine in 2 children, was reported in one study (Dummit et al., 1996).

Similar to the research on psychosocial treatments, many of the published pharmacological studies used samples of children who had a variety of different anxiety disorders. One of the earliest publications was not a controlled trial but a retrospective chart review of 21 children and adolescents treated with fluoxetine for overanxious disorder, avoidant disorder, and social phobia. Outcome data were based on prospective reports from attending nurses and patients' mothers. The results indicated that 81% of the children exhibited marked improvement in anxiety symptomatology, benefits that were achieved after 6–8 weeks of treatment. Furthermore, the results were consistent even after controlling for the presence and severity of depression. Of course, these results should be interpreted cautiously, given the biases associated with retrospective chart review.

Another open trial of fluoxetine examined its effects on 16 child outpatients with various anxiety disorders (Fairbanks et al., 1997). The children who participated in this trial had not responded to psychotherapy. Mean fluoxetine dose for children was 24 mg per day, and the mean dose for adolescents was 40 mg per day. Similar to findings from the Birmaher et al. (1994) study, treatment gains were evident after 6–9 weeks of treatment with fluoxetine, as measured by change scores on the Clinical Global Impression Scale. However, the outcome of this study is limited by the absence of blind evaluation and the lack of randomized procedures. Overall, children with only one anxiety disorder responded to lower doses of fluoxetine than did children with comorbid disorders. Only 10 children with social phobia were included in the trial; 80% were rated as clinically improved. Improvement rates were similarly high for children with other types of anxiety disorders. However, 62.5% of all children (not merely those with social phobia) still met diagnostic criteria for an anxiety disorder at posttreatment. Thus, although clinically improved, many children were still quite impaired at the end of treatment. Because of the high number of comorbid diagnoses among the children in this sample and the nonblind nature of the trial, only limited conclusions for the efficacy of fluoxetine for childhood social phobia can be drawn from this study.

Two other fluoxetine trials (one open and one double blind) have been conducted with selectively mute children, who shared similarities with children with social phobia. In a 9-week open trial, 21 children were treated with an average daily dose of 28.1 mg of fluoxetine (Dummit et al., 1996). All children referred for this trial met criteria for either avoidant disorder ($N = 18$) or social phobia ($N = 3$), in addition to selective mutism. The results indicated that 76% of the sample showed decreased anxiety and increased speech, as evaluated by psychiatrists at posttreatment. Although encouraging, these data are limited, as assessment of clinical improvement was made by the treating psychiatrist, not an independent evaluator. In the only double-blind study of fluoxetine to date (Black & Uhde, 1994), selectively mute children ages 6–12 years participated in a 12-week trial (average dose 21.4 mg per day). All children also had comorbid diagnoses of either social phobia or avoidant disorder. At posttreatment, parents rated the children treated with fluoxetine as significantly improved, compared with the children in the placebo group. However, clinician and teacher reports did not reveal any significant group differences. Overall, the authors reported that treatment effects were modest. Most of the children treated with fluoxetine were still symptomatic at the end of the trial. Thus the only placebo-controlled trial resulted in only minimal support for fluoxetine efficacy in selective mutism, and, by extension, social phobia and avoidant disorder. Furthermore, the results of these studies with selective mutism do not address the treatment of children with social phobia but without selective mutism.

Fourteen children and adolescents with social phobia participated in an 8-week open trial of sertraline (Compton et al., 2001). The mean age of the children was 13.57 years, and the mean dosage of sertraline was 123 mg. At posttreatment, 36% were judged as responders and 29% as partial responders. Overall, the group showed significant decreases on self-report measures of social anxiety. It is notable that for this study, a behavioral assessment test was used as part of the outcome for the pharmacological treatment trial. In both tasks (talking about themselves in front of a small audience and having a one-on-one conversation with a confederate), the children's distress was significantly lower at posttreatment. Of course, a randomized controlled trial is necessary in order to fully determine the efficacy of sertraline for this population.

In the largest controlled trial of SSRI treatment for childhood anxiety disorders to date, 128 children (ages 6–17) were randomly assigned to either 8 weeks of fluvoxamine or placebo (RUPP Anxiety Study Group, 2001). The average maximum dose of fluvoxamine was 300 mg per day. As with other studies cited, children in the sample had primary diagnoses of social phobia, separation anxiety disorder, or generalized anxiety disorder. Fluvoxamine demonstrated superior anxiety symptom reduction, as measured by the Pediatric Anxiety Rating Scale. According to the preestablished treatment-responder criteria, 76% (48 of 63) of those treated with fluvoxamine showed marked clinical improvement, in comparison with 29% (19 of 65) of children in the placebo group.

Two clinical trials examined alprazolam in children with social anxiety. In an initial 6-week open trial, 20 children (ages 8.8–16.5) with overanxious and avoidant disorder were treated with 0.5 mg to 1.5 mg of alprazolam daily. Only 6 children were rated as moderately improved in terms of overall clinical status, even though specific ratings of anxiety by both clinicians and parents suggested significant improvement (Simeon & Ferguson, 1987). Based on these findings, a 4-week double-blind controlled trial with 30 children (ages 8.4–16.9) diagnosed with either overanxious disorder or avoidant disorder was conducted. Average daily dose of alprazolam was 1.57 mg. There were no group differences at post-treatment. Thus both studies suggest that alprazolam response is low, at least over 4–6 weeks of treatment.

Benzodiazepines should be considered for the treatment of childhood anxiety disorders only after all other medications have failed to show improvement in symptomatology (Kratochvil et al., 1999; Pine & Grun, 1998; Velosa & Riddle, 2000), primarily because the side effects tend to be more serious and more common. Side effects include drowsiness, irritability, oppositional behavior, disinhibition, fatigue, nausea, headaches, ataxia, slurred speech, diplopia, and tremors (Kratochvil et al., 1999; Velosa & Riddle, 2000). The incidence and prevalence of benzodiazepine dependency in children is unknown, but because of the known risk of dependence in adults, these drugs are best used for the short term (Velosa & Riddle, 2000).

Family Treatment

Using the intervention developed by Kendall and his colleagues (Kendall, 1994), Barrett and colleagues (Barrett, Dadds, & Rapee, 1996) evaluated the addition of a family component. Seventy-nine children (27% with social phobia), ages 7–14, were randomly assigned to either 12-week CBT, CBT plus family management, or a wait-list control group. The family intervention included both parents and focused on training in reinforcement and contingency management strategies, coping techniques to deal with parental emotionality, and communication and problem-solving skills. Based on the presence or absence of a diagnosis at posttreatment, CBT and CBT plus parental involvement were effective (in comparison with the wait-list control condition). However, the CBT-plus-family-involvement condition was significantly superior to CBT alone (84% vs. 57% did not have a diagnosis at posttreatment, respectively) and to the wait-list control condition (26%). Among the children with social phobia, 61.5% of those in the active treatment groups no longer had a diagnosis at posttreatment. Interestingly, younger children (ages 7–10) responded better to the combined condition than to CBT alone (100% vs. 55.6% without a diagnosis, respectively). The percentage of younger children with social phobia was not reported.

Following this study, Barrett (1998) examined the effectiveness of CBT plus family intervention when presented in a group format. Sixty children were randomly assigned to GCBT, GCBT plus family involvement, or a wait-list control condition. Results indicated that 55.9% of children in the GCBT group did not meet diagnostic criteria at posttreatment, compared with 70.7% in the GCBT-plus-family-management condition, a nonsignificant difference. In fact, there were few significant differences between active treatment conditions at posttreatment. However, over follow-up, children in the GCBT-plus-family-management condition continued to improve when compared with children in the GCBT condition. However, because only 4 of the 60 children had primary diagnoses of social phobia (4% of children also had comorbid diagnoses of avoidant disorder), the effectiveness of this intervention specifically for children with social phobia is unclear. Finally, a 6-year follow-up of children treated with CBT found that treatment gains made at 12-month follow-up were maintained (Barrett, Duffy, Dadds, & Rapee, 2001). Among the sample of 52 patients who were able to be contacted 6 years later, 10 had social phobia at pretreatment. Among those 10 children, 9 (90%) did not meet criteria for a diagnosis 6 years later.

Tracy and colleagues (1998) compared cognitive-behavioral group treatment of social phobia for adolescents (CBGT-A) with CBGT-A plus parental involvement (CBGT-A/P) in 27 clinically referred adolescents. Parental involvement included taking part in four treatment sessions, receiving exposure to the theoretical rationale, skill-building sessions, and instructions in assisting the adolescent in exposure sessions. Both interventions resulted in significant improvement in social anxiety symptoms, but no change on measures of general anxiety and depression was apparent. Furthermore, there was no additive effect of parental involvement. These findings appear consistent with those of Barrett and colleagues (1996), who found that parental involvement was more effective with preadolescent children. Given that adolescents are more physically, mentally, and emotionally mature, parental involvement in the intervention may be less necessary than it is for preadolescent children.

Another controlled trial using only children with social phobia examined group CBT with parental involvement (CBT-PI), group CBT with no parental involvement (CBT-PNI), and a wait-list control condition (Spence et al., 2000). CBT included social skills training, relaxation techniques, social-problem solving, positive self-instruction, cognitive challenging, and exposure to social situations. The CBT-PI condition also included a component that taught parents to properly model and reinforce children's use of newly acquired social skills and to encourage children's participation in social activities outside of sessions. It is important to note that this parental intervention is different from that of Barrett and colleagues (1996) but similar to that of Tracy and colleagues (1998). Whereas Barrett and colleagues focused primarily on parental emotional concerns and issues, the intervention of Spence and colleagues (2000), like that of Tracy and colleagues (1998), focuses specifically on helping parents deal with their children's difficulties. At posttreatment, parental report indicated that 87.5% of the CBT-PI group and 58% of the CBT-PNI group no longer met diagnostic criteria for social phobia, compared with 7% of the wait-list control group. Similar results were reported for child self-report measures of social anxiety symptoms. Although there was a trend toward greater improvement in children in the CBT-PI group, differences were not statistically significant. Effects were maintained at 6- and 12-month follow-up. Additionally, both treatment conditions showed improvement in social skills from pretreatment to 12-month follow-up, based on parent reports, but no significant differences were found between the three groups on children's total number of peer interactions, on parental reports of competence with peers, or on independent observer ratings of assertiveness during behavioral observation from pre- to posttreatment. This finding suggests that the intervention was quite effective for social anxiety symptoms but did not substantially affect social behavior.

FUTURE DIRECTIONS

Although our understanding of social phobia has advanced significantly across the past two decades, much work remains to be done. Prospective studies of children with social phobia are needed in order to advance our knowledge of long-term consequences and phenomenological changes in symptom presentation that may occur across developmental transitions. Little is known about the day-to-day social experience of children with social phobia. We must conduct more complex daily diary studies, analogue social-skills assessment, peer ratings, and observations of interaction in multiple settings in natural environments to obtain a more comprehensive understanding of the antecedents, consequences, and corollaries of social anxiety.

Several models have been proposed to guide research on etiological processes in child anxiety. Research on the developmental psychopathology of social anxiety is expanding at an accelerated pace, particularly in terms of family variables. However, as yet few studies have investigated the mechanisms of information transfer. Patterns of familial communication must be examined in laboratory and naturalistic settings, with a goal toward expanding the limtied roster of variables that have been investigated thus far (e.g., warmth, control). With few exceptions, research on parent–child interaction and child psychopathology has included mothers as the sole parental representative. Greater effort must be made to include fathers in all research investigations. Furthermore, sibling relationships practically have been ignored. If we are to attempt to understand family dynamics as they relate to social anxiety, we must attempt to include all members of the family whenever possible.

The literature on the treatment of social phobia in children is in a more advanced stage than that on etiological processes. Exposure has been identified as a prime effective, perhaps necessary, component of successful treatment. It is important that we work to educate physicians, clinicians, and school counselors as to the positive benefits that may be obtained through short-term behavior therapy. Future research should investigate modes of delivery of exposure in an effort to provide relevant treatment guidelines. For instance, parents might be trained to assist with *in vivo* exposure activities, given limits on the out-of-office work that may be conducted under therapist direction. No matter the form of intervention—behavioral, pharmacological, or combined—long-term posttreatment follow-up investigation is needed to more thoroughly evaluate treatment efficacy. Likewise, the potential necessity for—and optimal timing of—booster sessions warrants examination. Importantly, it is time for treatment research to move beyond the specialty clinic. Transportability studies are greatly needed. We must find ways to export effective treatments to rural and school settings to reach the greatest number of children. Additionally, school settings would seem the optimal entry point for efforts directed at screening and early intervention.

SUMMARY

Since the release of the first edition of this book, significant advances have been made in the assessment and treatment of social phobia in children. In an effort to expand our understanding of the disorder, research on factors related to the development and maintenance of social phobia is receiving increased attention. Temperament, parent–child interaction, peer socialization, and traumatic conditioning all have been implicated in the development of social phobia, although it is widely acknowledged that the disorder results from the interplay of multiple factors.

As social phobia largely has been found to be an early-onset, comorbid, and chronic disorder, early detection and intervention could help avert a lifetime of personal distress and social maladjustment. The first controlled behavioral and pharmacological treatment trials recently have been conducted. A manualized multicomponent treatment program has been developed and is being made available to therapists, thus expanding the number of competent professionals available to provide effective treatment for children with social phobia. Behavioral interventions have been expanded to include parents and peers, attesting to increased developmental sensitivity to the needs of children and adolescents. Undoubtedly, the next decade will give witness to continued acceleration in the empirical exploration of the nature of social phobia and the means by which to remediate the disorder.

ACKNOWLEDGMENTS

Work on this chapter was supported in part by NIMH Grant Nos. 53503 and 60332 to Deborah C. Beidel and 61518 to Tracy L. Morris.

REFERENCES

Albano, A. M., Marten, P. A., Holt, C. S., Heimberg, R. G., & Barlow, D. H. (1995). Cognitive-behavioral group treatment for social phobia in adolescents: A preliminary study. *Journal of Nervous and Mental Disease, 183*, 649–656.

American Psychiatric Association. (1980). *Diagnostic and statistical manual of mental disorders* (3rd ed.). Washington DC: Author.

American Psychiatric Association. (1987). *Diagnostic and statistical manual of mental disorders* (3rd ed., rev.). Washington DC: Author.

American Psychiatric Association. (1994). *Diagnostic and statistical manual of mental disorders* (4th ed.). Washington, DC: Author.

Anderson, J. C., Williams, S., McGee, R., & Silva, P. A. (1987). DSM-III disorders in preadolescent children. *Archives of General Psychiatry, 44*, 69–76.

Andrews, G., Stewart, G., Allen, R., & Henderson, A. S. (1990). The genetics of six anxiety disorders: A twin study. *Journal of Affective Disorders, 19*, 23–29.

Barrett, P. M. (1998). Evaluation of cognitive-behavioral group treatments for childhood anxiety disorders. *Journal of Clinical Child Psychology, 27*, 459–468.

Barrett, P. M., Dadds, M. R., & Rapee, R. M. (1996). Family treatment of childhood anxiety: A controlled trial. *Journal of Consulting and Clinical Psychology, 64*, 333–342.

Barrett, P. M., Duffy, A. L., Dadds, M. R., & Rapee, R. M. (2001). Cognitive-behavioral treatment of anxiety disorders in children: Long-term (6–year) follow-up. *Journal of Consulting and Clinical Psychology, 69*, 135–141.

Barrios, B., & O'Dell, S. (1989). Fear and anxieties. In E. J. Mash & R. A. Barkley (Eds.), *Treatment of childhood disorders* (pp. 167–221). New York: Guilford Press.

Beidel, D. C. (1991). Social phobia and overanxious disorder in school-age children. *Journal of the American Academy of Child and Adolescent Psychiatry, 30*, 545–552.

Beidel, D. C., Christ, M. A. G., & Long, P. J. (1991). Somatic complaints in anxious children. *Journal of Abnormal Child Psychology, 19*, 659–670.

Beidel, D. C., & Turner, S. M. (1988). Comorbidity of test anxiety and other anxiety disorders in children. *Journal of Abnormal Child Psychology, 16*, 275–287.

Beidel, D. C., & Turner, S. M. (1998). *Shy children, phobic adults: The nature and treatment of social phobia.* Washington DC: American Psychological Association.

Beidel, D. C., & Turner, S. M. (1993, October). *Social phobia in children and adults.* Paper presented at the meeting of the American Academy of Child and Adolescent Psychiatry, Washington, DC.

Beidel, D. C., Turner, S. M., & Morris, T. L. (1999). Psychopathology of childhood social phobia. *Journal of the American Academy of Child and Adolescent Psychiatry, 38,* 643–650.

Beidel, D. C., Turner, S. M., & Morris, T. L. (2000). Behavioral treatment of childhood social phobia. *Journal of Consulting and Clinical Psychology, 68,* 1072–1080.

Birmaher, B., Waterman, G. S., Ryan, N., Cully, M., Balach, L., Ingram, J., & Brodsky, M. (1994). Fluoxetine for childhood anxiety disorders. *Journal of the American Academy of Child and Adolescent Psychiatry, 33,* 993–998.

Black, B., & Uhde, T. W. (1994). Treatment of elective mutism with fluoxetine: A double-blind placebo-controlled study. *Journal of the American Academy of Child and Adolescent Psychiatry, 33,* 1000–1006.

Broberg, A., Lamb, M. E., & Hwang, P. (1990). Inhibition: Its stability and correlates in sixteen- to forty-month-old children. *Child Development, 61,* 1153–1163.

Brown, J. B., & Lloyd, H. (1975). A controlled study of children not speaking at school. *Journal of the Association of Workers for Maladjusted Children, 3,* 49–63.

Bruch, M. A., Giordano, S., & Pearl, L. (1986). Differences between fearful and self-conscious shy subtypes in background and current adjustment. *Journal of Research in Personality, 20,* 172–186.

Bruch, M. A., & Heimberg, R. G. (1994). Differences in perceptions of parental and personal characteristics between generalized and nongeneralized social phobics. *Journal of Anxiety Disorders, 8,* 155–168.

Bruch, M. A., Heimberg, R. G., Berger, P., & Collins, T. M. (1989). Social phobia and perceptions of early parental and personal characteristics. *Anxiety Research, 2,* 57–63.

Buss, A. H., & Plomin, R. (1984). *Temperament: Early developing personality traits.* Hillsdale, NJ: Erlbaum.

Caspi, A., Edler, G. H., & Bem, D. J. (1988). Moving away from the world: Life-course patterns of shy children. *Developmental Psychology, 24,* 824–831.

Cheek, J. M., & Buss, A. H. (1981). Shyness and sociability. *Journal of Personality and Social Psychology, 41,* 330–339.

Clark, D. B. (1993, March). *Assessment of social anxiety in adolescents.* Paper presented at the Anxiety Disorders Association of America annual convention, Charleston, SC.

Compton, S. N., Grant, P. J., Chrisman, A. K., Gammon, P. J., Brown, V. L., & March, J. S. (2001). Sertraline in children and adolescents with social anxiety disorder: An open trial. *Journal of the American Academy of Child and Adolescent Psychiatry, 40,* 564–571.

Davidson, J. (1993, March). *Childhood histories of adult social phobics.* Paper presented at the Anxiety Disorders Association annual convention, Charleston, SC.

DeWit, D. J., MacDonald, K., & Offord, D. R. (1999). Childhood stress and symptoms of drug dependence in adolescence and early adulthood. *American Journal of Orthopsychiatry, 69,* 61–72.

DeWit, D. J., Ogborne, A., Offord, D. R., & MacDonald, K. (1999). Antecedents of the risk of recovery from DSM-III-R social phobia. *Psychological Medicine, 29,* 569–582.

Dummit, E. S., Klein, R. G., Tancer, N. K., Asche, B., & Martin, J. (1996). Fluoxetine treatment of children with selective mutism: An open trial. *Journal of the American Academy of Child and Adolescent Psychiatry, 35,* 615–621.

Essau, C. A., Conradt, J., & Petermann, F. (1999). Frequency and comorbidity of social phobia and social fears in adolescents. *Behaviour Research and Therapy, 17,* 831–843.

Fairbanks, J. M., Pine, D. S., Tancer, N. K., Dummit, E. S., Kentgen, L. M., Martin, J., Asche, B. K., & Klein, R. G. (1997). Open fluoxetine treatment of mixed anxiety disorder in children and adolescents. *Journal of Child and Adolescent Psychopharmacology, 7,* 17–29.

Ferrell, C., Beidel, D. C., & Turner, S. M. (2001). *A scale to determine the effectiveness of treatment for childhood social phobia.* Unpublished manuscript, University of Maryland, College Park.

Flannery-Schroeder, E. C., & Kendall, P. C. (2000). Group and individual cognitive-behavioral treatments for youth with anxiety disorders: A randomized clinical trial. *Cognitive Therapy and Research, 24,* 251–278.

Francis, G., Last, C. G., & Strauss, C. C. (1992). Avoidant disorder and social phobia in children and adolescents. *Journal of the American Academy of Child and Adolescent Psychiatry, 31,* 1086–1089.

Fyer, A. J., Mannuzza, S., Chapman, T. F., Liebowitz, M. R., & Klein, D. F. (1993). A direct interview family study of social phobia. *Archives of General Psychiatry, 50,* 286–293.

Gest, S. D. (1997). Behavioral inhibition: Stability and associations with adaptation from childhood to early adulthood. *Journal of Personality and Social Psychology, 72,* 467–475.

Greco, L. A., & Morris, T. L. (2002). Paternal child-rearing style and child social anxiety: Investigation of child perceptions and actual father behavior. *Journal of Psychopathology and Behavioral Assessment, 24,* 259–267.

Hayward, C., Varady, S., Albano, A. M., Thienemann, M., Henderson, L., & Schatzberg, A. F. (2000). Cognitive-behavioral group therapy for social phobia in female adolescents: Results of a pilot study. *Journal of the American Academy of Child and Adolescent Psychiatry, 39,* 721–726.

Hofmann, S. G., Albano, A. M., Heimberg, R. G., Tracey, S., Chorpita, B. F., & Barlow, D. H. (1999). Subtypes of social phobia in adolescents. *Depression and Anxiety, 9,* 15–18.

Kagan, J. (1997). Temperament and the reactions to unfamiliarity. *Child Development, 68,* 139–143.

Kagan, J., Reznick, J., Clarke, C., Snidman, N., & Garcia-Coll, C. (1984). Behavioral inhibition to the unfamiliar. *Child Development, 55,* 2212–2225.

Kashani, J. H., & Orvaschel, H. (1990). A community study of anxiety in children and adolescents. *American Journal of Psychiatry, 147,* 313–318.

Kendall, P. C. (1994). Treating anxiety disorders in children: Results of a randomized clinical trial. *Journal of Consulting and Clinical Psychology, 62,* 100–110.

Kendall, P. C., Flannery-Schroeder, E., Panichelli-Mindel, S., Southam-Gerow, M., Henin, A., & Warman, M. (1997). Therapy for youths with anxiety disorders: A second randomized clinical trial. *Journal of Consulting and Clinical Psychology, 65,* 366–380.

Kendall, P. C., & Southam-Gerow, M. A. (1996). Long-term follow-up of a cognitive-behavioral therapy for anxious youth. *Journal of Consulting and Clinical Psychology, 62,* 724–730.

Kendall, P. C., & Warman, M. (1996). Anxiety disorders in youth: Diagnostic consistency across DSM-III-R and DSM-IV. *Journal of Anxiety Disorders, 10,* 453–463.

Kendler, K. S., Neale, M. C., Kessler, R. C., Heath, A. C., & Eaves, L. I (1992). The genetic epidemiology of phobias in women: The interrelationship of agoraphobia, social phobia, situational phobia, and simple phobia. *Archives of General Psychiatry, 49,* 273–281.

Kerr, M., Lambert, W. W., & Bem, D. J. (1996). Life course sequelae of childhood shyness in Sweden: Comparison with the United States. *Developmental Psychology, 32,* 1100–1105.

Kratochvil, C., Kutcher, S., Reiter, S., & March, J. S. (1999). Pharmacotherapy of pediatric anxiety disorders. In S. W. Russ & T. H. Ollendick (Eds.), *Handbook of psychotherapies with children and families* (pp. 345–366). New York: Kluwer Academic.

Last, C. G., Hersen, M., Kazdin, A., & Orvaschel, H. (1991). Anxiety disorders in children and their families. *Archives of General Psychiatry, 48,* 928–934.

Last, C. G., & Perrin, S. (1993). Anxiety disorders in African-American and white children. *Journal of Abnormal Child Psychology, 21,* 153–164.

Last, C. G., Perrin, S., Hersen, M., & Kazdin, A. E. (1992). DSM-III-R anxiety disorders in children: Sociodemographic and clinical characteristics. *Journal of the American Academy of Child and Adolescent Psychiatry, 31,* 928–934.

Last, C. G., Strauss, C. C., & Francis, G. (1987). Comorbidity among childhood anxiety disorders. *Journal of Nervous and Mental Disease, 175,* 726–730.

Liebowitz, M. R., Gorman, J., Fyer, A. J., & Klein, D. F. (1985). Social phobia: Review of a neglected anxiety disorder. *Archives of General Psychiatry, 42,* 729–736.

Mancini, C., Van Ameringen, M., Szatmari, P., Fugere, C., & Boyle, M. (1996). A high-risk pilot study of the children of adults with social phobia. *Journal of the American Academy of Child and Adolescent Psychiatry, 35,* 1511–1517.

Marks, I. M. (1985). Behavioral psychotherapy for anxiety disorders. *Psychiatric Clinics of North America, 8,* 25–45.

Masia, C. L., Klein, R. G., Storch, E. A., & Corda, B. (2001). School-based behavioral treatment for social anxiety disorder in adolescents: Results of a pilot study. *Journal of the American Academy of Child and Adolescent Psychiatry, 40,* 780–786.

Masia, C. L., & Morris, T. L. (1998). Parental factors associated with social anxiety: Methodological limitations and suggestions for integrated behavioral research. *Clinical Psychology Science and Practice, 5,* 211–228.

Mineka, S., & Cook, M. (1988). Social learning and the acquisition of snake fear in monkeys. In T. R. Zentall & B. G. Galef (Eds.), *Social learning: Psychological and biological perspectives* (pp. 51–73). Hillsdale, NJ: Erlbaum.

Öst, L. G. (1985). Ways of acquiring phobias and outcome of behavioral treatments. *Behaviour Research and Therapy, 23,* 683–689.

Pine, D. S., & Grun, J. B. S. (1998). Anxiety disorders. In T. B. Walsh (Ed.), *Child psychopharmacology* (1st ed., Vol. 17, pp. 115–144). Washington, DC: American Psychiatric Press.

Prior, M., Smart, D., Sanson, A., & Oberklaid, F. (2000). Does shy-inhibited temperament in childhood lead to anxiety problems in adolescence? *Journal of the American Academy of Child and Adolescent Psychiatry, 39,* 461–468.

Research Units of Pediatric Psychopharmacology Anxiety Group. (in press). Fluvoxamine treatment of anxiety disorders in children and adolescents. *New England Journal of Medicine, 344,* 171–181.

Rubin, K. H., & Asendorpf, J. B. (1993). *Social withdrawal, inhibition, and shyness in childhood.* Hillsdale, NJ: Erlbaum.

Rubin, K. H., Le Mare, L. J., & Lollis, S. P. (1990). Social withdrawal in childhood: Developmental pathways to peer rejection. In S. R. Asher & J. D. Coie (Eds.), *Peer rejection in childhood* (pp. 217–249). Cambridge, UK: Cambridge University Press.

Schneier, F. R., Johnson, J., Hornig, C. D., Liebowitz, M. R., & Weissman, M. M. (1992). Social phobia: Comorbidity and morbidity in an epidemiologic sample. *Archives of General Psychiatry, 49,* 282–288.

Silverman, W. K., Kurtines, W. M., Ginsburg, G. S., Weems, C. F., Lumpkin, P. W., & Carmichael, D. H. (1999). Treating anxiety disorders in children with group cognitive-behavioral therapy: A randomized clinical trial. *Journal of Consulting and Clinical Psychology, 67,* 995–1003.

Silverman, W. K., Kurtines, W. M., Ginsburg, G. S., Weems, C. F., Rabian, B., & Serafini, L. T. (1999). Contingency management, self-control, and education support in the treatment of childhood phobic disorders: A randomized clinical trial. *Journal of Consulting and Clinical Psychology, 67,* 675–687.

Simeon, J. G., & Ferguson, H. B. (1987). Alprazolam effects in children with anxiety disorders. *Canadian Journal of Psychiatry, 32,* 570–574.

Simeon, J. G., Ferguson, H. B., Knott, V., Roberts, N., Gauthier, B., Dubois, C., & Wiggins, D. (1992). Clinical, cognitive, and neurophysiological effects of alprazolam in children and adolescents with overanxious and avoidant disorders. *Journal of the American Academy of Child and Adolescent Psychiatry, 31,* 29–33.

Spence, S. H., Donovan, C., & Brechman-Toussaint, M. (1999). Social skills, social outcomes and cognitive features of childhood social phobia. *Journal of Abnormal Psychology, 108,* 211–221.

Spence, S. H., Donovan, C., & Brechman-Toussaint, M. (2000). The treatment of childhood social phobia: The effectiveness of a social skills training-based, cognitive-behavioral intervention, with and without parental involvement. *Journal of Child Psychology and Psychiatry, 41,* 713–726.

Stemberger, R. T., Turner, S. M., Beidel, D. C., & Calhoun, K. S. (1995). Social phobia: An analysis of possible developmental factors. *Journal of Abnormal Psychology, 104,* 526–531.

Strauss, C. C., & Last, C. G. (1993). Social and simple phobias in children. *Journal of Anxiety Disorders, 1,* 141–152.

Thomas, A., & Chess, S. (1977). *Temperament and development.* New York: Brunner/Mazel.

Torgersen, S. (1983). Genetic factors in anxiety disorders. *Archives of General Psychiatry, 40,* 1085–1089.

Tracy, S. A., Mattis, S. G., Chorpita, B. F., Albano, A. M., Heimberg, R. G., & Barlow, D. H. (1998, November). *Cognitive-behavioral group treatment of social phobia in adolescents: Preliminary examination of the contribution of parental involvement.* Poster presented at the Association for Advancement of Behavior Therapy annual convention, Washington, DC.

Turner, S. M., Beidel, D. C., Borden, J. W., Stanley, M. A., & Jacob, R. G. (1991). Social phobia: Axis I and II correlates. *Journal of Abnormal Psychology, 100,* 102–106.

Turner, S. M., Beidel, D. C., Dancu, C. V., & Keys, D. J. (1986). Psychopathology of social phobia and comparison to avoidant personality disorder. *Journal of Abnormal Psychology, 95,* 389–394.

Turner, S. M., Beidel, D. C., & Jacob, R. G. (1994). Social phobia: A comparison of behavior therapy and atenolol. *Journal of Consulting and Clinical Psychology, 62,* 350–358.

Turner, S. M., Beidel, D. C., Roberson-Nay, R., & Tervo, K. (2003). Parenting behaviors in parents with anxiety disorders. *Behaviour Research and Therapy, 41,* 541–554.

Velosa, J. F., & Riddle, M. A. (2000). Pharmacologic treatment of anxiety disorders in children and adolescents. *Psychopharmacology, 9,* 119–133.

Chapter 8

Separation Anxiety Disorder

WENDY K. SILVERMAN
ANDREAS DICK-NIEDERHAUSER

Separation anxiety disorder (SAD) is a common psychiatric disorder of childhood and early adolescence and is characterized by an unrealistic and excessive fear of separation from an attachment figure, usually the parent, which significantly interferes with daily activities and developmental tasks. Children and adolescents (hereafter referred to as children) with SAD are tremendously worried that harm may come to their parents or themselves when separated, so that they might never be reunited again.

The range of emotional, cognitive, somatic, and behavioral symptoms associated with the fear or threat of separation from an attachment figure cripples the child's enjoyment of life, his or her social and family relationships, and abilities to participate and progress in school and recreational and creative activities. Several studies have suggested that childhood SAD may be a risk factor for other anxiety disorders later in life (Keller et al., 1992; Last, Perrin, Hersen, & Kazdin, 1996; Moreau & Follet, 1993), but whether this link is specific to panic disorder and agoraphobia (Gittelman & Klein, 1984) or whether SAD represents a general factor of vulnerability for a broad range of anxiety disorders is still debated (Barlow, 2002; Silove & Manicavasagar, 2001).

Separation anxiety has been studied as a characteristic of normal development and as a symptom for many years (Bowlby, 1973; Freud,

164

1909/1955). Bowlby's influential attachment theory emphasizes the survival value of infants' proximity to their caretakers and of caregivers' tendency to behave reciprocally. When infants' proximity to their caretakers is inadequate (i.e., separation), an intense affective response is produced (separation distress or anxiety). Normal separation distress usually intensifies during early childhood, then gradually subsides at 3 to 5 years of age (Kagan, Kearsley, & Zelazo, 1978).

Separation anxiety became a distinct clinical diagnostic category with publication of the third edition of the *Diagnostic and Statistical Manual of Mental Disorders* (DSM-III; American Psychiatric Association) in 1980. In accordance with the DSM, when children's separation anxieties persist beyond the developmentally appropriate years, and if the anxieties cause significant distress or impairment in social, academic, family, or other important areas of youths' functioning, a specific psychological maladjustment as characterized by the diagnosis of SAD may be warranted.

EPIDEMIOLOGY AND COMORBIDITY

SAD is among the most common anxiety disorders in childhood. In a sample of children referred to an anxiety disorders specialty clinic, SAD was the most prevalent disorder, with a rate of 33% (Last, Francis, Hersen, Kazdin, & Strauss, 1987). Different epidemiological studies indicate a prevalence of 3 to 5% in children and adolescents (Anderson, Williams, McGee, & Silva, 1987; Benjamin, Costello, & Warren, 1990; Bird et al., 1988; Bowen, Offord, & Boyle, 1990; Costello, 1989b; Costello et al., 1988; Kashani et al., 1987; Lewinsohn, Hops, Roberts, Seeley, & Andrews, 1993; Prior, Sanson, Smart, & Oberklaid, 1999). The prevalence of reported SAD symptoms without significant impairment is much higher, with an estimate of up to 50% in 8-year-olds (Kashani & Orvaschel, 1990).

Several studies have found an overrepresentation of girls with SAD (Anderson et al., 1987; Costello, 1989b; Last, Francis, et al., 1987a), whereas other studies have reported equal frequency in girls and boys (Bird, Gould, Yager, Staghezza, & Canino, 1989; Francis, Last, & Strauss, 1987; Last, Perrin, Hersen, & Kazdin, 1992). Males and females seem to be indistinguishable in the expression of their SAD symptoms (Francis et al., 1987).

Even though most children with anxiety disorders are from middle- to upper-middle-class families, 50 to 75% of children with SAD come from low-socioeconomic-status homes (Last et al., 1992; Last, Francis, et al., 1987; Velez, Johnson, & Cohen, 1989) and tend to be of lower socioeconomic status than children with overanxious and phobic disorders (primarily school avoidant; Last, Francis, et al., 1987). In addition, although the research is sparse, among children referred to anxiety disorders specialty clinics, rates of SAD have not been found to vary between European American and African American children (Last & Perrin, 1993) or between European American and Hispanic American children (Ginsburg & Silverman, 1996).

Using a dimensional measure of anxiety, the Multidimensional Anxiety Scale for Children (MASC; March, Parker, Sullivan, Stallings, & Conners, 1997), sociodemographic variations have been found among community (N = 2,384; ages 8–19 years) and clinic (N = 227; ages 8–18 years) samples of children who report symptoms of SAD and social phobia (Compton, Nelson, & March, 2000). Children were divided into three age groups: 8–12 years, 13–15 years, and 16–19 years. Children's responses to symptoms of separation anxiety and social phobia were classified according to whether they were above (high) or below (low) the mean score on the respective subscales. Results indicated that children from the community who reported a high number of symptoms of SAD and social phobia tended to be between 8 and 12 years of age and female. Children from the community who reported a high number of SAD symptoms but minimal symptoms of social phobia also tended to be between 8 and 12 years of age and female. Children from the community sample who reported a high number of social phobia symptoms only tended to be in middle adolescence (ages 13–15 years old) and male. With respect to race, European American children reported a higher number of symptoms of social phobia than African American children; African American children reported a higher number of symptoms of SAD than European American children. Similar comparisons were conducted for the clinical sample (with the exception of race). Results indicated that children from the clinical sample who reported a high number of both SAD and social phobia symptoms tended to be between 8 and 12 years old. In terms of gender, females reported more symptoms of both SAD and social phobia than males.

In general, the prevalence of SAD seems to be higher in childhood than in adolescence (Breton et al., 1999; Kashani & Orvaschel, 1988, 1990; McGee et al., 1990). A community epidemiological study with 1,299 adolescents (ages 12–16 years; Bowen et al., 1990) yielded a prevalence of SAD of 2.4%, though other studies have found lower rates among adolescents (e.g., Kashani & Orvaschel, 1988). Peak age onset appears to be around 7 to 9 years (Bird et al., 1989; Last et al., 1992), but the disorder may develop during adolescence as well (Last et al., 1992).

Francis and colleagues (1987) observed age differences in the symptom expression of SAD among three age groups of 45 children and adolescents. Over one-half of young children (5–8 years) reported nightmares involving separation as compared with less than one-fourth of older children (9–12 years) and adolescents (13–16 years). In addition, although the majority of young and older children presented with excessive distress upon separation, very few of the adolescents presented with this particular symptom of SAD. Finally, all of the adolescents with SAD presented with physical complaints on school days; only about two-thirds of the young and older children reported this symptom. The most frequently coexisting symptoms were examined for each age group: Most adolescents complained of school reluctance and physical symptoms on school days. Older children were most likely to report excessive distress upon separation, as well as withdrawal, apathy, sadness, and poor concentration. Two equally likely symptom combinations were found for young children: (1) worry about attachment figures and calamitous events; (2) worry about attachment figures and school refusal.

In clinical samples of children with SAD, approximately one-half are diagnosed with another anxiety disorder—most often overanxious disorder under DSM-III or DSM-III-R criteria—or specific phobia, and one-third with depression (Benjamin et al., 1990; Hewitt et al., 1997; Last, Hersen, Kazdin, Finkelstein, & Strauss, 1987; Last, Strauss, & Francis, 1987). SAD also has been found to be comorbid with obsessive–compulsive disorder (Valleni-Basile, Garrison, Jackson, & Waller, 1994) and gender identity disorder (Zucker, Bradley, & Sullivan, 1996). However, because comorbidity is generally reported as very high among children with anxiety disorders (e.g., Last et al., 1992), according to Last, Strauss, and Francis (1987), children with a primary diagnosis of SAD are the anxious group least likely to meet criteria for a concurrent anxiety disorder. Studies of depressed children have found concurrent SAD diagnoses in 40 to 60% of participants, with SAD usually preceding the depression (Keller et al., 1992; Kovacs, Gatsonis, Paulauskas, & Richards, 1989; Ryan et al., 1987).

School-refusal behavior, or school phobia, itself not a separate diagnostic category, is a common associated clinical feature of children with SAD. The prevalence of school refusal behavior in the school-age population is reported to be approximately 5%, although rates of school absenteeism are much higher in some urban areas (King & Bernstein, 2001). Although early views were that SAD and school refusal were one and the same (see Kearney & Silverman, 1996), not all children with school refusal behavior suffer from SAD, and not all children with SAD manifest school refusal behavior. Last and Strauss (1990) investigated DSM-III-R anxiety disorder diagnoses in 63 school-refusing youths (ages 7–17 years). Although the most common primary diagnosis was SAD ($N = 24$), social phobia ($N = 16$) and simple phobia ($N = 14$) also were common. School-refusal behavior also may be the expression of other disorders, including specific phobia (e.g., the loud ringing of the school bell), a social phobia, a mood disorder, a disruptive behavior disorder, or family problems (see Kearney & Silverman; 1996; King & Bernstein, 2001). In general, although school-refusal behavior may be a manifestation of SAD, school-refusal behavior is currently conceptualized as a heterogenous set of emotional and behavioral disorders.

NATURAL HISTORY

Only a small number of prospective studies have been conducted that included samples of children with SAD (e.g., Cantwell & Baker, 1989; Keller et al.,1992; Last et al., 1996). A widely cited study is Cantwell and Baker's (1989) 4-year follow-up study of 151 children who had presented to a speech and language clinic. Nine of the children initially met DSM-III criteria for SAD (mean age = 3.6 years). At follow-up, SAD had the highest recovery rate and the lowest stability relative to the two other childhood anxiety disorders investigated in this study, avoidant and overanxious disorders. More specifically, 11% still had SAD; 44% had other disorders. Last and colleagues (1996) similarly found high recovery and low stability for SAD in their follow-up study of 102 children who had presented to an anxiety disorders specialty clinic: 96% of the children with initial SAD had recovered by the 3- to 4-year follow-up; 25% had developed a new psychiatric disorder (the specific disorders were not reported).

A main conclusion that can be drawn about the natural history of anxiety disorders in children in general, and SAD in particular, is that with the exception of obsessive–compulsive disorder and phobic disorders, which appear to be "true to form" (Flament et al., 1988; Milne et al., 1995; Newman et al., 1996)—that is, in children who have already manifested these particular conditions, subsequent illness episodes are more likely to represent these earlier diagnoses than new and unrelated conditions (Kovacs & Devlin, 1998)—other anxiety disorders, including SAD, are not true to form. However, the course of separation anxiety disorder, like the other anxiety disorders, tends to show homotypic continuity with respect to "any anxiety disorder" (Kovacs & Devlin, 1998). That is, although the child may not continue to meet the criteria for SAD that he or she previously met, it is likely that he or she will continue to meet criteria for an anxiety disorder.

Bowlby (1973) viewed agoraphobia in adulthood as a function of insecure attachments, and Klein (1964, 1980), drawing on Bowlby's views, postulated that "spontaneous panic attacks" might be an expression of a "protest–despair" mechanism in response to threats of separation among individuals with a biologically determined lowered threshold for this response. Because of these views, some further comments would be useful regarding whether there is a linkage between SAD and later panic disorder and/or agoraphobia in adulthood. Gittelman and Klein (1984) noted that evidence for a linkage comes from three different lines of research: (1) similar drug treatment response (i.e., to imipramine) among children with SAD and adults with agoraphobia; (2) family concordance for SAD and agoraphobia; and (3) history of childhood SAD in adults with agoraphobia. In recent summaries of this literature (Barlow, 2002; Silove & Manicavasagar, 2001), however, some of this evidence was found to be either not convincing or open to alternative interpretations. Consequently, based on the current knowledge base, possible linkage between SAD and later panic disorder and/or agoraphobia in adulthood remains inconclusive.

In addition to a linkage being postulated between SAD and later panic disorder and/or agoraphobia in adulthood, a linkage has been postulated between SAD in childhood and adolescence and SAD in adulthood (e.g., Manicavasagar & Silove, 1997; Manicavasagar, Silove, & Curtis, 1997; Manicavasagar, Silove, Curtis, & Wagner, 2000; Ollendick, Lease, & Cooper, 1993). Empirical support for this linkage comes from findings showing that adult patients who meet DSM criteria for SAD also report having had substantially higher levels of separation anxiety in their childhoods than adult patients who do not meet DSM criteria for SAD. The symptoms of these adults with SAD also predate such comorbid disorders as panic disorder–agoraphobia and generalized anxiety disorder. Based on such findings, Manicavasagar and colleagues have suggested that a revised developmental model of SAD may be warranted. That is, although SAD may remit (or become a different type of anxiety disorder with development), some children and adolescents, perhaps those who encounter continued insecurities in their primary bonds and/or are biologically vulnerable, may experience the persistence of SAD into adulthood (Manicavasagar et al., 2000).

Although the above-mentioned findings are tantalizing, it is important to consider that they are based on participants' retrospective reports, as well as on measures (regarding past and current SAD) that were not thoroughly evaluated for validity. Consequently, just as it appears inconclusive to state that a firm linkage exists between SAD and later panic disorder and/or agoraphobia in adulthood, it also appears inconclusive to state that a firm linkage exists between SAD in childhood and adolescence and SAD in adulthood. Moreover, in any discussion about the natural history or developmental course of a childhood psychopathological condition, including SAD, it is important to recognize the basic tenets of developmental psychopathology (see Cichetti & Cohen, 1995). Although SAD in childhood may lead to panic disorder and/or agoraphobia in adulthood in some individuals, this is not necessarily true in all cases. This is the principle of multifinality, which states that any given factor (e.g., SAD) will function differently and can lead to multiple outcomes depending on the system in which the factor operates. Similarly, although panic disorder and/or agoraphobia in adulthood may have been reached via a single pathway (e.g., via separation distress or SAD), other pathways also may have led to the adults' panic disorder and/or agoraphobia. This is the principle of equifinality, which states that a diversity of paths may lead to the same outcome (for further discussion of these issues, see Cichetti & Cohen, 1995; Silverman & Ollendick, 1999; Vasey & Dadds, 2001).

ETIOLOGY

As just noted, a considerable body of research has investigated SAD and separation distress as risk factors for the development of anxiety disorders, particularly with regard to agoraphobia and panic disorder (see also Battaglia et al., 1995; Gittelman & Klein, 1984; Manassis & Bradley, 1994; Raskin, Peeke, Dickman, & Pinsker, 1982; Silove, Manicavasagar, Curtis, & Blaszczynski, 1996; Yeragani, Meiri, Balon, Patel, & Pohl, 1989). In contrast, sparse research exists on presumable risk factors and developmental pathways leading to SAD. In this section, we attempt to draw a preliminary picture of the main etiologically relevant factors of SAD.

Biological Factors and Temperament

In the Virginia Twin Study, with 1,412 twin pairs ages 8–16 years, Topolski and colleagues (1997) reported that genetic variation did not appear to be a major contributor to the explanation of individual differences in symptoms of SAD. The estimate of heredity for SAD was only 4%, whereas the influence of the shared environment, especially family factors, was 40%. Based on the same sample, marked gender differences in the contributions of genes and environment to parental ratings of SAD were found: Eaves and colleagues (1997) reported a heritability estimate for boys of nearly zero and for girls of approximately 75% in the data pooled across ages. Accordingly, Silove, Manicavasagar, O'Connell, and Morris-Yates (1995), in a sample of 200 normal adolescent twin and adult twin pairs, found a substantial genetic contribution to symptoms of separation anxiety in females but not in males, with unique environmental influences being important in both groups. However, the latter study was based on participants' retrospective reports of early separation anxiety using the Separation Anxiety Symptom Inventory (Silove et al., 1993). The findings suggesting heritability of SAD in girls could not be replicated by results obtained from interviews with the children, in which no genetic contribution to SAD was found (Eaves et al., 1997).

Kagan, Reznik, and Snidman (1988) first analyzed the physiological basis of shyness and inhibited behavior in childhood and proposed the concept of behavioral inhibition as a stable temperamental trait across childhood. Kagan and colleagues' influential work stemmed in part from the rather consistent observation that anxious individuals rapidly experience a high physiological arousal in certain situations, which raises the probability of their being receptive to conditioning processes (Barlow, 2002). In a longitudinal study with 44 inhibited children and 32 uninhibited children (ages 2–8 years), Biederman and colleagues (1993) found that behaviorally inhibited children had higher rates of SAD, as well as other anxiety disorders, than noninhibited children. Among those children without a disorder at baseline, at follow-up inhibited children had higher rates of anxiety disorders, including SAD, than uninhibited children. Biederman and colleagues is, however, the only study so far linking behavioral inhibition specifically to SAD (see Oosterlaan, 2001, for review).

Cognitive Factors

The notion of normative stability of a temperamental trait may be put into question. Cognitive approaches emphasize children's self-regulatory mechanisms that contribute to the change of temperamental traits in the course of development. Studies using an information-processing approach show that selective attention mechanisms influence children's processing of threatening information and may play an important role in the regulation of childhood anxiety (e.g., Dalgleish et al., 1997; Vasey, El-Hag, & Daleiden, 1996). Boegels and Zigterman (2000) investigated whether clinic-referred children, ages 9–18 years, with SAD ($N = 7$), social phobia ($N = 5$), and generalized anxiety disorder ($N = 3$) display such a bias, compared with a clinic-referred group of children with externalizing disorders and a nonclinic control group. Children with anxious disorders indeed reported more negative cognitions than children in both of the two comparison groups and judged ambiguous situations as more dangerous. Anxious children also had lower estimations of their own competency to cope with danger than the comparison groups. The results further indicated that children with SAD had characteristic dysfunctional cognitions about ambiguous situations similar to most children with anxiety disorders (e.g., Vasey et al.,1996). However, as far as the authors are aware, the question of whether the cognitive processes or contents of children with SAD might be distinguishable from those of children suffering from other anxiety disorders or other (non-anxiety-related) psychiatric disorders has so far not been directly studied.

Recently the concept of anxiety sensitivity, the belief about the negative consequences of anxious symptoms (Reiss, 1991), has come to the attention of researchers interested in the development of anxiety in children (for reviews, see Reiss, Silverman, & Weems, 2001; Silverman & Weems,

1999). Anxiety sensitivity has been found to differentiate between children with and without panic attacks and panic disorder (Kearney, Albano, Eisen, Allan, & Barlow, 1997; Lau, Calamari, & Waraczynski, 1996). In a large prospective study (Hayward, Killen, Kraemer, & Taylor, 2000) in which 2,365 students were evaluated on entrance into high school and then prospectively for up to 4 years, although SAD was not predictive of initial panic attacks, both anxiety sensitivity and negative affectivity predicted the onset of panic attacks in univariate analyses. However, because in multivariate analyses negative affectivity was a more robust predictor than anxiety sensitivity, the authors concluded that the former is a more fundamental vulnerability for anxiety disorders and the latter is a more specific vulnerability for panic disorder to develop, given negative affect and the occurrence of panic attacks. Weems, Berman, Silverman, and Rodriguez (2002) recently examined the relation between attachment beliefs and anxiety sensitivity in a sample of high school students ($N = 203$; mean age 15.7 years) and university students ($N = 324$; mean age 21.7 years). The Experiences in Close Relationships Scale (Brennan, Clark, & Shaver, 1998) was used to assess attachment beliefs and to classify participants into attachment groups. Results indicated that individuals with insecure attachment, specifically those classified as preoccupied and fearful, had significantly higher anxiety sensitivity scores than securely attached individuals in both the high school and university samples. Just how attachment styles may relate to SAD remains an issue, however, that requires further research and clarity (see the next section).

Finally, Muris, Schmidt, Merckelbach, and Schouten (2001) also found that anxiety sensitivity was most strongly related to panic symptoms as assessed by the Spence Children's Anxiety Scale (SCAS; Spence, 1998) in a non-clinic-referred sample of adolescents ($N = 819$; ages 13–16 years). Significant relations were found as well, however, with SCAS's subscale scores of SAD, social phobia, generalized anxiety disorder, and obsessive–compulsive disorder. As far as we are aware, studies specifically designed to explore for possible linkages between anxiety sensitivity in children with and without SAD have not been conducted.

Family Processes and Attachment

According to case illustrations of families with children with SAD, father and child are seen as being in competition with each other for the mother's interest and attention. Familial conflict is supposedly a result of this competition and lack of marital coalition, as mother and child remain enmeshed in their alliance with each other. Often mothers of children with SAD indicate being frightened about letting their child go anywhere without them, and these mothers display the same dependence on their own mothers as their children display toward them (Gardner, 1992; Hamilton, 1994; Zamudio &Wolfe, 1996). Gardner (1985) discusses other possible psycho-dynamics existing between the child with SAD and his or her mother, including notions of sexual-inhibition problems in the mother (and so, for example, the milder sexuality of the mother–son relationship is preferred over the mother–father relationship by the mother), as well as maternal displacement and projection of anger. To date, however, empirical research investigating these hypothesized psychodynamic mechanisms among children with SAD and their parents is sparse.

In contrast, growing empirical research has investigated the link between family processes and the development of SAD in relation to attachment and parental rearing styles, with the latter conceptualized along two orthogonal dimensions: warmth versus hostility and control versus autonomy (Boer, 1998; Cassidy, 1995; Dadds, Barrett, Rapee, & Ryan, 1996; Lutz & Hock, 1995; Manassis, Bradley, Goldberg, Hood, & Swinson, 1994; Rapee, 1997; Siqueland, Kendall, & Steinberg, 1996; Warren, Huston, Egeland, & Sroufe, 1997). Insecure mother–child attachment has been consistently linked with both clinical and subclinical anxiety in children. All four of the attachment styles classified by Ainsworth, Blehar, Waters, and Wall (1978) and Main and Solomon (1990)—secure, insecure–avoidant, insecure–ambivalent, and insecure–disorganized—have been found to be represented in children with anxiety disorders, but the highest risks for developing an anxiety disorder come from disorganized attachment, which is associated with unresolved trauma or loss, and ambivalent attachment (Cassidy, 1995; Manassis et al., 1994; Warren et al., 1997). As far as we are aware, however, the specificity of an association between disorganized attachment and SAD (rather than anxiety disorders in general) has not been established.

Lutz and Hock (1995) explored how adult mental representations of attachment relationships and memories of childhood experiences with parents contributed to a mother's anxiety about separation from her own infant. Mothers with insecure attachment representations, when asked to remember details of their own childhoods, reported more negative recollections of early parental caregiving, particularly rejection and discouragement of independence. When their own infants were 2 months old, these mothers experienced heightened levels of maternal separation anxiety. It has also been found that about 80% of children whose mothers have been diagnosed with an anxiety disorder show an insecure attachment to their mothers (Manassis et al., 1994).

Manassis (2001) has suggested two specific pathways that lead to the development and maintenance of SAD. A first hypothetical pathway would predispose temperamentally difficult children to an ambivalent caregiver–child attachment, with the caregiver being only intermittently available for the child and thus constantly reinforcing attachment behavior in the child. Such a child would become preoccupied with obtaining comfort from the parent and would reduce his or her exploratory behavior, which also reduces exposure to new situations and to possible enhancements of coping skills. The parent's selective attention to negative affect in his or her ambivalent child would lead to an escalating cycle of anxiety between parent and child, with the child attempting to alleviate anxiety by being close to the parent but then experiencing parental hostility resulting in increased anxiety. SAD is maintained through preoccupation with obtaining parental comfort, reducing the opportunity for desensitization, and exaggerated displays of negative affect that fail to elicit reassurance from others.

A second hypothetical pathway would lead from a psychological affliction of the child's caregiver due to unresolved loss or trauma to a disorganized attachment, providing the child with no consistent model for coping with distress. Often these parents are physically and mentally ill, which may lead to SAD in their children, because they fear for the well-being and the lives of their parents.

Empirical support for these hypothetical pathways comes from studies examining the influence of parental rearing styles on the development of anxiety (Rapee, 1997). A consistent positive relation between parental rejection and control and later anxiety has been found, especially for adults with an insecure–preoccupied attachment style, which corresponds to the anxious–ambivalent attachment in childhood. Anxious children report more maternal control than their healthy siblings (Boer, 1998), and parents of anxious children grant less autonomy than parents of control children (Siqueland et al., 1996). Dadds and colleagues (1996) found that parents of anxious children are less likely to grant autonomy of thought and action than are controls. They also found that these parents influence the child to be more cautious and to avoid taking risks. These findings were recently replicated and extended by Hudson and Rapee (2002), who found, in studying 57 children (37 with anxiety disorders and 20 non-clinic-referred children, ages 7–16 years), that mothers and fathers were not only overly involved with the anxious child but also with the siblings of the anxious child. Such findings suggest that overinvolvement does not occur exclusively in the context of relationships with the child who has an anxiety disorder.

There are, however, no studies on parental rearing styles conducted exclusively with children who suffer from SAD. Furthermore, most studies do not allow conclusions about the direction of the effect. A model of reciprocal determinism in which the child's and parent's behaviors are seen as interlinked probably explains the findings best (Boer & Lindhout, 2001).

Parental Anxiety and Depression

An increased prevalence of anxiety disorders and depression has been demonstrated in families of children with SAD, relative to controls. Last, Hersen, and colleagues (1987) found that 68% of mothers of SAD children had a lifetime diagnosis of an anxiety disorder, 53% had a lifetime diagnosis of major depression, and 47% had a current anxiety disorder diagnosis. Offspring of parents with panic disorder have been shown to have a threefold greater risk of SAD, and offspring of parents with panic disorder plus major depression have more than a tenfold greater risk (Leckman et al., 1985; Weissman, Leckman, Merikangas, Gammon, & Prusoff, 1984). The occurrence of avoidance behavior due to anxious symptomatology in parents has been found to be a strong predictor of anxiety problems in the child; parental avoidance behavior could be interpreted as parental modeling of caution and fearfulness observed by the child (Silverman, Cerny, Nelles, & Burke, 1988). In an at-risk sample of 4- to 10-year-olds (i.e., offspring of mothers with panic disorder or family history of panic disorder), maternal expressed emotion assessed via a 5-minute speech sample indicated that mothers' display of emotional overinvolvement was highly related to SAD in the at-risk sample (Hirshfeld, Biederman, Brody, Faraone, & Rosenbaum, 1997).

Maternal depression also has been associated with an increased risk of insecure mother–child attachment, with depressed mothers showing less facilitation of their children's attempts to approach unfamiliar situations (Kochanska, 1991). In a study with 16 children (mean age 11 years) of mothers with agoraphobia and 16 children of mothers with no history of psychopathology matched by age, gender, and socioeconomic status, the mothers with agoraphobia reported more maternal separation anxiety with regard to their child than the control group. Maternal separation anxiety correlated negatively with children's perceived control (Capps, Sigman, Sena, & Henker, 1996). As mentioned previously, the effect probably is best interpreted as the result of a reciprocal relation between caregiver and child: When a child is more anxious, there may be greater cause for the parent's anxiety about separation. Parental anxious symptoms also may serve as a source of threat itself. Turner, Beidel, and Costello (1987) observed that children of parents with anxiety disorders, especially those who experienced panic, exhibited considerable concern about the welfare of their parent.

Caregiver's Stressors and Resources

Other risk factors for the development of SAD include the caregiver's social supports, his or her life stresses, and the marital relationship. Parents with few social supports and high levels of stress have an increased risk of developing insecure attachments with their infants (Jacobson & Frye, 1991; Vaughn, Egeland, Sroufe, & Waters, 1979; Waters, Merrick, Treboux, Corwell, & Albersheim, 2000). Last and colleagues (1992) found that the presence of two parents reduces the risk of SAD, allowing one to compensate for parenting difficulties in the other, provided the marital relationship is supportive. Stifter, Coulehan, and Fish (1993) examined the effects of maternal employment and separation anxiety on maternal interactive behavior and infant attachment. Alhough mothers' employment status was not directly related to the children's attachment style assessed at 18 months in the Strange Situation, infants of employed mothers with high anxiety levels developed anxious–avoidant attachments. Fein, Gariboldi, and Boni (1993) examined antecedents of maternal separation anxiety in mothers prior to the entry of their infants or toddlers into center-based infant care. Anxious mothers were younger and less educated, received less support, had infants with negative temperaments, and provided less varied stimulation in the home. For infants, only parent background and social support predicted anxiety, but for toddlers, negative temperament and social isolation were predictive.

Life Events and Chronic Stress

According to Bowlby's (1973) clinical observations, a child's actual experiences of separation from his or her primary caregiver, as well as parental threats of leaving the child or giving him or her away, are the foundations on which SAD may develop. There are yet no studies on the relation between stressful life events and the development of SAD. However, in a study of an English inner-city population of working-class and single mothers at risk for both depression and anxiety conditions in adult life due to adverse experiences in childhood, the onset of depression and anxiety both appeared to be provoked by life events: loss and lack of hope tended to lead to depression, and danger and lack of security led to anxiety (Brown & Harris, 1993; Brown, Harris, & Eales, 1993). Conditions of chronic stress affecting the child that may lead to SAD include physical and mental illness of family members and family violence (Bowler, 1996; Turner et al., 1987).

   In summary, many questions concerning the etiology of SAD remain unanswered. It has not yet been systematically studied how cultural norms of parenting and of parent–child relationships influence the development of SAD. Further research should also try to differentiate more clearly between predisposing risk factors and events that may trigger the manifestation of SAD under the conditions in which a predisposition has previously developed. As often is the case in developmental psychopathology, a lack of prospective studies can be observed. An important challenge for researchers is to disentangle the relations among the different risk factors and to improve understanding about the developmental pathways of SAD.

TREATMENT

There appears to be general consensus in the field that exposure-based cognitive-behavioral treatments (CBT) are the methods of choice for anxiety disorders (see Silverman & Berman, 2001, for review). CBT has been found to be efficacious in treating anxiety disorders in children, including SAD, whether delivered using an individual-child format (e.g., Kendall, 1994; Kendall et al., 1997), a format that uses increased parental involvement (Barrett, Dadds, & Rapee, 1996; Cobham, Dadds, & Spence, 1998; Silverman, Kurtines, Ginsburg, Weems, Rabian, & Serafini, 1999), or a format that emphasizes increased peer involvement (i.e., group CBT; Barrett, 1998; Flannery-Schroeder & Kendall, 2000; Silverman, Kurtines, Ginsburg, Weems, Lumpkin, & Carmichael, 1999).

The randomized controlled clinical trials of anxiety disorders in children have not found specificity or differential response for SAD relative to the other anxiety disorders (e.g., Barrett et al.,1996; Kendall, 1994; Kendall et al., 1997; Silverman, Kurtines, Ginsburg, Weems, Lumpkin, & Carmichael, 1999; Silverman, Kurtines, Ginsburg, Weems, Rabian, & Serafini, 1999). The presence of comorbid conditions, including the additional diagnosis of SAD, also has not been shown to lead to differential response to CBT (Kendall, Brady, & Verduin, 2001). Limited sample sizes, however, preclude a full and systematic evaluation of either one of these two issues.

In terms of treatment studies that have used only youths with SAD, several single-case-study designs have been conducted showing that behavioral and/or CBT procedures effectively reduce children's symptoms of SAD and associated behaviors, such as school refusal behavior and nighttime fears (e.g., Hagopian & Slifer, 1993; Neisworth, Madle, & Goeke, 1975; Ollendick, Hagopian, & Huntzinger, 1991; Phillips & Wolpe, 1981). For example, Hagopian and Slifer (1993) reported the successful use of graded exposure plus positive reinforcement in decreasing a 6-year-old girl's school refusal behavior and SAD. Treatment emphasized fading out the mother's proximity and presence in the classroom while increasing the girl's time spent in school. There have been no randomized clinical trials using only youths with SAD (see Barrett, 2001, who reached similar conclusion in her review).

Although a few clinical trials on CBT use samples of children with school refusal behavior (King et al., 1998; Last, Hansen, & Franco, 1998), in light of what was said earlier regarding the heterogeneity among children with school refusal behavior, we are wary about calling these "SAD studies." Moreover, on the one hand, in light of recent evidence showing that CBT appears to be efficacious in treating a heterogenous set of anxiety disorders, including SAD, with a group approach (Lumpkin, Silverman, Weems, Markham, & Kurtines, 2002), perhaps a specific intervention for use with SAD is not needed. On the other hand, the issue is probably complicated by the nature of the developmental pathway particular to a specific SAD case. For example, a child may develop an ambivalent attachment relationship toward his or her caregiver, characterized by a preoccupation with obtaining the parent's comfort, which tends to reduce the child's exploratory behavior, leading to a deficit in coping skills. If the parent at the same time is concerned about the child becoming more and more independent in the course of the child's development (e.g., because the presence of the child may help the parent compensate for an unsatisfactory marital relationship), it is unlikely that a treatment that does not aim at a transformation of the attachment relationship and the family processes specific to this case could achieve a stable improvement of this child's SAD. However, so far attachment theory has had little impact on either case conceptualization or treatment of SAD patients (Greenberg, 1999). We are currently in the process of investigating the relevance of parent–child attachment to the treatment of SAD, especially with regard to those children with SAD who do not improve following exposure-based CBT.

The pharmacological literature for the treatment of childhood anxiety disorders, including SAD, is in its infancy when compared with the treatment literature on exposure-based CBT (see Stock, Werry, & McClellan, 2001, for review). The available literature consists of a small number of open-label trials and case studies. Although some research shows that benzodiazepines, selective serotonin reuptake inhibitors (SSRIs), and tricyclic antidepressants (TCAs) may be effective in treating SAD in children and adolescents, firm inferences cannot be drawn from the findings in light of methodological constraints (see Kearney & Silverman, 1998). Antidepressants that include SSRIs and TCAs are most often used with adults and youths (Stock et al., 2001). Results on the use of TCAs for reducing SAD have been mixed. For example, in an early study (Gittelman-Klein & Klein, 1971), imipramine was shown to be effective. More recent studies, however, have not replicated these findings (Bernstein, Garfinkel, & Borchardt, 1990; Klein, Koplewitz, & Kanner, 1992). In a study examining the efficacy of the antidepressant fluoxetine (i.e., Prozac) in 21 patients with overanxious disorder, social phobia, and SAD (Birmaher et al., 1994), 81% of the children displayed moderate to marked improvement of their anxiety symptoms, and no side effects were reported by any of the children. In addition, results from open-label trials suggest that benzodiazepines, which are typically used in adults with anxiety disorders—specifically, panic disorder—can be helpful for children with panic disorder (D'Amato, 1962; Simeon et al., 1992). Overall, however, pharmacological intervention has been recommended with more difficult or "resistant" cases rather than as a front-line intervention to be used with all cases (American Academy of Child and Adolescent Psychiatry, 1997; Stock et al., 2001).

SUMMARY

Although SAD is among the most prevalent disorders of childhood and adolescence, many questions remain about the disorder, and this chapter has served to highlight these questions. Some of these relate to the etiology of SAD and the prognosis for children with the disorder (e.g., do they develop panic disorder as adults? SAD as adults?). In addition, although considerable strides in knowledge have been made with respect to developing and evaluating CBT for anxiety disorders in children, there remains the question of whether more specialized or focused interventions might be needed for SAD, or at least for certain types or subtypes of SAD cases. If so, which cases? Furthermore, even more questions arise concerning pharmacological treatment of SAD.

It is our hope that this chapter serves to sharpen investigators' research focus in the years to come. We hope that future research will move beyond "lumping" various anxiety disorders together, which is what is done in the majority of studies conducted to date. Rather, future research would benefit from asking those research questions most relevant to SAD, as highlighted in this chapter, and using samples of carefully diagnosed children with SAD, and examining the influence, if any, of other comorbid conditions. It is this type of research that is most likely to be most successful in advancing and refining understanding about SAD.

REFERENCES

Ainsworth, M. D. S., Blehar, M. C., Waters, E., & Wall, E. (1978). *Patterns of attachment: A psychological study of the strange situation.* Hillsdale, NJ: Erlbaum.

American Academy of Child and Adolescent Psychiatry. (1997). AACAP official action: Practice parameters for the assessment and treatment of children and adolescents with anxiety disorders. *Journal of the American Academy of Child and Adolescent Psychiatry, 36,* 9–20.

American Psychiatric Association. (1980). *Diagnostic and statistical manual of mental disorders* (3rd ed.). Washington, DC: Author.

Anderson, J. C., Williams, S., McGee, R., & Silva, P. (1987). DSM-III disorders in preadolescent children: Prevalence in a large sample from the general population. *Archives of General Psychiatry, 44,* 69–76.

Barlow, D. H. (2002). *Anxiety and its disorders: The nature and treatment of anxiety and panic* (2nd ed.). New York: Guilford Press.

Barrett, P. M. (1998). Evaluation of cognitive-behavioral group treatments for childhood anxiety disorders. *Journal of Clinical Child Psychology, 27,* 459–468.

Barrett, P. M. (2001). Current issues in the treatment of childhood anxiety. In M. W. Vasey & M. R. Dadds (Eds.), *The developmental psychopathology of anxiety* (pp. 304–324). New York: Oxford University Press.

Barrett, P. M., Dadds, M. R., & Rapee, R. M. (1996). Family treatment of childhood anxiety: A controlled trial. *Journal of Consulting and Clinical Psychology, 64,* 333–342.

Battaglia, M., Bertella, S., Politi, E., Bernardeschi, L., Perna, G., Gabriele, A., Bellodi, L. (1995). Age at onset of panic disorder: Influence of familial liability to the disease and of childhood separation anxiety disorder. *American Journal of Psychiatry, 152,* 1362–1364.

Benjamin, R. S., Costello, E. J., & Warren, M. (1990). Anxiety disorders in a pediatric sample. *Journal of Anxiety Disorders, 4,* 293–316.

Bernstein, G. A., Garfinkel, B. D., & Borchardt, C. M. (1990). Comparative studies of pharmacotherapy for school refusal. *Journal of the American Academy of Child and Adolescent Psychiatry, 29,* 773–781.

Biederman, J., Rosenbaum, J. F., Bolduc-Murphy, E. A., Faraone, S. V., Charloff, J., Hirshfeld, D. R., & Kagan, J. (1993). A 3-year follow-up of children with and without behavioral inhibition. *Journal of the American Academy of Child and Adolescent Psychiatry, 32,* 814–821.

Bird, H. R., Canino, G., Rubio-Stipec, M., Gould, M. S., Ribera, J., Sesman, M., Woodbury, M., Huertas-Goldman, S., Pagan, A., Sanchez-Lacay, A., et al. (1988). Estimates of the prevalence of childhood maladjustment in a community survey in Puerto Rico: The use of combined measures. *Archives of General Psychiatry, 45,* 1120–1126.

Bird, H. R., Gould, M. S., Yager, T., Staghezza, B., & Canino, G. (1989). Risk factors for maladjustment in Puerto Rican children. *Journal of the American Academy of Child and Adolescent Psychiatry, 28,* 847–850.

Birmaher, B., Waterman, G. S., Ryan, N., Cully, M., Balach, L., Ingram, J., & Brodsky, M. (1994). Fluoxetine for childhood anxiety disorders. *Journal of the American Academy of Child and Adolescent Psychiatry, 33,* 993–1000.

Boegels, S. M., & Zigterman, D. (2000). Dysfunctional cognitions in children with social phobia, separation anxiety disorder, and generalized anxiety disorder. *Journal of Abnormal Child Psychology, 28,* 205–211.

Boer, F. (1998). Anxiety disorders in the family: The contribution of heredity and family interactions. In P. D. A. Treffers (Ed.), *Emotionale stoornissen en somatoforme stoornissen bij kinderen en adolescenten: de stand van zaken* [Emotional disorders and somatoform disorders in children and adolescents: The current state of research] (pp. 109–114). Leiden, The Netherlands: Boerhaave Commissie.

Boer, F., & Lindhout, I. (2001). Family and genetic influences: Is anxiety "all in the family"? In W. K. Silverman & P. D. A. Treffers (Eds.), *Anxiety disorders in children and adolescents. Research, assessment, and intervention* (pp. 235–254). Cambridge, UK: Cambridge University Press.

Bowen, R. C., Offord, D. R., & Boyle, M. H. (1990). The prevalence of overanxious disorder and separation anxiety disorder: Results from the Ontario child health study. *Journal of the American Academy of Child and Adolescent Psychiatry, 29,* 753–758.

Bowlby, J. (1973). *Attachment and loss: Vol. 2. Separation anxiety and anger.* New York: Basic Books.

Bowler, J. (1996). An attachment theory approach to the treatment of separation anxiety beyond infancy. *Psychotherapy in Private Practice, 15,* 71–79.

Brennan, K. A., Clark, C. L., & Shaver, P. R. (1998). Self-report measurement of adult attachment: An integrative overview. In J. A. Simpson & W. S. Rholes (Eds.), *Attachment theory and close relationships* (pp. 46–76). New York: Guilford Press.

Breton, J. J., Bergeron, L., Valla, J. P., Berthiaume, C., Gaudet, N., Lambert, J., St.-Georges, M., Houde, L., & Lepine, S. (1999). Quebec child mental health survey: Prevalence of DSM-III-R mental health disorders. *Journal of Child Psychology and Psychiatry, 40,* 375–384.

Brown, G. W., & Harris, T. O. (1993). Etiology of anxiety and depressive disorders in an inner-city population: 1. Early adversity. *Psychological Medicine, 23,* 143–154.

Brown, G. W., Harris, T. O., & Eales, M. J. (1993). Etiology of anxiety and depressive disorders in an inner-city population: 2. Comorbidity and adversity. *Psychological Medicine, 23,* 155–165.

Cantwell, D. P., & Baker, L. (1989). Stability and natural history of DSM-III childhood diagnoses. *Journal of the American Academy of Child and Adolescent Psychiatry, 28,* 691–700.

Capps, L., Sigman, M., Sena, R., & Henker, B. (1996). Fear, anxiety, and perceived control in children of agoraphobic parents. *Journal of Child Psychology and Psychiatry, 37,* 445–452.

Cassidy, J. (1995). Attachment and generalized anxiety disorder. In D. Cicchetti & S. Toth (Eds.), *Emotion, cognition, and representation: Rochester Symposium on Developmental Psychopathology* (Vol. 6, pp. 343–370). Rochester, NY: University of Rochester Press.

Cicchetti, D., & Cohen, D. J. (1995). Perspectives on developmental psychopathology. In D. Cicchetti & D. J. Cohen (Eds.), *Development and psychopathology: Vol. 1. Theory and methods* (pp. 3–22). New York: Wiley.

Cobham, V. E., Dadds, M. R., & Spence, S. H. (1998). The role of parental anxiety in the treatment of childhood anxiety. *Journal of Consulting and Clinical Psychology, 66,* 893–905.

Compton, S. N., Nelson, A. H., & March, J. S. (2000). Social phobia and separation anxiety symptoms in community and clinical samples of children and adolescents. *Journal of the American Academy of Child and Adolescent Psychiatry, 39,* 1040–1046.

Costello, E. J. (1989a). Child psychiatric disorders and their correlates: A primary care pediatric sample. *Journal of the American Academy of Child and Adolescent Psychiatry, 28,* 851–855.

Costello, E. J. (1989b). Developments in child psychiatric epidemiology. *Journal of the American Academy of Child and Adolescent Psychiatry, 28,* 836–841.

Costello, E. J., Costello, A. J., Edelbrock, C., Burns, B. J., Dulcan, M. K., Brent, D., & Janiszewski, S. (1988). Psychiatric disorders in pediatric primary care: Prevalence and risk factors. *Archives of General Psychiatry, 45,* 1107–1116.

Dadds, M. R., Barrett, P. M., Rapee, R. M., & Ryan, S. (1996). Family process and child anxiety and aggression: An observational analysis. *Journal of Abnormal Child Psychology, 24,* 715–734.

Dalgleish, T., Taghavi, R., Neshat-Doost, H., Moradi, A., Yule, W., & Canterbury, R. (1997). Information processing in clinically depressed and anxious children and adolescents. *Journal of Child Psychology and Psychiatry, 38,* 535–541.

D'Amato, G. (1962). Chlordiazepoxide in the management of school phobia. *Diseases of the Nervous System, 23,* 292–295.

Eaves, L. J., Silberg, J. L., Meyer, J. M., Maes, H. H., Simonoff, E., Pickles, A., Rutter, M., Neale, M. C., Reynolds, C. A., Erikson, M. T., Heath, A. C., Loeber, R., Truett, K. R., & Hewitt, J. K. (1997). Genetics and developmental psychopathology: 2. The main effects of genes and environment on behavioral problems in the Virginia Twin Study of Adolescent Behavioral Development. *Journal of Child Psychology and Psychiatry, 38,* 965–980.

Fein, G. G., Gariboldi, A., & Boni, R. (1993). Antecedents of maternal separation anxiety. *Merrill–Palmer Quarterly, 39,* 481–495.

Flament, M. F., Whitaker, A., Rapoport, J. L., Davies, M., Berg, C. Z., Kalikow, K., Sceery, W., & Shaffer, D. (1988). Obsessive compulsive disorder in adolescence: An epidemiological study. *Journal of the American Academy of Child and Adolescent Psychiatry, 27,* 764–771.

Flannery-Schroeder, E. C., & Kendall, P. C. (2000). Group versus individual cognitive behavioral treatment for youth with anxiety disorders: A randomized clinical trial. *Cognitive Therapy and Research, 24,* 251–278.

Francis, G., Last, C. G., & Strauss, C. C. (1987). Expression of separation anxiety disorder: The roles of age and gender. *Child Psychiatry and Human Development, 18,* 82–89.

Freud, S. (1955). Analysis of a phobia in a five-year-old boy. In J. Strachey (Ed. & Trans.), *The standard edition of the complete psychological works of Sigmund Freud* (Vol. 10, pp. 1–149). London: Hogarth Press. (Original work published 1909)

Gardner, R. A. (1985). *Separation anxiety disorder: Psychodynamics and psychotherapies.* Cresskill, NJ: Creative Therapeutics.

Gardner, R. A. (1992). Children with separation anxiety disorder. In J. D. O'Brien, D. J. Pilowsky, & O. W. Lewis (Eds.), *Psychotherapies with children and adolescents: Adapting the psychodynamic process* (pp. 3–25). Washington, DC: American Psychiatric Press.

Ginsburg, G. S., & Silverman, W. K. (1996). Phobic and anxiety disorders in Hispanic and Caucasian youth. *Journal of Anxiety Disorders, 10,* 517–528.

Gittelman, R., & Klein, D. F. (1984). Relationship between separation anxiety and panic and agoraphobia disorders. *Psychopathology, 17,* 56–65.

Gittelman-Klein, R., & Klein, D. F. (1971). Controlled imipramine treatment of school phobia. *Archives of General Psychiatry, 25,* 204–207.

Greenberg, M. T. (1999). Attachment and psychopathology in childhood. In J. Cassidy & P. R. Shaver (Eds.), *Handbook of attachment: Theory, research, and clinical applications* (pp. 469–496). New York: Guilford Press.

Hagopian, L. P., & Slifer, K. J. (1993). Treatment of separation anxiety disorder with graduated exposure and reinforcement targeting school attendance: A controlled case study. *Journal of Anxiety Disorders, 7,* 271–280.

Hamilton, B. (1994). A systematic approach to a family and school problem: A case study in separation anxiety disorder. *Family Therapy, 21,* 149–152.

Hayward, C., Killen, J. D., Kraemer, H. C., & Taylor, C. B. (2000). Predictors of panic attacks in adolescents. *Journal of the American Academy of Child and Adolescent Psychiatry, 39,* 207–214.

Hewitt, J. K., Silberg, J. L., Rutter, M., Simonoff, E., Meyer, J. M., Maes, H., Pickles, A., Neale, M. C., Loeber, R., Erickson, M. T., Kendler, K. S., Heath, A. C., Truett, K. R., Reynolds, C. A., & Eaves, L. J. (1997). Genetics and developmental psychopathology: 1. Phenotypic assessment in the Virginia Twin Study of Adolescent Behavioral Development. *Journal of Child Psychology and Psychiatry, 38,* 943–963.

Hirshfeld, D. R., Biederman, J., Brody, L., Faraone, S. V., & Rosenbaum, J. F. (1997). Associations between expressed emotion and child behavioral inhibition and psychopathology: A pilot study. *Journal of the American Academy of Child and Adolescent Psychiatry, 36,* 205–214.

Hudson, J. L., & Rapee, R. M. (2002). Parent–child interactions in clinically anxious children and their siblings. *Journal of Clinical Child and Adolescent Psychology, 31,* 548–555.

Jacobson, S. W., & Frye, K. F. (1991). Effect of maternal social support on attachment: Experimental evidence. *Child Development, 62,* 572–582.

Kagan, J., Kearsley, R., & Zelazo, P. (1978). *Infancy: Its place in human development.* Cambridge, MA: Harvard University Press.

Kagan, J., Reznick, J. S., & Snidman, N. (1988). Biological bases of childhood shyness. *Science, 240,* 167–173.

Kashani, J. H., Beck, N. C., Hoeper, E. W., Fallahi, C., Corcoran, C. M., McAllister, J. A., Risenberg, T. K., & Reid, J. C.(1987). Psychiatric disorders in a community sample of adolescents. *American Journal of Psychiatry, 144,* 584–589.

Kashani, J. H., & Orvaschel, H. (1988). Anxiety disorders in mid-adolescence: A community sample. *American Journal of Psychiatry, 145,* 960–964.

Kashani, J. H., & Orvaschel, H. (1990). A community study of anxiety in children and adolescents. *American Journal of Psychiatry, 147,* 313–318.

Kearney, C. A., Albano, A. M., Eisen, A. R., Allan, W. D., & Barlow, D. H. (1997). The phenomenology of panic disorder in youngsters: An empirical study of a clinical sample. *Journal of Anxiety Disorders, 11,* 49–62.

Kearney, C. A., & Silverman, W. K. (1996). The evolution and reconciliation of taxonomic strategies for school refusal behavior. *Clinical Psychology: Science and Practice, 3,* 339–354.

Kearney, C. A., & Silverman, W. K. (1998). Pharmacological treatment for anxiety disorders in children: It's not what it seems. *Journal of Anxiety Disorders, 12,* 83–102.

Keller, M. B., Lavori, P. W., Wunder, J., Beardslee, W. R., Schwartz, C. E., & Roth, J. (1992). Chronic course of anxiety disorders in children and adolescents. *Journal of the American Academy of Child and Adolescent Psychiatry, 31,* 595–599.

Kendall, P. C. (1994). Treating anxiety disorders in children: Results of a randomized clinical trial. *Journal of Consulting and Clinical Psychology, 62,* 100–110.

Kendall, P. C., Brady, E. U., & Verduin, T. L. (2001). Comorbidity in childhood anxiety disorders and treatment outcome. *Journal of the American Academy of Child and Adolescent Psychiatry, 40,* 787–794.

Kendall, P. C., Flannery-Schroeder, E., Panichelli-Mindel, S. M., Southham-Gerow,

M., Henin, A., & Warman, M. (1997). Therapy for youths with anxiety disorders: A second randomized clinical trial. *Journal of Consulting and Clinical Psychology, 65,* 366–380.

King, N. J., & Bernstein, G. A. (2001). School refusal in children and adolescents: A review of the past 10 years. *Journal of the American Academy of Child and Adolescent Psychiatry, 40,* 197–205.

King, N. J., Tonge, B. J., Heyne, D., Pritchard, M., Rollings, S., Young, D., Myerson, N., & Ollendick, T. H. (1998). Cognitive-behavioral treatment of school-refusing children: A controlled evaluation. *Journal of the American Academy of Child and Adolescent Psychiatry, 37,* 395–403.

Klein, D. (1964). Delineation of two drug-responsive anxiety syndromes. *Psychopharmacologia, 5,* 397–408.

Klein, D. (1980). Anxiety reconceptualized: Early experience with imipramine and anxiety. *Comprehensive Psychiatry, 21,* 411–427.

Klein, R.G., Koplewitz, H. S., & Kanner, A. (1992). Imipramine treatment of children with separation anxiety disorder. *Journal of the American Academy of Child and Adolescent Psychiatry, 31,* 21–28.

Kochanska, G. (1991). Patterns of inhibition to the unfamiliar in children of normal and affectively ill mothers. *Child Development, 62,* 250–263.

Kovacs, M., & Devlin, B. (1998). Internalizing disorders. *Journal of Child Psychology and Psychiatry, 39,* 47–63.

Kovacs, M., Gatsonis, C., Paulauskas, S. L., & Richards, C. (1989). Depressive disorders in childhood: 4. A longitudinal study of comorbidity with and risk for anxiety disorders. *Archives of General Psychiatry, 46,* 776–782.

Last, C. G., Francis, G., Hersen, M., Kazdin, A. E., & Strauss, C. C. (1987). Separation anxiety and school phobia: A comparison using DSM-III criteria. *American Journal of Psychiatry, 144,* 653–657.

Last, C. G., Hansen, C., & Franco, N. (1998). Cognitive-behavioral treatment of school phobia. *Journal of the American Academy of Child and Adolescent Psychiatry, 37,* 404–411.

Last, C. G., Hersen, M., Kazdin, A. E., Finkelstein, R., & Strauss, C. (1987). Comparison of DSM-III separation anxiety and overanxious disorders: Demographic characteristics and patterns of comorbidity. *Journal of the American Academy of Child and Adolescent Psychiatry, 26,* 527–531.

Last, C. G., & Perrin, S. (1993). Anxiety disorders in African-American and white children. *Journal of Abnormal Child Psychology, 21,* 153–164.

Last, C. G., Perrin, S., Hersen, M., & Kazdin, A. E. (1992). DSM-III-R anxiety disorders in children: Sociodemographic and clinical characteristics. *Journal of the American Academy of Child and Adolescent Psychiatry, 31,* 1070–1076.

Last, C. G., Perrin, S., Hersen, M., & Kazdin, A. E. (1996). A prospective study of childhood anxiety disorders. *Journal of the American Academy of Child and Adolescent Psychiatry, 35,* 1502–1510.

Last, C. G., & Strauss, C. C. (1990). School refusal in anxiety-disordered children and adolescents. *Journal of the American Academy of Child and Adolescent Psychiatry, 29,* 31–35.

Last, C. G., Strauss, C. C., & Francis, G. (1987). Comorbidity among childhood anxiety disorders. *Journal of Nervous and Mental Disease, 175,* 726–730.

Lau, J. J., Calamari, J. E., & Waraczynski, M. (1996). Panic attack symptomatology and anxiety sensitivity in adolescents. *Journal of Anxiety Disorders, 10*, 355–364.

Leckman, J. F., Weissman, M. M., Merikangas, K. R., Pauls, D. L., Prusoff, B. A., & Kidd, K. K. (1985). Major depression and panic disorder: A family study perspective. *Psychopharmacology Bulletin, 21*, 543–545.

Lewinsohn, P. M., Hops, H., Roberts, R. E., Seeley, J. R., & Andrews, J. A. (1993). Adolescent psychopathology: 1. Prevalence and incidence of depression and other DSM-III-R disorders in high school students. *Journal of Abnormal Psychology, 102*, 133–144.

Lumpkin, P. W., Silverman, W. K., Weems, C. F., Markham, M. R., & Kurtines, W. M. (2002). Treating a heterogeneous set of anxiety disorders in youths with group cognitive behavioral therapy: A partially nonconcurrent multiple-baseline evaluation. *Behavior Therapy, 33*, 163–177.

Lutz, W. J., & Hock, E. (1995). Maternal separation anxiety: Relations to adult attachment representations in mothers of infants. *Journal of Genetic Psychology, 156*, 57–72.

Main, M., & Solomon, J. (1990). Procedures for identifying infants as disorganized/disoriented during the Ainsworth Strange Situation. In M. T. Greenberg, D. Cicchetti, & E. M. Cummings (Eds.), *Attachment in the preschool years: Theory, research, and intervention* (pp. 121–160). Chicago: University of Chicago Press.

Manassis, K. (2001). Child–parent relations: Attachment and anxiety disorders. In W. K. Silverman & P. D. A. Treffers (Eds.), *Anxiety disorders in children and adolescents: Research, assessment, and intervention* (pp. 255–272). Cambridge, UK: Cambridge University Press.

Manassis, K., & Bradley, S. J. (1994). The development of childhood anxiety disorders: Toward an integrated model. *Journal of Applied and Developmental Psychology, 15*, 345–366.

Manassis, K., Bradley, S. J., Goldberg, S., Hood, J., & Swinson, R. P. (1994). Attachment in mothers with anxiety disorders and their children. *Journal of the American Academy of Child and Adolescent Psychiatry, 33*, 1106–1113.

Manicavasagar, V., & Silove, D. (1997). Is there an adult form of separation anxiety disorder? A brief clinical report. *Australian and New Zealand Journal of Psychiatry, 31*, 299–303.

Manicavasagar, V., Silove, D., & Curtis, J. (1997). Separation anxiety in adulthood: A phenomenological investigation. *Comprehensive Psychiatry, 38*, 274–282.

Manicavasagar, V., Silove, D., Curtis, J., & Wagner, R. (2000). Continuities of separation anxiety from early life into adulthood. *Journal of Anxiety Disorders, 14*, 1–18.

March, J. S., Parker, J. D. A., Sullivan, K., Stallings, P., & Conners, K. (1997). The Multidimensional Anxiety Scale for Children (MASC): Factor structure, reliability, and validity. *Journal of the American Academy of Child and Adolescent Psychiatry, 36*, 554–565.

McGee, R., Feehan, M., Williams, S., Partridge, F., Silva, P. A., & Kelly, J. (1990). DSM-III disorders in a large sample of adolescents. *Journal of the American Academy of Child and Adolescent Psychiatry, 29*, 611–619.

Milne, J. M., Garrison, C. Z., Addy, C. L., McKeown, R. E., Jackson, K. L., Cuffe, S. P., & Waller, J. L. (1995). Frequency of phobic disorder in a community sample of young adolescents. *Journal of the American Academy of Child and Adolescent Psychiatry, 34,* 1202–1211.

Moreau, D. M., & Follet, C. (1993). Panic disorder in children and adolescents. *Child and Adolescent Psychiatric Clinics of North America, 2,* 581–602.

Muris, P., Schmidt, H., Merckelbach, H., & Schouten, E. (2001). Anxiety sensitivity in adolescents: Factor structure and relationships to trait anxiety and symptoms of anxiety disorders and depression. *Behaviour Research and Therapy, 39,* 89–100.

Neisworth, J. T., Madle, R. A., & Goeke, K. E. (1975). "Errorless" elimination of separation anxiety: A case study. *Journal of Behavior Therapy and Experimental Psychiatry, 6,* 79–82.

Newman, D. L., Moffitt, T. E., Caspi, A., Magdol, L., Silva, P. A., & Stanton, W. R. (1996). Psychiatric disorder in birth cohort of young adults: Prevalence, comorbidity, clinical significance, and new case incidence from ages 11 to 21. *Journal of Consulting and Clinical Psychology, 64,* 552–562.

Ollendick, T. H., Hagopian, L. P., & Huntzinger, R. M. (1991). Cognitive behavior therapy with nighttime fearful children. *Journal of Behavior Therapy and Experimental Psychiatry, 22,* 112–121.

Ollendick, T. H., Lease, C. A., & Cooper, C. (1993). Separation anxiety in young adults: A preliminary examination. *Journal of Anxiety Disorders, 7,* 293–305.

Oosterlaan, J. (2001). Behavioural inhibition and the development of childhood anxiety disorders. In W. K. Silverman & P. D. A. Treffers (Eds.), *Anxiety disorders in children and adolescents: Research, assessment and intervention* (pp. 45–71). Cambridge, UK: Cambridge University Press.

Phillips, D., & Wolpe, S. (1981). Multiple behavioral techniques in severe separation anxiety of a twelve-year-old. *Journal of Behavior Therapy and Experimental Psychiatry, 12,* 329–332.

Prior, M., Sanson, A., Smart, D., & Oberklaid, F. (1999). Psychological disorders and their correlates in an Australian community sample of preadolescent children. *Journal of Child Psychology and Psychiatry, 40,* 563–580.

Rapee, R. M. (1997). Potential role of childrearing practices in the development of anxiety and depression. *Clinical Psychology Review, 17,* 47–67.

Raskin, M., Peeke, H. V. S., Dickman, W., & Pinsker, H. (1982). Panic and generalized anxiety disorders: Developmental antecedents and precipitants. *Archives of General Psychiatry, 39,* 687–689.

Reiss, S. (1991). Expectancy model of fear, anxiety, and panic. *Clinical Psychology Review, 11,* 141–153.

Reiss, S., Silverman, W. K., & Weems, C. F. (2001). Anxiety sensitivity. In M. W. Vasey & M. R. Dadds (Eds.), *The developmental psychopathology of anxiety* (pp. 92–111). London: Oxford University Press.

Ryan, N. D., Puig-Antich, J., Ambrosini, P., Rabinovich, H., Robinson, D., Nelson, B., et al. (1987). The clinical picture of major depression in children and adolescents. *Archives of General Psychiatry, 44,* 854–861.

Silove, D., & Manicavasagar, V. (2001). Early separation anxiety and its relationship to adult anxiety disorders. In M. W. Vasey & M. R. Dadds (Eds.), *The developmental psychopathology of anxiety* (pp. 459–480). New York: Oxford University Press.

Silove, D., Manicavasagar, V., Curtis, J., & Blaszczynski, A. (1996). Is early separation anxiety a risk factor for adult panic disorder? A critical review. *Comprehensive Psychiatry, 37,* 167–179.

Silove, D., Manicavasagar, V., O'Connell, D., Blaszczynski, A., Wagner, R., & Henry, J. (1993). The development of the Separation Anxiety Symptom Inventory (SASI). *Australian and New Zealand Journal of Psychiatry, 27,* 477–488.

Silove, D., Manicavasagar, V., O'Connell, D., & Morris-Yates, A. (1995). Genetic factors in early separation anxiety: Implications for the genesis of adult anxiety disorders. *Acta Psychiatrica Scandinavica, 92,* 17–24.

Silverman, W. K., & Berman, S. L. (2001). Psychosocial interventions for anxiety disorders in children: Status and future directions. In W. K. Silverman & P. D. A. Treffers (Eds.), *Anxiety disorders in children and adolescents: Research, assessment and intervention* (pp. 313–334). Cambridge, UK: Cambridge University Press.

Silverman, W. K., Cerny, J. A., Nelles, W. B., & Burke, A. E. (1988). Behavior problems in children of parents with anxiety disorders. *Journal of the American Academy of Child and Adolescent Psychiatry, 27,* 779–784.

Silverman, W. K., Kurtines, W. M., Ginsburg, G. S., Weems, C. F., Lumpkin, P. W., & Carmichael, D. H. (1999). Treating anxiety disorders in children with group cognitive-behavioral therapy: A randomized clinical trial. *Journal of Consulting and Clinical Psychology, 67,* 995–1003.

Silverman, W. K., Kurtines, W. M., Ginsburg, G. S., Weems, C. F., Rabian, B., & Serafini, L. T. (1999). Contingency management, self-control, and educational support in the treatment of childhood phobic disorders: A randomized clinical trial. *Journal of Consulting and Clinical Psychology, 67,* 675–687.

Silverman, W. K., & Ollendick, T. H. (Eds.). (1999). *Developmental issues in the clinical treatment of children.* Needham Heights, MA: Allyn & Bacon.

Silverman, W. K., & Weems, C. F. (1999). Anxiety sensitivity in children. In S. Taylor (Ed.), *Anxiety sensitivity: Theory, research, and treatment of the fear of anxiety* (pp. 239–268). Mahwah, NJ: Erlbaum.

Simeon, J. G., Ferguson, H. B., Knott, V., Roberts, N., Gauthier, B., Dubois, C., & Wiggins, D. (1992). Clinical, cognitive, and neurophysiological effects of alprazolam in children and adolescents with overanxious and avoidant disorders. *Journal of the American Academy of Child and Adolescent Psychiatry, 31,* 29–33.

Siqueland, L., Kendall, P. C., & Steinberg, L. (1996). Anxiety in children: Perceived family environments and observed family interaction. *Journal of Clinical Child Psychology, 25,* 225–237.

Spence, S. H. (1998). A measure of anxiety symptoms among children. *Behaviour Research and Therapy, 36,* 545–566.

Stifter, C. A., Coulehan, C. M., & Fish, M. (1993). Linking employment to attachment: The mediating effects of maternal separation anxiety and interactive behavior. *Child Development, 64,* 1451–1460.

Stock, S. L., Werry, J. S., & McClellan, J. M. (2001). Pharmacological treatment of pediatric anxiety. In W. K. Silverman & P. D. A. Treffers (Eds.), *Anxiety disorders in children and adolescents: Research, assessment, and intervention* (pp. 335–367). Cambridge, UK: Cambridge University Press.

Topolski, T. D., Hewitt, J. K., Eaves, L. J., Silberg, J. L., Meyer, J. M., Rutter, M., Pickles, A., & Simonoff, E. (1997). Genetic and environmental influences on child reports of manifest anxiety and symptoms of separation anxiety and overanxious disorder: A community-based twin study. *Behavior Genetics, 27,* 15–28.

Turner, S. M., Beidel, D. C., & Costello, A. (1987). Psychopathology in the offspring of anxiety disordered parents. *Journal of Consulting and Clinical Psychology, 55,* 229–235.

Valleni-Basile, L. A., Garrison, C. Z., Jackson, K. L., & Waller, J. L. (1994). Frequency of obsessive–compulsive disorder in a community sample of young adolescents. *Journal of the American Academy of Child and Adolescent Psychiatry, 33,* 782–791.

Vasey, M. W., & Dadds, M. R. (Eds.). (2001). *The developmental psychopathology of anxiety.* London: Oxford University Press.

Vasey, M. W., El-Hag, N., & Daleiden, E. L. (1996). Anxiety and the processing of emotionally threatening stimuli: Distinctive patterns of selective attention among high- and low-test-anxious children. *Child Development, 67,* 1173–1185.

Vaughn, B., Egeland, B., Sroufe, L. A., & Waters, E. (1979). Individual differences in infant–mother attachment at 12 and 18 months: Stability and change in families under stress. *Child Development, 50,* 971–975.

Velez, C. N., Johnson, J., & Cohen, P. A. (1989). A longitudinal analysis of selected risk factors for childhood psychopathology. *Journal of the American Academy of Child and Adolescent Psychiatry, 28,* 861–864.

Warren, S. L., Huston, L., Egeland, B., & Sroufe, L. A. (1997). Child and adolescent anxiety disorders and early attachment. *Journal of the American Academy of Child and Adolescent Psychiatry, 36,* 637–644.

Waters, E., Merrick, S., Treboux, D., Corwell, J., & Albersheim, L. (2000). Attachment security in infancy and early adulthood: A twenty-year longitudinal study. *Child Development, 71,* 684–689.

Weems, C. F., Berman, S. L., Silverman, W. K., & Rodriguez, E. (2002). The relation between anxiety sensitivity and attachment style in adolescence and early adulthood. *Journal of Behavioral Assessment and Psychopathology, 24,* 159–168.

Weissman, M. M., Leckman, L. F., Merikangas, K. R., Gammon, G. D., & Prusoff, B. A. (1984). Depression and anxiety disorders in parents and children: Results from the Yale family study. *Archives of General Psychiatry, 41,* 845–852.

Yeragani, V. K., Meiri, P. C., Balon, R., Patel, H., & Pohl, R. (1989). History of separation anxiety in patients with panic disorder and depression and normal controls. *Acta Psychiatrica Scandinavica, 79,* 550–556.

Zamudio, A., & Wolfe, N. L. (1996). Case illustration of Henry: A 10–year-old Latino child. In F. H. McClure & E. Teyber (Eds.), *Child and adolescent therapy: A multicultural–relational approach* (pp. 251–286). Orlando, FL: Harcourt Brace College.

Zucker, K. J., Bradley, S. J., & Sullivan, C. B. L. (1996). Traits of separation anxiety in boys with gender identity disorder. *Journal of the American Academy of Child and Adolescent Psychiatry, 35,* 791–798.

Chapter 9

Panic Disorder

THOMAS H. OLLENDICK
BORIS BIRMAHER
SARA G. MATTIS

The prevalence of child and adolescent psychiatric disorders throughout the world has been estimated to be between 15 and 25% (Kazdin, 2000; Ollendick & Hersen, 1999). Anxiety disorders are among the most common of these psychiatric disorders. As defined by the fourth edition of the *Diagnostic and Statistical Manual of Mental Disorders* (DSM-IV; American Psychiatric Association [APA], 1994), the *International Classification of Diseases* (ICD-10; World Health Organization, 1992), and their earlier variants, the anxiety disorders constitute approximately 20% of all childhood and adolescent disorders. Although specific phobia, separation anxiety disorder, and social phobia are among the most common anxiety disorders in childhood and adolescence, panic disorder (PD) also occurs in a significant minority of these youths. For example, in child and adolescent community samples, PD has been reported to range between 0.5 and 5.0% (e.g., Essau, Conradt, & Petermann, 1999; Hayward et al., 1997; Hayward, Killen, Kraemer, & Barr-Taylor, 2000; Macaulay & Kleinknecht, 1989; Moreau & Follet, 1993; Verhulst, van der Ende, Ferdinand, & Kasius, 1997) and in pediatric psychiatric clinics from 0.2 to 10% (Biederman et al., 1997; Kearney, Albano, Eisen, Allan, & Barlow, 1997; Last & Strauss, 1989). Although most cases of PD occur in adolescent females, they also occur in children and adolescents of both sexes (Ollendick, Mattis, & King, 1994). Moreover, retrospective studies have found that up to 40% of adults with PD report that their disorders began before they were 20 years old (Moreau & Follet, 1993). The peak onset of PD in these studies has been reported to be between 15 and 19 years of age; however, 10–18% report that their first panic attack (PA) occurred before they were 10 years of age (Thyer, Parrish, Curtis, Nesse, & Cameron, 1985; Von Korff, Eaton, & Keyl, 1985). These prevalence rates, along with emerging evidence that there may be a decrease in age of onset of PD in successive generations (Battaglia, Bertella, Bajo, Binaghi, & Bellodi, 1998), indicate the obvious need to study the symptom picture, developmental course, etiology, and treatment of PD in children and adolescents.

PD is a disabling condition accompanied by psychosocial, family, peer, and academic difficulties (Birmaher & Ollendick, 2003; Moreau & Weissman, 1992; Ollendick, Mattis, & King, 1994). In addition, PD is associated with increased risk for other anxiety disorders, major depressive disorder (MDD), and substance abuse (Birmaher & Ollendick, 2003; Moreau & Weissman, 1992; Ollendick et al., 1994; Strauss et al., 2000). Moreover, such adverse outcomes are more prevalent in adults whose PD starts early in life (before17 years of age; see Weissman et al., 1997). Nevertheless, it takes on average 12.7 years from the onset of reported symptoms for adults to initiate and seek treatment (Moreau & Follet, 1993), and, unfortunately, it appears that very few youngsters with PD seek help at all (Essau et al., 1999, 2000; King, Gullone, Tonge, & Ollendick, 1993; Ollendick, 1995).

In this chapter we review the current literature on the symptom picture, developmental course, etiology, and treatment of PD in children and adolescents. In addition, we suggest directions for future research and clinical practice. Elsewhere, we review the assessment of PD and recent efforts aimed at preventing its development and onset in childhood (Birmaher & Ollendick, 2003; Mattis & Ollendick, 2002; Ollendick, 1998).

SYMPTOM PICTURE

In order to meet diagnostic criteria for PD, the child or adolescent must experience recurrent PAs. Therefore, we first describe the symptom picture of PAs and then the picture of PD in children and adolescents.

Panic Attacks

A PA is an acute anxiety episode in which the child or adolescent experiences a set of emotional, cognitive, and somatic symptoms—in the absence of real danger—that are similar to those triggered by objectively life-threatening situations. The episode is typically intense and is accompanied by at least 4 of 13 symptoms described in DSM-IV (APA, 1994): emotional symptoms (e.g., feelings of unreality or being detached from oneself, feelings of choking), somatic symptoms (e.g., palpitations, chest pain, tingling sensations, chills or hot flushes, dizziness, nausea, sweating, trembling, or shaking), and cognitive symptoms (e.g., fear of losing control or going crazy, fear of dying). The PA usually reaches its peak in intensity within a few minutes (i.e., 5 to 10 minutes) before gradually subsiding (i.e., 15 to 30 minutes later). The child feels that something is wrong or that something bad is going to happen but does not know exactly what is going to happen, when it will happen, where it will happen, and, perhaps most of all, why it will happen. As a consequence, the young person might believe that he or she is going to go crazy, lose control, faint, develop a severe illness, or even die. The previously noted symptoms, by themselves, can increase the youngster's level of anxiety and create a vicious circle, which serves to worsen and maintain PA frequency, intensity, and duration (American Psychiatric Association, 1998).

There are three types of PAs: (1) *uncued*, (2) *situationally bound*, and (3) *situationally predisposed* (American Psychiatric Association, 1994). Uncued PAs are unexpected and spontaneous and come seemingly "out of the blue." Situationally bound PAs almost always occur immediately on exposure to, or in anticipation of, a specific triggering event (e.g., the presence of a phobic object). Situationally predisposed PAs, although also triggered by certain situations (e.g., a threatening or embarrassing situation), do not always occur immediately after exposure to the external trigger (American Psychiatric Association, 1998). It is important to note that PAs may initially be uncued but, over time, may become paired with specific stimuli (e.g., elevators, shopping centers, crowed places) and may subsequently result in situationally bound or situationally predisposed attacks. Frequently, regardless of the type of PA, avoidance behaviors develop.

Community studies using structured psychiatric interviews have found that 2–18% of adolescents between 12 and 18 years of age have experienced at least one four-symptom PA during their lives (Essau et al., 1999; Hayward et al., 1997, 2000). Studies using self-report questionnaires have yielded considerably higher prevalence rates, reaching to between 43 and 60% (King et al., 1993; King, Ollendick, Mattis, Yang, & Tonge, 1997; Lau, Calamari, & Waraczynski, 1996; Macaulay & Kleinknecht, 1989); however, reliance on self-report questionnaires alone tends to produce increased rates of false positive cases (Hayward et al., 1997). That is, many of these cases turn out not to be true cases of PA when followed up with structured psychiatric interviews. PAs tend to be equally prevalent in males and females (Essau et al., 1999; Hayward et al., 2000; King et al., 1993) but tend to be more severe in females (Hayward, Killen, & Taylor, 1989;

Hayward et al., 2000; King et al., 1997; Macaulay & Kleinknecht, 1989). PAs can and do occur in children but are much less prevalent than in adolescents (Hayward et al., 1989; King et al., 1997; Ollendick et al., 1994).

In community samples approximately 20 to 50% of PAs are reported to be uncued (Essau et al., 1999; King et al., 1997; Macaulay & Kleinknecht, 1989). Similar to findings in adult studies, adolescents usually experience somatic and emotional symptoms, including palpitations, trembling/shaking, nausea, abdominal distress, chills, hot flushes, sweating, and dizziness (Essau et al., 1999; Macaulay & Kleinknecht, 1989). However, cognitive symptoms (e.g., fear of losing control, going crazy, or dying) are less frequently reported than somatic symptoms (Ollendick et al., 1994).

Between 10 and 30% of youngsters with PA develop moderate to severe avoidance behaviors (e.g., agoraphobia) of specific situations (e.g., school, restaurants, malls, crowds) for fear they might have another attack (Essau et al., 1999; Hayward et al., 2000; King et al., 1993). Similar to adults (American Psychiatric Association, 1994, 1998), youths with more severe and intense PAs tend to have other anxiety and depressive symptoms or disorders (Essau et al., 1999; Hayward et al., 1989; 2000; King et al., 1993; Macaulay & Kleinknecht, 1989). They also report less social support from their family members and more family-related psychosocial stressors (King et al., 1993, 1997; Macaulay & Kleinknecht, 1989). PAs can also affect the well-being and self-esteem of these children and adolescents because they may see the PA as a sign of emotional weakness or believe the PAs are an indicator of a life-threatening illness or possibly even death (Birmaher & Ollendick, 2003).

Panic Disorder

PD is characterized primarily by recurrent, unexpected, or *uncued* PAs. In addition, it is characterized by at least one month of persistent concern about having another PA (anticipatory anxiety), worry about the implications and consequences of the PA, and/or significant impairment in functioning (American Psychiatric Association, 1994, 1998). In addition, for a diagnosis of PD, the PA should not be accounted for primarily by other physical or psychiatric illnesses. The ICD-10 (World Health Organization, 1992) includes similar diagnostic criteria.

Clinical studies (Alessi & Magen, 1988; Alessi, Robbins, & Dilsaver, 1987; Biederman et al., 1997; Kearney et al., 1997; Last & Strauss, 1989; Moreau & Follet, 1993; Ollendick, 1995) have shown that older adolescents who are European American, female, and of middle class are more likely to present to outpatient clinics for treatment of PD. Similar to findings with adults, more than half of these adolescents report palpitations, tremor, dizziness, shortness of breath, faintness, sweating, chest pressure and pain, and fear of dying.

Although PD in children has been reported in the clinical literature, it appears that this disorder is less frequent and perhaps less severe in this age range. It has been suggested by some that PD is less frequent because children do not have the cognitive ability to make internal, catastrophic misinterpretations of the somatic symptoms associated with PD (e.g., thoughts of losing control, going crazy, or dying in response to the somatic symptoms; see Nelles & Barlow, 1988). However, these notions have not been supported empirically. On the contrary, although children of varying ages tend to make noncatastrophic interpretations of their panic-like symptoms (e.g., "I am catching a cold or the flu"), they are *capable* of making internal, catastrophic cognitions (e.g., "I must be dying like my grandfather"; see Mattis & Ollendick, 1997a). Rarely, however, do young children attribute the somatic symptoms they experience to "going crazy"; rather, they are more likely to think something is wrong with them physically and that they might be catching a severe disease. It has been shown that children as young as 8 years of age report high levels of anxiety sensitivity (i.e., fear of anxiety symptoms) and elevated internal attributions of responsibility in response to negative outcomes; these cognitive processes, in turn, may serve as important risk factors for future development of PD (Ginsburg & Drake, 2002; Mattis & Ollendick, 1997a; Ollendick, 1998).

Diagnosis

Up to 90% of children and adolescents with PD have other, comorbid anxiety disorders (e.g., separation anxiety disorder, social phobia, general anxiety disorder) and/or depressive disorders (Alesi et al., 1987; Alessi & Magen, 1988; Biederman et al., 1997; Essau et al., 2000). PD has also been shown to be comorbid with other psychiatric disorders in children and adolescents, including attention-deficit/hyperactivity disorder, oppositional defiant disorder, and bipolar disorder (Biederman et al., 1997; Last & Strauss, 1989). It has also been reported that individuals with PD are at high risk for suicide, but it is not clear whether this tendency is due to the high comorbidity with mood or other disorders (American Psychiatric Association, 1998). PD has also been associated with medical and neurological conditions such as migraine and, more controversially, with mitral valve prolapse (American Psychiatric Association, 1998). Unfortunately, little research on these possibilities has been conducted with children and adolescents to date.

Differential diagnosis is also important in children and adolescents who present primarily with other disorders. For example, youngsters with primary mood disorders and other anxiety disorders (e.g., social phobia, separation anxiety disorder, specific phobia) can also experience PAs (American Psychiatric Association, 1994, 1998). In such instances, a differential diagnosis is imperative, and the secondary diagnosis of PD would be made only if the PA is not explained by the other psychiatric disorder. For example, if socially anxious or separation anxious youths experience PAs *only* when they are exposed to potentially embarrassing or evaluative situations or situations in which they might be separated from their parent(s), respectively, the diagnosis of PD would not be made.

Children and adolescents with certain medical conditions (e.g., hyperthyroidism, hyperparathyroidism) may also experience anxiety symptoms secondary to their medical condition that resemble PAs, and they can be misdiagnosed with PD. On the other hand, inasmuch as PD is frequently accompanied by a number of somatic symptoms, youths with PD can be and frequently are misdiagnosed with a spate of medical conditions, including pulmonary (e.g., asthma), cardiovascular (e.g., angina, arrhythmias, myocardial infarction), neurological (e.g., seizures, vestibular dysfunctions, syncope), and gastrointestinal illnesses (e.g., irritable bowel syndrome; American Psychiatric Association, 1998). Therefore, clinicians need to be aware of these conditions and to show good clinical judgment when these medical illnesses need to be ruled out (Birmaher & Ollendick, 2003).

Substances, including street drugs (e.g., cocaine, caffeine) and over-the-counter medications, and acute withdrawal from prescribed medications and other substances (e.g., benzodiazepines, alcohol) can also induce PAs. In these instances, PD would be diagnosed only if the PAs have occurred before or lasted long enough after the substance has been discontinued (American Psychiatric Association, 1994). Finally, a child can be experiencing anxiety symptoms and PAs due to exposure to real current or past threatening situations, such as violence or sexual or physical abuse. Such possibilities should be routinely explored in the clinical interview prior to commencement of psychosocial or pharmacological treatment.

DEVELOPMENTAL COURSE

No longitudinal studies of children and adolescents with PD have been published, so the developmental course of this disorder is unknown. In adults, however, PD has been reported to wax and wane, with periods of frequent PAs and periods in which the PAs diminish in frequency or seemingly disappear altogether. In longitudinal studies of adults who present at medical centers and hospitals, approximately one-third show improvement, one-third remain subsyndromal, and one-third continue to fulfill criteria for PD. Even if the persons improve, however, they frequently continue to have some episodes with some symptoms of PAs, even though they might not meet full criteria for a PA (e.g., "limited symptom attacks" of less than four symptoms; American Psychiatric Association, 1994, 1998).

Although the developmental course of PAs and PD has not yet been tracked with children and adolescents, female sex, puberty, negative affectivity (NA; an increased sensitivity to negative stimuli, with resulting distress and fearfulness), anxiety sensitivity (AS; an increased tendency to respond fearfully to anxiety symptoms), internal attributions of responsibility in response to negative events, and presence of MDD have been associated with the onset of full-blown PAs in both African American and European American youths (Ginsburg & Drake, 2002; Hayward et al., 1997, 2000; Kearney et al., 1997; Lau et al., 1996; Mattis & Ollendick, 1997a). Although less conclusive, family conflict and stress have also been shown to be predictive of PAs in adolescents (King et al., 1997; Macaulay & Kleinknecht, 1989).

Female sex, MDD, high AS, and family history of MDD and PD have been associated with higher rates of PD as well (e.g., Biederman et al., 2001; Goldstein, Wickramarante, Horwath, & Weissman, 1997; Horesh, Amir, Kedem, Goldberger, & Kotler, 1997; Kearney et al., 1997). Earlier studies suggested that childhood separation anxiety disorder might herald the development of PD during late adolescence and adulthood (see reviews by Ollendick & Huntzinger, 1990, and Silove, Manicavasagar, Curtis, & Blaszczynski, 1996). However, more recent studies have failed to affirm this intuitive relationship (Craske, Poulton, Tsao, & Plotkin, 2001; Essau et al., 1999; Hayward et al., 2000).

Thus, although longitudinal studies have not yet been conducted, we know much about the risk factors that might serve to occasion the development and onset of PAs and PD in children and adolescents (see the preceding and the review by Hirshfeld, Rosenbaum, Smoller, Fredman, & Bulzacchelli, 1998). Inasmuch as the field of developmental psychopathology has emphasized the identification of specific risk factors and protective factors that confer vulnerability or resiliency to child and adolescent psychiatric disorders at varying ages, this approach is likely to be of considerable utility in the identification of specific developmental pathways (Hirshfeld et al., 1998; Lease & Ollendick, 2000; Ollendick & Hirshfeld-Becker, 2002; Ollendick & Vasey, 1999; Vasey & Ollendick, 2000).

ETIOLOGY

Several groups of children and adolescents are at risk to develop anxiety disorders, including PD. These children include offspring of parents who are anxious or depressed or both; so-called behaviorally inhibited children (Kagan, Reznick, & Snidman, 1988); and, more controversially, children with psychological characteristics that portend anxiety outcomes (Mattis & Ollendick, 1997a).

As noted by Hirshfeld and colleagues (1998), considerable evidence exists that anxiety can and does run in families. Family history studies, for example, show that PD can be familial, although the relative contributions of genes and environment to that familiality is difficult to determine. Because family members share environments as well as genes, disorders such as PD may run in families for reasons that have little to do with genetics. Family and twin studies, however, suggest that genetic factors influence liability to PD (heritability estimates range from 32 to 46%). Still, and as is evident in these heritability estimates, environmental factors explain a somewhat larger portion of the variance. Model fitting of genetic and environmental components of variance in the Virginia Twin Registry study (Kendler, Neale, Kessler, Heath, & Eaves, 1993) indicate that the liability to PD is primarily due to additive-genetic and individual-specific environmental effects rather than to family environment more broadly. Investigations are currently underway to sort out these influences and, using the methods of molecular genetics, to map genes that influence anxiety disorders more generally and PAs and PD in particular. In all probability, PD, like many other psychiatric disorders, may be influenced by several genes (oligogenic) or many genes (polygenic), each exerting a small but nontrivial effect. Multifactorial inheritance is likely (Hirshfeld et al., 1998).

Behavioral inhibition (BI) occurs in 10–15% of European American children and is manifested by the tendency to withdraw, to seek a parent, and to inhibit play and vocalization following encounter with unfamiliar events or people (Kagan et al., 1988). As infants, these children tend to be irritable and overly reactive; as toddlers, they tend to be introverted and quiet and to show increased vigilance and reduced exploratory behavior. In contrast to uninhibited children, these children have low thresholds for arousal in the amygdala and hypothalamic circuits, resulting in increased sympathetic arousal (Hirshfeld et al., 1998). Parents of children with BI usually have anxiety disorders themselves, including—but not limited to—PD (Biederman et al., 2001; Hirshfeld et al., 1998). Moreover, offspring of parents with PD and agoraphobia (as well as MDD) tend to have high rates of BI. Children with *persistent* BI have higher rates of anxiety disorders than children who are not inhibited and children who do not show persistent inhibition. Other studies have shown that monozygotic twins are more concordant for BI than dyzygotic twins are (DiLalla, Kagan, & Reznick, 1994; Matheny, 1989; Robinson, Kagan, Reznick, & Corley, 1992). Heritability estimates of BI approach .50. These findings suggest a significant genetic contribution to BI, which, in turn, appears to signal development of anxiety disorder. It is important to note, however, that not all children characterized as behaviorally inhibited develop PD (or other anxiety disorders). In addition, it appears that BI itself may be preceded by high reactivity (high negative affect and irritability in infancy). Kagan and Snidman (1991), for example, have reported that a number of children with BI have histories of high reactivity and, conversely, that about two-thirds of high-reactive infants go on to become behaviorally inhibited in toddlerhood.

Children who have high stress reactivity and poor self-regulatory ability and who fail to regulate distress through caregiver contact and comfort may also be at increased risk to develop PAs and eventual PD (Mattis & Ollendick, 1997a; Ollendick, 1998). After repeated experiences of separation, these children may begin to view separation and associated alarms as frightening experiences and develop anxious apprehension over the possibility that they will recur. Over time, such instances are hypothesized to lead to increased AS and attributions of internal responsibility for the negative outcomes associated with these experiences (Mattis & Ollendick, 1997a; Ollendick, 1998). Anxiety sensitivity, in particular, has been shown to be associated with the development of anxiety disorders, including PD in both adults (Rapee, Ancis, & Barlow, 1988) and in children and adolescents (Mattis & Ollendick, 1997b; Rabian, Peterson, Richters, & Jensen, 1993). Finally, avoidance behaviors (agoraphobia) may develop in the absence of safety signals (a secure base) and the absence of effective coping skills and self-efficacy for the mastery of such stressful situations (Ollendick, 1995, 1998). Such an "experiential" and "cognitive" pathway remains to be demonstrated prospectively, however.

Although space in this chapter does not permit a full explication of etiological pathways to the onset of PAs and PD, it appears safe to conclude that multiple pathways exist, including those associated with genetic, temperamental, cognitive, familial, and environmental risk factors. Moreover, it appears that any one pathway, including the one associated with any one of these risk factors, does not necessarily result in PD. Such a conclusion is consistent with the tenets of developmental psychopathology: namely, that multiple pathways can lead to any one disorder (the principle of equifinality) and that any one pathway can result in a diversity of outcomes, only one of which is PD (the principle of multifinality; Ollendick & Hirshfeld-Becker, 2002; Toth & Cicchetti, 1999).

TREATMENT

This section reviews psychosocial and pharmacological treatments for PD. Most of the studies with adults and all of the available studies with children and adolescents address the acute treatment of PD. Studies evaluating the effects of continuation (to avoid relapses) and maintenance (to avoid recurrences, i.e., new episodes) of treatment are scarce in the adult literature and do not exist in the child and adolescent literature. Given the paucity of studies with children and adolescents, most of the treatments described in this section are extrapolated from the adult literature. Accordingly, appropriate caution should be exercised, because adult treatments do not always take into account developmental factors and because children may respond differently to psychological and pharmacological treatments than their adult counterparts do (Birmaher & Ollendick, 2003; Ollendick & Vasey, 1999).

Psychoeducation

For both psychosocial and pharmacological treatments, education about the problem or disorder is indicated. Children and their parents should be educated about the symptom picture, the developmental course (if known), the etiology (again, if known), and the assessment and treatment of that disorder. Psychoeducation can increase compliance with treatment, reduce anxiety, and improve the child's self-esteem (e.g., the child can understand that having PAs is not a sign of weakness) and family relationships (e.g., parents understand that child is not pretending; parents may diminish self-blame). Although no studies have been published on the effects of psychoeducation alone for children and adolescents with PD, for other disorders—including depression, bipolar disorder, and even schizophrenia—psychoeducation alone and in combination with active treatments has been found to be helpful (e.g., Brent, Poling, McKain, & Baugher, 1993). The American Psychiatric Association's (1998) *Practice Guidelines for the Treatment of Patients with Panic Disorder* also stress the importance of psychoeducation, whether or not psychosocial or pharmacological interventions are implemented subsequently.

Acute Treatment

Psychosocial Interventions

Psychosocial treatments for the successful treatment of PD have been based largely on cognitive and cognitive-behavioral theories (Chambless & Ollendick, 2001). The primary proponents of the cognitive model have been Beck and Clark (Beck & Emery, 1985; Clark, Salkovskis, & Chalkley, 1985). In its simplest form, this model suggests that the insidious spiral into panic is due to catastrophic misinterpretations of otherwise normal bodily sensations. Implicit in this theory is the notion that nothing particularly unique is occurring in the individual from a neurobiological perspective; rather, it is primarily a "psychological" account of the development and maintenance of panic. Mild chest pain experienced after exercise, for example, might be interpreted by an at-risk or psychologically vulnerable youngster as an impending heart attack from which the young person believes he or she might actually die. Individual differences in the tendency to misinterpret somatic events would differentiate the child or adolescent who develops PAs and the one who does not. Youngsters high in AS (i.e., anxiety sensitivity) might more likely be vulnerable to the onset of PAs and the development of PD. Treatment, according to this theory, consists largely of a mixture of cognitive techniques and behavioral experiments designed to modify the faulty misinterpretations of bodily sensations and the processes that serve to maintain them. Considerable support for this model has been garnered in recent years for the treatment of PAs and PD, at least with adults (cf. Clark, 1996; Clark et al., 1999). To our knowledge, this approach has not been used nor evaluated with children and adolescents, however.

The primary proponent of the cognitive-behavioral model has been Barlow (2002), and the treatment evolving from this perspective has come to be called Panic Control Treatment (PCT). According to Barlow, several risk factors are required in order for PAs and PD to develop. First, a person must have the tendency to be neurobiologically overreactive to stress. In particular, some individuals seem to react to the stress of negative life events with considerable apprehension, believing that some drastic or terrible thing will happen to them. Such apprehension leads to a fight-or-flight response that is, in all likelihood, triggered prematurely and unnecessarily. That is, the response exceeds the stimulus event. Barlow refers to this premature, unnecessary, and extreme response as a "false alarm." Over time, through a process of conditioning, false alarms become associated with bodily sensations (e.g., rapid heartbeat, difficulty breathing), and PAs follow. After repeated conditioning trials, the person becomes extremely sensitive to the physical sensations so that even slight bodily changes associated with exercise or fatigue, for example, trigger an alarm reaction and a resultant PA. Subsequently, the individual develops anxious apprehension over the possibility that future alarms or PAs will occur. This tendency to develop anxious apprehension is viewed as a psychological vulnerability that arises from developmental experiences in which predictability and control are largely absent. Finally, avoidance behavior may develop depending on the person's coping skills and perceptions of safety.

Treatment from this model is composed of three primary strategies: relaxation training and breathing retraining to address neurobiological sensitivities to stress; interoceptive exposure to address heightened somatic symptoms; and cognitive restructuring to address faulty misinterpretations associated with the somatic symptoms. In effect, this model consists of cognitive therapy (similar to that espoused by Beck and Emery [1985] and

Clark et al. [1985]), as well as behavioral therapy (relaxation training, breathing retraining, interoceptive exposure). Considerable support for this cognitive-behavioral model has been garnered in recent years in the treatment of PAs and PD, especially with adults (Barlow, Gorman, Shear, & Woods, 2000; Barlow & Lehman, 1996).

Mattis and Ollendick (1997b) adapted Barlow's model of panic to children and suggested a pathway through which stressful separation experiences, in combination with individual differences in temperament characteristics and attachment styles, result in development of panic. They propose that children respond to stressful separation experiences differently depending on their temperaments (in particular, behavioral inhibition) and the nature of their attachment relationships with significant adults (in particular, insecure-ambivalent or resistant relationships). According to this model, children who are characterized by this constellation of variables and events are at high risk for the development of PAs and eventual PD. Inasmuch as these children have difficulty being soothed and comforted by their caregivers in times of stress (e.g., separations), they experience intense alarm reactions and have little sense of predictability or control over these stressors. These at-risk children learn to associate distress in these situations with physical or somatic symptoms (e.g., pounding heart, shaky hands), resulting in a cascade of false alarms. Next, as suggested by Mattis and Ollendick (1997b), the child begins to display anxious apprehension over the possibility of future alarms or panic attacks. Anxious apprehension is viewed as a psychological vulnerability, encapsulated in the notion of AS (anxiety sensitivity). PA symptoms are likely to occur when these at-risk children perceive little control over what will happen to them and little ability to predict what will happen to them in the future. Agoraphobic avoidance develops when the children begin to withdraw from unfamiliar people and situations as a way of coping with and reducing their distress (Mattis & Ollendick, 2002).

Treatment studies based on Barlow's (2002) model and Mattis and Ollendick's (2002) adaptation of it have been sparse; however, two single-case studies lend initial support to its use, and one randomized, large-scale treatment outcome study appears promising. In the first study, Barlow and Seidner (1983) treated three adolescent agoraphobics with an early rendition of PCT. The adolescents were treated in a 10-session group-therapy format and were accompanied by their mothers, who were enlisted to facilitate behavior change. Treatment consisted of panic-management procedures, cognitive restructuring, and instructions to engage in structured homework sessions, which involved graduated exposure to feared situations. Parents were instructed in the nature of agoraphobia and procedures for dealing with anxiety that were neither reinforcing of anxiety-related behaviors nor punishing to the adolescent. Parents encouraged and supported their teens in practicing between sessions, and they practiced with them at least once a week. Following treatment, two of the three adolescents showed marked improvement in their symptoms; however, the other adolescent did not show significant change. In fact, treatment resulted in a slight increment in phobic avoidance for this adolescent. Barlow and Seidner (1983) suggested that treatment outcome was related to level of parent–adolescent conflict; that is, for the two families in which a reasonably good parent–adolescent relationship was evident, treatment was successful; for the remaining family, the presence of parent–adolescent conflict appeared to interfere with treatment outcome. Although this single-case group study was uncontrolled and only two of the three adolescents responded positively, the treatment appeared promising.

In the second study, Ollendick (1995) used a controlled multiple-baseline design across four adolescents with panic disorder with agoraphobia (PDA) to illustrate the controlling effects of the adapted version of PCT. The adolescents ranged in age from 13 to 17 years of age; however, their PAs began when they were between 9 and 13 years of age—nearly 4 years, on average, prior to the beginning of treatment. Adolescents were treated individually and alone but, as in Barlow and Seidner (1983), their mothers were enlisted to facilitate behavior change. Treatment consisted of information about panic (i.e., psychoeducation), relaxation training and breathing retraining, cognitive restructuring, interoceptive exposure, participant modeling (e.g., the therapist and then the parent demonstrated approach behavior in agoraphobic situations), *in vivo* exposure, and profuse praise and social reinforcement. Treatment varied in duration but lasted between 10 and 12 sessions. Treatment was effective for all four adolescents in eliminating panic attacks, reducing agoraphobic avoidance, decreasing accompanying negative mood states, and increasing self-efficacy for coping with previously avoided situations and panic attacks should they occur in the future. Follow-up over a 6-month interval affirmed the lasting effects of the treatment. As noted by Ollendick, this single-case-design study did not allow the mechanisms of change to be detected. Multiple cognitive-behavioral treatment components were used, and parents were recruited to facilitate and encourage change in their adolescents. Any one of these components, either alone or in concert with other components, might have been responsible for the changes observed. Future research will need to identify the effective ingredients in randomized clinical control trials with children and adolescents.

Presently, Mattis and her colleagues are undertaking a randomized controlled trial of a developmental adaptation of Panic Control Treatment (PCT-A) and a self-monitoring control condition in the treatment of PD in adolescents (Mattis, personal communication, 2002). Three aspects of PD are addressed in this intervention: (1) the cognitive aspect of PD, or the tendency to misinterpret physical sensations as catastrophic; (2) the tendency to hyperventilate or overbreathe, thus creating and/or intensifying physical sensations of panic; and (3) conditioned fear reactions to the physical sensations. Key components of treatment include correcting misinformation about panic, breathing retraining, cognitive restructuring, and interoceptive and *in vivo* exposure. In the interoceptive exposure component of treatment, the adolescents are taught to face their primary fear; namely, the physical sensations of panic. Exercises such as shaking their heads from side to side for 30 seconds, running in place for 1 minute, holding their breath for 30 seconds, spinning in a chair for 1 minute, hyperventilating for 1 minute, and breathing through a thin straw for 2 minutes are used to facilitate exposure to the interoceptive physical sensations. Adolescents are informed that they will be learning different "tools" or ways to address their panic and resultant anxiety. Specifically, "Changing My Breathing" is described as a tool for reducing the frequency and intensity of unwanted or undesired physical sensations; "Being a Detective" is introduced as the process of evaluating and changing anxious, worrisome, and nonproductive thoughts; and "Facing My Fears" is the strategy for reducing avoidance through interoceptive and graduated *in vivo* exposure exercises. The adolescent is further informed that the goal of using these tools is to break the cycle of panic by reducing physical panic sensations, anxious thoughts, and avoidance, while also altering the relations among the components. For example, reducing physical sensations through breathing retraining will also change anxious thoughts associated with the sensations and, in turn, reduce the likelihood that avoidance of the situation will be necessary or desired. Eleven sessions, all manualized, are enacted. Although the randomized trial is still underway, initial findings show significant reduction in severity of PAs and PD, as well as AS, in those adolescents receiving PCT-A relative to those in the monitoring control group (Mattis et al., 2001). These preliminary findings appear to support the efficacy of this innovative adaptation of PCT.

At this point in time, it is obvious that psychosocial treatments have been used only sparingly with adolescents and not at all with children who present with PD. The reasons for this state of affairs are not at all clear, especially as very similar procedures have been used effectively with children and adolescents with other forms of phobic and anxiety disorders (see Ollendick & King, 1998, 2000, for reviews). Many of these cognitive-behavioral treatments enjoy empirically validated status. It is perhaps even more alarming that no other psychosocial treatments (i.e., interpersonal psychotherapy, psychodynamic therapy, family therapy) have been evaluated with children and adolescents who present with PAs or PD. Clearly, the development and evaluation of psychosocial treatments for PAs and PD in children and adolescents are in an embryonic stage and are sorely in need of systematic inquiry.

Phamacological Interventions

As with psychosocial treatments, no randomized controlled trials (RCTs) for the pharmacological treatment of PD in children and adolescents have yet been completed (Birmaher & Ollendick, 2003; Kutcher & Mackenzie, 1988). In adults, RCTs comparing the following classes of medications with placebo have been found to be relatively effective in the treatment of PD: the selective serotonin reuptake inhibitors (SSRIs; 60–80% vs. 36–60%); the tricyclic antidepressants (TCAs; 45–70% vs. 15–50%); and the high-potency benzodiazepines (55–75% vs. 15–50%). The SSRIs have been the first choice because of their easier administration and side-effects profile and because they are thought to be less dangerous in case of an overdose. Although the monoamine oxidase inhibitors (MAOIs) are also efficacious in the treatment of PD in adults (APA, 1998), they are used primarily for those patients who have not responded well to other treatments; however, they also carry the risk of hypertensive crisis and require dietary restrictions.

Anecdotal case reports have shown that benzodiazepines (e.g., Biederman, 1987; Kutcher & Mackenzie, 1988; Lepola, Leinonen, & Koponen, 1996; Simeon & Ferguson, 1987; Simeon et al., 1992) and the SSRIs (e.g., Fairbanks et al., 1997; Renaud, Birmaher, Wassick, & Bridge, 1999) may be efficacious treatments for PD in children and adolescents. For example, in a prospective open trial, Renaud and colleagues (1999) treated 12 children and adolescents with PD with SSRIs for a period of 6–8 weeks. The youths were followed for 6 months and evaluated periodically with clinician-based and self-report rating scales for anxiety and depression, global functioning, and side effects. Nearly 75% of the youths showed much to very much improvement with SSRIs without experiencing significant side effects. At the end of the trial, eight (67%) no longer fulfilled criteria for PD, whereas four (33%) continued to have significant and persisting residual symptoms.

On the basis of the adult literature, clinical experience, results of several open trials, and the fact that SSRIs have been effective in the treatment of children and adolescents with other anxiety disorders (Research Units of Pediatric Psychopharmacology Anxiety Study Group [RUPP], 2001) and major depressive disorders (e.g., Emslie et al., 1997), Birmaher and Ollendick (2003) suggest that the SSRIs are a safe and promising treatment for children and adolescents with PD as well. However, they also note that RCTs evaluating the effects of SSRIs in youths are sorely needed at this time.

Until these studies are carried out and more evidence is accumulated, it appears that the pharmacological treatment of choice to treat PD in youngsters is the SSRIs. As recommended by Birmaher and Ollendick (2003), these medications should be initiated with low doses (e.g., fluoxetine 5 mg per day, fluvoxamine 12.5 mg per day, paroxetine 10 mg per day, sertraline 25 mg per day) to avoid the potential exacerbation of panic symptoms that sometimes have been observed in adults with PD (American Psychiatric Association, 1998). Starting with low doses also diminishes the risk of producing side effects, especially in youngsters who are known to be highly sensitive to experiencing somatic symptoms and whose parents also have anxiety disorder and may be overanxious about the appearance of minor side effects.

For an appropriate acute trial, the SSRIs should be administered for at least 12 weeks (American Psychiatric Association, 1998). Youths who have not shown improvement within 6–8 weeks should be reevaluated with regard to diagnosis, compliance with treatment, presence of comorbid disorders or medical, neurological, and psychosocial problems. These youngsters may require changes in medications or combination treatment with psychotherapy (e.g., CBT, as discussed previously).

For children and adolescents who do not tolerate or respond to at least two trials with SSRIs, other types of medications that have been found useful for the treatment of adults with PD, such as venlafaxine, nefazodone, or the TCAs, can be tried (APA, 1998; Birmaher & Ollendick, 2003). If TCAs are used, close monitoring of blood pressure, pulse, and heart rate, as well the development of other TCA side effects (e.g, anticholinergic), is required.

As described previously, the high-potency benzodiazepines (e.g., alprazolam) are also efficacious for the treatment of adults with PD (American Psychiatric Association, 1998). However, due to the risk of developing tolerance and dependence after long-term use, it is better to consider the temporary use of these medications for situations in which rapid control of symptoms is necessary (e.g., a youngster with severe PAs who requires frequent visits to the medical or psychiatric emergency room; a child adamantly refusing to go to school because he is afraid of having a PA at school; or an adolescent with recurrent fainting episodes in theaters or malls). When these circumstances occur, it is recommended that the benzodiazepine be combined with the SSRIs, then, after several weeks, the benzodiazepines tapered down for several weeks (e.g., 12 weeks) at rates no higher than 10% of the dose per week (American Psychiatric Association, 1998; Birmaher & Ollendick, 2003). The benzodiazepines are generally contraindicated in youths with substance abuse. Because some SSRIs (e.g., fluvoxamine) may interfere with the metabolism of the benzodiazepines and increase blood levels (Leonard, March, Rickler, & Allen,

1997), caution is recommended. In this case, lower doses of benzodiaze-pines may suffice.

As noted earlier, PD is accompanied frequently by a variety of other psychiatric disorders. Treatment of these comorbid conditions is essential to improving the youngster's functioning. Fortunately, two of the common comorbid disorders, depression and other anxiety disorders, may also re-spond to SSRIs, CBT, or both (Birmaher et al., 1994; Brent et al., 1997; Emslie et al. 1997; Kendall et al., 1997; Ollendick & King, 1998, 2000; RUPP, 2001).

Finally, given that children and adolescents are frequently dependent on their parents; that PD, as well as other anxiety disorders and depression, run in families (e.g., Biederman et al., 2001); and that parental psychiatric disorders may affect the treatment response and course of several psychiat-ric illnesses, it is important to offer treatment to parents as well (Birmaher & Ollendick, 2003).

Combined Interventions

To date, no controlled clinical trials have examined the joint efficacy of psychosocial and pharmacological treatments with children or adolescents. Given the independent promise of both treatments, however, there is reason to believe that synergistic effects will occur, as has been evidenced in the treatment of other anxiety disorders with children and adolescents, as well as with adults. Still, research into their combinatorial effects, like that pur-sued in adult populations, is needed (e.g., Barlow et al., 2000) before firm conclusions can be drawn.

Continuation and Maintenance Treatments

Similar to other psychiatric and medical illnesses, after achieving a thera-peutic response, it is important to continue the same treatment (CBT and/ or medications) to prevent relapses. During these phases, depending on the youngster's clinical status, she or he may need to be seen less frequently. Unfortunately, very little research in adults (American Psychiatric Associa-tion, 1998) and none in youths regarding the continuation and mainte-nance treatment phases for PD have been carried out. In adults, it has been recommended to continue the medications for at least 12–18 months and, thereafter, if the person is judged to be stable, to reduce the medications very slowly to avoid withdrawal side effects that may mimic the relapse of PAs and to avoid relapses or recurrences (American Psychiatric Associa-tion, 1998). Although it is unknown at this time, it is conceivable that at least some children and adolescents will require treatment for years, consis-tent with findings from the adult literature.

FUTURE DIRECTIONS AND CONCLUSIONS

The study of PAs and PD in children and adolescents is truly in its own stage of early development (Birmaher & Ollendick, 2003; Mattis & Ollendick, 2002). Although it was initially thought that children could not develop PAs and PD due to cognitive limitations, it now seems clear that children (and adolescents) can and do develop these disorders. Moreover, as with adults, these disorders are frequently comorbid with other anxiety and affective disorders and, albeit less frequently, comorbid with externalizing disorders, such as substance abuse and conduct disturbance. The effects of these disorders on the developing child are considerable; many of these children experience academic, behavioral, emotional, and social difficulties. Still, the developmental course of PD is poorly understood at this time and is in need of careful examination and inquiry. Treatment, especially treatment guided by a stages-of-treatment model, is unfortunately not well established at this time. Yet promising psychosocial and pharmacological interventions exist. However, RCTs with children and adolescents are lacking, and little has been done in terms of the combination of psychosocial and pharmacological treatments. Hence, although we know much about PAs and PD in children and adolescents, much remains to be learned.

REFERENCES

Alessi, N. E., & Magen, J. (1988). Panic disorders in psychiatrically hospitalized children. *American Journal of Psychiatry, 145*,1450–1452.

Alessi, N. E., Robbins, D. R., & Dilsaver, S. C. (1987). Panic and depressive disorders among psychiatrically hospitalized adolescents. *Psychiatry Research, 20,* 275–283.

American Psychiatric Association. (1994). *Diagnostic and Statistical Manual of Mental Disorders* (4th ed.). Washington, DC: Author.

American Psychiatric Association. (1998). Practice guidelines for the treatment of patients with panic disorder. *American Journal of Psychiatry, 155,* 1–34.

Barlow, D. H. (2002). *Anxiety and its disorders: The nature and treatment of anxiety and panic* (2nd ed.). New York: Guilford Press.

Barlow, D. H., Gorman, J. M., Shear, M. K., & Woods, S. W. (2000). Cognitive-behavioral therapy, imipramine, or their combination for panic disorder: A randomized controlled trial. *Journal of the American Medical Association, 283*(19), 2529–2536.

Barlow, D. H., & Lehman, C. L. (1996). Advances in the psychosocial treatment of anxiety disorders: Implications for national health care. *Archives of General Psychiatry, 53,* 727–735.

Barlow, D. H., & Seidner, A. L. (1983). Treatment of adolescent agoraphobics: Effects on parent-adolescent relations. *Behaviour Research and Therapy, 21,*519–526.

Battaglia, M., Bertella, S., Bajo, S., Binaghi, F., & Bellodi, L. (1998). Anticipation of age at onset in panic disorder. *American Journal of Psychiatry, 155*, 590–595.

Beck, A. T., & Emery, G. (1985). *Anxiety disorders and phobias: A cognitive perspective.* Philadelphia: Center for Cognitive Therapy.

Biederman, J. (1987). Clonazepam in the treatment of prepubertal children with panic-like symptoms. *Journal of Clinical Psychiatry, 48*(Suppl.), 38–41.

Biederman, J., Faraone, S. V., Hirshfeld-Becker, D. R., Friedman, D., Robin, J. A., & Rosenbaum, J. F. (2001). Patterns of psychopathology and dysfunction in high-risk children of parents with panic disorder and major depression. *American Journal of Psychiatry, 158*(1), 49–57.

Biederman, J., Faraone, S. V., Marrs, A., Moore, P., Garcia, J., Ablon, S., Mick, E., Gershon, J., & Kearns, M. E. (1997). Panic disorder and agoraphobia in consecutively referred children and adolescents. *Journal of the American Academy of Child and Adolescent Psychiatry, 36*, 214–223.

Birmaher, B., & Ollendick, T. H. (2003). Childhood onset panic disorder. In T. H. Ollendick & J. S. March (Eds.), *Phobic and anxiety disorders in children and adolescents: A clinician's guide to effective psychosocial and pharmacological interventions* (pp. 110–132). New York: Oxford University Press.

Birmaher, B., Waterman, G. S., Ryan, N. D., Cully, M., Balach, L., Ingram, J., & Brodsky, M. (1994). Fluoxetine for childhood anxiety disorders. *Journal of the American Academy of Child and Adolescent Psychiatry, 33*, 993–999.

Brent, D. A., Holder, D., Kolko, D., Birmaher, B., Baugher, M., Roth, C., Iyengar, S., & Johnson, B. A. (1997). A clinical psychotherapy trial for adolescent depression comparing cognitive, family, and supportive therapy. *Archives of General Psychiatry, 54*, 877–885.

Brent, D. A., Poling, K., McKain, B., & Baugher, M. (1993). A psychoeducational program for families of affectively ill children and adolescents. *Journal of the American Academy of Child and Adolescent Psychiatry, 32*, 770–774.

Chambless, D. L., & Ollendick, T. H. (2001). Empirically supported psychological interventions: Controversies and evidence. *Annual Review of Psychology, 52*, 685–716.

Clark, D. M. (1996). Panic disorder: From theory to therapy. In P. M. Salkovskis (Ed.), *Frontiers of cognitive therapy: The state of the art and beyond* (pp. 318–344). New York: Guilford Press.

Clark, D. M., Salkovskis, P. M., & Chalkley, A. J. (1985). Respiratory control as a treatment for panic attacks. *Journal of Behavior Therapy and Experimental Psychiatry, 16*, 23–30.

Clark, D. M., Salkovskis, P. M., Hackmann, A., Wells, A., Ludgate, J., & Gelder, M. (1999). Brief cognitive therapy for panic disorder: A randomized controlled trial. *Journal of Consulting and Clinical Psychology, 67*, 583–589.

Craske, M. G., Poulton, R., Tsao, J. C., & Plotkin, D. (2001). Paths to panic disorder/agoraphobia: An exploratory analysis from age 3 to 21 in an unselected birth cohort. *Journal of the American Academy of Child and Adolescent Psychiatry, 40*, 556–563.

DiLalla, K., Kagan, J., & Reznick, J. (1994). Genetic etiology of behavioral inhibition among 2-year-old children. *Infant Behavior and Development, 17*, 405–412.

Emslie, G. J., Rush, A. J., Weinberg, W. A., Kowatch, R. A., Hughes, C. W., Carmody,

T., & Rintelmann, J. (1997). A double-blind, randomized, placebo-controlled trial of fluoxetine in children and adolescents with depression. *Archives of General Psychiatry, 54*, 1031–1037.

Essau, C. A., Conradt, J., & Petermann, F. (1999). Frequency of panic attacks and panic disorder in adolescents. *Depression and Anxiety, 9*, 19–26.

Essau, C. A., Conradt, J., & Petermann, F. (2000). Frequency, comorbidity, and psychosocial impairment of anxiety disorders in German adolescents. *Journal of Anxiety Disorders, 14*, 263–279.

Fairbanks, J. M., Pine, D. S., Tancer, N. K., Dummit E. S., III, Kentgen, L. M., Asche, B. K., & Klein, R. G. (1997). Open fluoxetine treatment of mixed anxiety disorders in children and adolescents. *Journal of the American Academy of Child and Adolescent Psychiatry, 7*, 17–29.

Ginsburg, G. S., & Drake, K. L. (2002). Anxiety sensitivity and panic attack symptomatology among low-income African-American adolescents. *Journal of Anxiety Disorders, 16*, 83–96.

Goldstein, R. B., Wickramarante, P. J., Horwath, E., & Weissman, M. M. (1997). Familial aggregation and phenomenology of "early"-onset (at or before age 20 years) panic disorder. *Archives of General Psychiatry, 54*, 271–278.

Hayward, C., Killen, J. D., Kraemer, H. C., & Barr Taylor, C. (2000). Predictors of panic attacks in adolescents. *Journal of the American Academy of Child and Adolescent Psychiatry, 39*, 207–214.

Hayward, C., Killen, J. D., Kraemer, H. C., Blair-Greiner, A., Strachowski, D., Cunning, D., & Barr Taylor, C. (1997). Assessment and phenomenology of nonclinical panic attacks in adolescent girls. *Journal of Anxiety Disorders, 11*, 17–32.

Hayward, C., Killen, J. D., & Taylor, C. B. (1989). Panic attacks in young adolescents. *American Journal of Psychiatry, 146*, 1061–1062.

Hirshfeld, D. R., Rosenbaum, J. F., Smoller, J. W., Fredman, S. J., & Bulzacchelli, M. T. (1998). Early antecedents of panic disorder. In J. F. Rosenbaum & M. W. Pollack (Eds.), *Panic disorder and its treatment* (pp. 93–151). New York: Dekker.

Horesh, N., Amir, M., Kedem, P., Goldberger, Y., & Kotler, M. (1997). Life events in childhood, adolescence and adulthood and the relationship to panic disorder. *Acta Psychiatrica Scandinavica, 96*, 373–378.

Kagan, J., Reznick, J. S., & Snidman, N. (1988). Biological bases of childhood shyness. *Science, 240*, 167–171.

Kagan, J., & Snidman, N. (1991). Infant predictors of inhibited and uninhibited profiles. *Psychological Science, 2*, 40–44.

Kazdin, A. E. (2000). *Psychotherapy for children and adolescents: Directions for research and practice*. New York: Oxford University Press.

Kearney, C. A., Albano, A. M., Eisen, A. R., Allan, W. D., & Barlow, D. H. (1997). The phenomenology of panic disorder in youngsters: An empirical study of a clinical sample. *Journal of Anxiety Disorders, 11*, 49–62.

Kendall, P. C., Flannery-Schroeder, E., Panichelli-Mindel, S., Southam-Gerow, M., Henin, A., & Warman, M. (1997). Therapy for youth with anxiety disorders: A second randomized clinical trial. *Journal of Consulting and Clinical Psychology, 65*, 366–380.

Kendler, K. S., Neale, M. C., Kessler, R. C., Heath, A. C., & Eaves, L. J. (1993). Panic disorder in women: A population-based twin study. *Psychological Medicine, 23,* 397–406.

King, N. J., Gullone, E., Tonge, B. J., & Ollendick, T. H. (1993). Self-reports of panic attacks and manifest anxiety in adolescents. *Behaviour Research and Therapy, 31,*111–116.

King, N. J., Ollendick, T. H., Mattis, S. G., Yang, B., & Tonge, B. (1997). Nonclinical panic attacks in adolescents: Prevalence, symptomatology and associated features. *Behaviour Change, 13,*171–183.

Kutcher, S., & Mackenzie, S. (1988). Successful clonazepam treatment of adolescents with panic disorder. *Journal of Clinical Psychopharmacology, 8,* 299–301.

Last, C. G., & Strauss, C. C. (1989). Panic disorder in children and adolescents. *Journal of Anxiety Disorders, 3,* 87–95.

Lau, J. J., Calamari, J. E., & Waraczynski, M. (1996). Panic attack symptomatology and anxiety sensitivity in adolescents. *Journal of Anxiety Disorders, 10,* 355–364.

Lease, C. A., & Ollendick, T. H. (2000). Development and psychopathology. In A. S. Bellack & M. Hersen (Eds.), *Psychopathology in adulthood* (pp. 131–149). Boston: Allyn & Bacon.

Leonard, H. L., March, J., Rickler, K. C., & Allen, A. J. (1997). Pharmacology of the selective serotonin reuptake inhibitors in children and adolescents. *Journal of the American Academy of Child and Adolescent Psychiatry, 36,* 725–736.

Lepola, U., Leinonen, E., & Koponen, H. (1996). Citalopram in the treatment of early-onset panic disorder and school phobia. *Pharmacopsychiatry, 29,* 30–32.

Macaulay, J. L., & Kleinknecht, R. A. (1989). Panic and panic attacks in adolescents. *Journal of Anxiety Disorders, 3,* 221–241.

Matheny, A. P. (1989). Children's behavioral inhibition over age and across situations: Genetic similarity for a trait during change. *Journal of Personality, 57,*215–235.

Mattis, S. G., Hoffman, E. C., Cohen, E. M., Pincus, D. B., Choate, M. L., & Micco, J. A. (2001, March). Cognitive-behavioral treatment of panic disorder in adolescence. In C. L. Masia & E. A. Stroch (Chairs), *Treatment of childhood anxiety: Innovative interventions and future directions.* Symposium conducted at the meeting of the Anxiety Disorders Association of America, Atlanta, GA.

Mattis, S. G., & Ollendick, T. H. (1997a) Children's cognitive responses to the somatic symptoms of panic. *Journal of Abnormal Child Psychology, 25,* 47–57.

Mattis, S. G., & Ollendick, T. H. (1997b). Panic in children and adolescents: A developmental analysis. In T. H. Ollendick & R. J. Prinz (Eds.), *Advances in clinical child psychology* (Vol. 19, pp. 27–74). New York: Plenum Press.

Mattis, S. G., & Ollendick, T. H. (2002). *Panic disorder and anxiety in adolescents.* London: British Psychological Society.

Moreau, D. L., & Follet, C. (1993). Panic disorder in children and adolescents. *Child and Adolescent Psychiatric Clinics North America, 2,* 581–602.

Moreau, D. L., & Weissman, M. M. (1992). Panic disorder in children and adolescents: A review. *American Journal of Psychiatry, 149,* 1306–1314.

Nelles, W. B., & Barlow, D. H. (1988). Do children panic? *Clinical Psychology Review, 8,* 359–372.

Ollendick, T. H. (1995). Cognitive-behavioral treatment of panic disorder with agoraphobia in adolescents: A multiple baseline design analysis. *Behavior Therapy*, *26*, 517–531.

Ollendick, T. H. (1998). Panic disorder in children and adolescents: New developments, new directions. *Journal of Clinical Child Psychology*, *27*, 234–245.

Ollendick, T. H., & Hersen, M. (Eds.). (1999). *Handbook of child psychopathology* (3rd ed.). New York: Plenum Press.

Ollendick, T. H., & Hirshfeld-Becker, D. R. (2002). The developmental psychopathology of social anxiety disorder. *Biological Psychiatry*, *51*, 44–58.

Ollendick, T. H., & Huntzinger, R. M. (1990). Separation Anxiety Disorders in children. In M. Hersen & C. G. Last (Eds.), *Handbook of child and adult psychopathology: A longitudinal perspective* (pp. 133–149). New York: Pergamon Press.

Ollendick, T. H., & King, N. J. (1998). Empirically supported treatments for children with phobic and anxiety disorders: Current status. *Journal of Clinical Child Psychology*, *27*,156–167.

Ollendick, T. H., & King, N. J. (2000). Empirically supported treatments for children and adolescents. In P. C. Kendall (Ed.), *Child and adolescent therapy: Cognitive-behavioral procedures* (2nd ed., pp. 386–425). New York: Guilford Press.

Ollendick, T. H., Mattis, S. G., & King, N. J. (1994). Panic in children and adolescents: A review. *Journal of Child Psychology and Psychiatry*, *35*,113–134.

Ollendick, T. H., & Vasey, M. W. (1999). Developmental theory and the practice of clinical child psychology. *Journal of Clinical Child Psychology*, *28*, 457–466.

Rabian, B., Peterson, R. A., Richters, J., & Jensen, P. S. (1993). Anxiety sensitivity among anxious children. *Journal of Clinical Child Psychology*, *22*, 441–446.

Rapee, R., Ancis, J., & Barlow, D. (1988). Emotional reactions to physiological sensations: Panic disorder patients and non-clinical subjects. *Behaviour Research Therapy*, *26*, 265–269.

Renaud, J., Birmaher, B., Wassick, S. C., & Bridge, J. (1999). Use of selective serotonin reuptake inhibitors for the treatment of childhood panic disorder: A pilot study. *Journal of Child and Adolescent Psychopharmacology*, *9*, 73–83.

Research Units of Pediatric Psychopharmacology Anxiety Study Group. (2001). Fluvoxamine for anxiety in children. *New England Journal of Medicine*, *344*, 1279–1285.

Robinson, J. L., Kagan, J., Reznick, J. S., & Corley, R. (1992). The heritability of inhibited and uninhibited behavior: A twin study. *Developmental Psychology*, *28*, 1030–1037.

Silove, D., Manicavasagar, V., Curtis, J., & Blaszczynski, A. (1996). Is early separation anxiety a risk factor for adult panic disorder? A critical review. *Comprehensive Psychiatry*, *37*,167–179.

Simeon, J., & Ferguson, B. (1987). Alprazolam effects in children with anxiety disorders. *Canadian Journal of Psychiatry*, *32*, 570–574.

Simeon, J., Ferguson, B., Knott, V., Roberts, N., Gauthier, B., Dubois, C., & Wiggins, D. (1992). Clinical, cognitive and neurophysiological effects of alprazolam in children with overanxious and avoidant disorders. *Journal of the American Academy of Child and Adolescent Psychiatry*, *31*, 29–33.

Strauss, J., Birmaher, B., Bridge, J., Axelson, D., Chiappetta, L., Brent, D., & Ryan, N.

(2000). Anxiety disorders in suicidal youth. *Canadian Journal of Psychiatry—Revue Canadienne de Psychiatrie, 45*(8), 739–745.

Thyer, B. A., Parrish, R. T., Curtis, G. C., Nesse, R. M., & Cameron, O. G. (1985). Ages of onset of DSM-III anxiety disorders. *Comprehensive Psychiatry, 26,*113–122.

Toth, S. L., & Cicchetti, D. (1999). Developmental psychopathology and child psychotherapy. In S. W. Russ & T. H. Ollendick (Eds.), *Handbook of psychotherapies with children and families.* New York: Kluwer Academic/Plenum.

Vasey, M. W., & Ollendick, T. H. (2000). Anxiety. In A. J. Sameroff, M. Lewis, & S. M. Miller (Eds.), *Handbook of developmental psychopathology* (2nd ed., pp. 511–529). New York: Kluwer Academic/Plenum Press.

Verhulst, F. C., van der Ende, J., Ferdinand, R. F., & Kasius, M. C. (1997). The prevalence of DSM-III-R diagnoses in a national sample of Dutch adolescents. *Archives of General Psychiatry, 54,* 329–336.

Von Korff, M., Eaton, W., & Keyl, P. (1985). The epidemiology of panic attacks and panic disorder: Results of three community surveys. *American Journal of Epidemiology, 122,* 970–981.

Weissman, M. M., Bland, R. C., Canino, G. J., Faravelli, C., Greenwald, S., Hwu, H., Joyce, P. R., Karam, E. G., Lee, C., Lellouch,. J., Lipine, J., Newman, S. C., Oakley-Browne, M. A., Rubio-Stipec, M., Wells, J. E., Wickramaratne, P. J., Wittchen, H., & Yeh, E. (1997). The Cross-National Epidemiology of Panic Disorder study. *Archives of General Psychiatry, 54,* 305–309.

World Health Organization. (1992). *International statistical classification of diseases and related health problems.* Geneva: Author.

Chapter 10

Obsessive–Compulsive Disorder

John S. March
Martin E. Franklin
Henrietta L. Leonard
Edna B. Foa

At any given time, between 0.5 and 1% of children and adolescents suffer from clinically significant obsessive–compulsive disorder (OCD; Flament et al., 1988). Though some children persevere in the face of OCD, the disorder typically disrupts academic, social, and vocational functioning (Adams, Waas, March, & Smith, 1994). Hence, besides reducing morbidity associated with pediatric OCD, improvements in treating the disorder early in life have the potential to reduce adult morbidity. Taking these recent improvements in our understanding of the diagnosis and treatment of pediatric OCD as our text, we review the epidemiology, diagnostic criteria, phenomenology and natural history, neurobiology, and treatment of young persons with OCD.

EPIDEMIOLOGY

As with adults, OCD is substantially more common in children and adolescents than once thought, with a 6-month prevalence of clinically significant OCD in approximately 1 in 200 children and adolescents (Flament et al., 1988; Rutter, Tizard, & Whitmore, 1970), though some think that the prevalence is somewhat higher (Valleni-Basile et al.,

1996). Among adults with OCD, one-third to one-half develop the disorder during childhood (Rasmussen & Eisen, 1990), implying that the childhood-onset form of OCD foreshadows considerable adult morbidity. Unfortunately, children and adolescents with the disorder often go unrecognized. In Flament's epidemiological survey, only 4 of the 18 children found to have OCD were under professional care (Flament et al., 1988). Not 1 of the 18 had been correctly identified as suffering from OCD, including the 4 children in mental health treatment, perhaps confirming Jenike's character-ization of OCD as a "hidden epidemic" (Jenike, 1989). Reasons that have been advanced for underdiagnosis and undertreatment include OCD-specific factors (secretiveness and lack of insight), health care provider fac-tors (such as incorrect diagnosis and either lack of familiarity or unwilling-ness to use proven treatments), and general factors (such as lack of access to treatment resources).

DIAGNOSIS, PHENOMENOLOGY, AND COURSE

Diagnosis

As described in DSM-IV (American Psychiatric Association, 1994), OCD is characterized by recurrent obsessions, compulsions, or both that cause marked distress or interference in one's life. Key features of the DSM-IV di-agnosis of OCD include the following:

- To merit a diagnosis of OCD, an affected youngster must have either obsessions or compulsions, although the great majority have both. *Obsessions* are recurrent and persistent thoughts, images, or impulses that are ego-dystonic, intrusive, and, for the most part, acknowledged as senseless. Obsessions are generally accompanied by dysphoric affects, such as fear, disgust, doubt, or a feeling of incompleteness, and so are distressing to the affected individual.
- Like adults, young persons with OCD typically attempt to ignore, suppress, or neutralize obsessive thoughts and associated feelings by per-forming *compulsions*, which are repetitive, purposeful behaviors done in response to an obsession, often according to certain rules or in a stereo-typed fashion. Compulsions, which can be observable repetitive behaviors, such as washing, or covert mental acts, such as counting, exist at least in part because they serve to neutralize or alleviate obsessions and accompa-nying dysphoric affects over the short run.
- Because many normal behaviors may resemble OCD sympyoms, DSM-IV specifies that OCD symptoms be distressing or time-consuming (more than an hour a day) or significantly interfere with school, social ac-tivities, or important relationships.

• DSM-IV specifies that affected individuals recognize at some point in the illness that obsessions originate within the mind and are not simply excessive worries about real problems; similarly, compulsions must be seen as excessive or unreasonable. Persons of all ages who lack insight receive the designation "poor insight type." Most children and adolescents recognize the senselessness of OCD; however, the requirement that insight be preserved is waived for children because of the general (but not necessarily correct) perception that children and adolescents more frequently see OCD symptoms as reasonable.

• Finally, to be clear about the origin of the symptoms, DSM-IV also requires that the specific content of the obsessions cannot be related to another Axis I diagnosis, such as thoughts about food that result from an eating disorder or guilty thoughts (ruminations) that originate with depression.

Phenomenology

Common obsessions and compulsions seen in pediatric OCD are presented in Table 10.1. In the pediatric population, the most common obsessions are fear of contamination, fear of harm to self or to a familiar person, and symmetry or exactness urges. Corresponding compulsions in children are washing and cleaning, followed by checking, counting, repeating, touching, and straightening (Swedo, Rapoport, Leonard, Lenane, & Cheslow, 1989). In almost every case, these symptoms can be driven by one or more dysphoric affects, including fear, doubt, disgust, rudimentary urges, and "just so" feelings, which some have labeled sensory incompleteness (Goodman, Rasmussen, Foa, & Price, 1994). For example, washing rituals may be a reaction to contamination fears or a response to feeling "sticky." The former is

TABLE 10.1. Common Symptoms of
Obsessive–Compulsive Disorder

Common obsessions	Common compulsions
Contamination	Washing
Harm to self or others	Repeating
Aggressive themes	Checking
Sexual ideas/urges	Touching
Scrupulosity/religiosity	Counting
Symmetry urges	Ordering/arranging
Need to tell, ask, confess	Hoarding
	Praying

cognitive-phobic in origin; the latter may occur in response to a sensori-motor dysesthesia or without an obvious trigger. Whatever their origin, most children experience washing and checking rituals at some time during the course of the illness.

OCD symptoms frequently change over time, often with no clear progression pattern. Many if not most children have more than one OCD symptom at any one time, and many will have experienced almost all the classic OCD symptoms by the end of adolescence (Rettew, Swedo, Leonard, Lenane, & Rapoport, 1992). Those with only obsessions or compulsions are very rare (Swedo et al., 1989). This is especially so now that DSM-IV makes a clear distinction between mental rituals and mental compulsions, thereby reducing the number of patients misclassified as pure obsessionals but who in fact have mental rituals.

A clinically useful detailed symptom checklist accompanies the Yale–Brown Obsessive Compulsive Scale (Y-BOCS) and should be a regular part of the initial assessment and maintenance care of every patient with OCD.

Comorbidity

Children with a variety of psychiatric disorders may exhibit obsessions or ritualistic behaviors, confounding the diagnosis of OCD in some patients. In addition, more than one disorder may be diagnosed in a single patient, as the diagnosis of OCD is not exclusionary. Tic disorders, anxiety disorders, the disruptive behavior disorders, and learning disorders are common in clinical (Riddle et al., 1990; Swedo et al., 1989) and epidemiological samples of children with OCD (Flament et al., 1988). For unknown reasons, comorbid major depression, although not uncommon in clinical and epidemiological samples of youths with OCD (Swedo et al., 1989; Valleni-Basile et al., 1994), may be less common as a comorbid condition than it is in adult OCD (Rasmussen, 1994). Clinically, comorbid obsessive–compulsive (OC) spectrum disorders, such as trichotillomania, body dysmorphic disorder, and habit disorders such as nail biting, are not uncommon in patients with OCD. A surprisingly small number of children exhibit obsessive–compulsive personality disorder (OCPD), implying that obsessive–compulsive personality traits, although overrepresented among children with OCD, are neither necessary nor sufficient for the diagnosis, although the relationship between OCD and OCPD merits further study (Swedo et al., 1989).

Age, Gender, and Race

In clinical samples, the modal age of onset of OCD was 7, and the mean age at onset was 10 (Swedo et al., 1989). Boys appear more likely to have a prepubertal onset and to have a family member with OCD or Tourette's disorder (TD), whereas girls are more likely to develop OCD during adolescence. In the Flament et al. epidemiological study, the ratio of males to females was 1:1 (Flament et al., 1988), implying that the male-to-female ratio equalizes in adolescence, or that there is an ascertainment bias in the clinical samples, or both. In general, comorbid internalizing and externalizing symptoms are more common in boys (earlier onset) than in girls (later onset) as well (Swedo et al., 1989; Valleni-Basile et al., 1994). For unclear reasons, OCD is more common in European American than in African American children in clinical samples, although epidemiological data in adults suggest no differences in prevalence as a function of ethnicity or geographic region (Rasmussen, 1994).

Developmental Considerations

Most, if not all, children exhibit normal age-dependent obsessive–compulsive behaviors. For example, young children frequently like things done "just so" or insist on elaborate bedtime rituals. Such behaviors often can be understood in terms of developmental issues involving mastery and control, and they are usually gone by middle childhood, replaced by collecting, hobbies, and focused interests. Clinically, normative OC behaviors can be reliably discriminated from OCD on the basis of timing, content, and severity (Leonard, Goldberger, Rapoport, Cheslow, & Swedo, 1990). Developmentally sanctioned obsessive–compulsive behaviors occur early in childhood, are rare during adolescence, are common to large numbers of children, and are associated with mastery of important developmental transitions. In contrast, OCD occurs somewhat later, appears "bizarre" to adults and to other children, if not to the affected child, and always produces dysfunction rather than mastery. The common belief that children and adolescents with OCD often lack insight into the senseless nature of their behaviors may in part represent an artifact of (1) difficulty maintaining insight during acute "attacks" of OCD or (2) confounding of insight and secretiveness due to fear of punishment or simple embarrassment. Clinically, how the child talks with himself and with others and they with him about OCD has an important impact on whether insight *appears to be* (in contrast to *is*) preserved.

Natural History

Before the arrival of modern pharmacotherapy and cognitive behavior therapy, the outcome of treatment was dismal. Currently, although OCD often remains a chronic mental illness in adult (Rasmussen & Eisen, 1990) and pediatric (Leonard et al., 1993) patients, most patients achieve meaningful symptom relief with well-delivered comprehensive treatment. Interestingly, young boys with OCD and no tics are at clear risk for later development of tic disorders (Leonard et al., 1992). Those who develop tics evidence greater anxiety, a younger age at onset of OCD, and a higher likelihood of having a family member with a tic disorder than those without tics, suggesting that OCD and TD may be alternative manifestations of the same underlying illness. Finally, successful treatment by definition interrupts, even if only temporarily, the natural history of OCD. Though the relative merits of pharmacotherapy and cognitive-behavioral treatment (CBT) have not been resolved, CBT seems the more durable treatment (Franklin, Tolin, March, & Foa, 2001; March & Mulle, 1995; March, Mulle, & Herbel, 1994). Because relapse commonly follows medication discontinuation (Leonard et al., 1991), adding CBT may limit relapse when medications are discontinued (March et al., 1994).

PEDIATRIC OBSESSIVE–COMPULSIVE DISORDER AS A NEUROPSYCHIATRIC DISORDER

Successful treatment of OCD with serotonin reuptake inhibitors initially led to a neurobehavioral explanation for OCD in the form of the "serotonin hypothesis" (reviewed in Barr, Goodman, Price, McDougle, & Charney, 1992). Later, phenomenological similarities between obsessive–compulsive symptoms (washing, picking, and licking), coupled with studies of trichotillomania, led to the hypothesis that OCD is (in some patients) a "grooming behavior gone awry" (Swedo, 1989). Taken in this context, Esman, reviewing the psychoanalytic understanding of OCD, noted that insight-oriented psychotherapy has proven disappointing at best in ameliorating OCD symptoms (Esman, 1989). Although some argue that some OCD symptoms have underlying dynamic meaning, it is doubtful whether specific OCD symptoms really represent derivatives of intrapsychic conflicts, because there are a finite number of OCD symptoms that are universally experienced in typical patterned fashion. Moreover, there is no reason to suggest that OCD patients are any more conflicted about sexual matters than other psychiatric patients (Staebler, Pollard, & Merkel, 1993).

On the contrary, OCD is often cited as an example of the quintessential neuropsychiatric disorder (March & Leonard, 1998). Evidence favoring a neuropsychiatric model of the etiopathogenesis of OCD includes (1) family genetic studies that suggest that OCD and TD may, in some but not all cases, represent alternate expressions of the same gene(s), may represent different genes, or may arise spontaneously (Pauls, Alsobrook, Goodman, Rasmussen, & Leckman, 1995; Pauls, Towbin, Leckman, Zahner, & Cohen, 1986); (2) neuroimaging studies that implicate abnormalities in circuits linking basal ganglia to cortex (Rosenberg & Keshavan, 1998), with these circuits "responding" to either cognitive-behavioral or pharmacological treatment with an SSRI (Baxter, 1992; Rosenberg, MacMillan, & Moore, 2001); and (3) neurotransmitter and neuroendocrine abnormalities in childhood-onset OCD (Hamburger, Swedo, Whitaker, Davies, & Rapoport, 1989; Swedo & Rapoport, 1990).

Of these lines of evidence, the relationship between OCD and TD is particularly relevant (Cohen & Leckman, 1994). It is now well documented that individuals with OCD show an increased rate of tic disorders; the converse is also true (Pauls et al., 1995). Additionally, in systematic family genetic studies of probands with TD or other tic disorders, first-degree relatives show an increased rate of both tic disorders and OCD (Pauls et al., 1986). Similar findings are present in first-degree relatives of OCD probands (Leonard et al., 1992). Interestingly, Pauls and colleagues note that early onset may indicate a greater degree of genetic vulnerability (Pauls et al., 1995).

As with adults, children and adolescents with OCD frequently exhibit subtle neurological (Denckla, 1989) and neuropsychiatric (Cox, Fedio, & Rapoport, 1989) abnormalities often involving nonverbal reasoning skills, which may place them at risk for specific learning problems, such as dysgraphia, dyscalculia, poor expressive written language, and slow processing speed and efficiency. Although some have speculated that these neurocognitive impairments may adversely affect the outcome of pharmacotherapy for OCD (Hollander et al., 1990; March et al., 1990), others have found no such association (Leonard & Rapoport, 1989; Swedo, Leonard, & Rapoport, 1990). Clinically, the overlap between OCD and learning disorders should prompt a careful neuropsychological evaluation in patients with OCD who are having trouble with academic tasks rather than a reflexive acceptance that school problems are due to OCD alone.

OCD and tic symptoms that arise or exacerbate in the context of group A beta-hemolytic streptococcal infection (GABHS), which Leonard and Swedo (2001) have labeled "pediatric autoimmune neuropsychiatric disorder associated with strep" (PANDAS), may define a singular subgroup of children with OCD or tic disorders (Leonard & Swedo, 2001). Obsessive–compulsive symptoms are not uncommon in pediatric patients with Sydenham's chorea, which is a neurological variant of rheumatic fever (RF). Moreover, OCD is far more common in patients with chorea than in those without it. Like rheumatic carditis, Sydenham's is believed to represent an autoimmune inflammation of the basal ganglia triggered by antistreptococcal antibodies. Thus Swedo and colleagues have theorized that OCD in the context of Sydenham's chorea may provide a medical model for the etiopathogenesis of OCD and tic disorders (Swedo et al., 1998). In this model, antineuronal antibodies that formed against group A beta-hemolytic strep cell wall antigens are seen to cross-react with caudate neural tissue, with consequent initiation of OC symptoms. In turn, this would suggest that acute onset or dramatic exacerbation of OCD or tic symptoms should prompt investigation of GABHS infection, especially as immunomodulatory treatments, including antibiotic therapies, plasmapheresis, or intravenous immuniglobulin, may be of benefit to some patients (Perlmutter et al., 1999).

The interested reader is referred to recent reviews for a more detailed discussion of these and related topics (Leonard & Swedo, 2001; Rosenberg & Keshavan, 1998; Sallee & March, 2001).

ASSESSMENT

An adequate assessment of pediatric OCD should include a comprehensive evaluation of current and past OCD symptoms, current OCD symptom severity and associated functional impairment, and a survey of comorbid psychopathology. In addition, the strengths of the child and family should be evaluated, as well as their knowledge of OCD and its treatment. Many self-report and clinician-administered instruments can be used to guide this type of assessment. We typically mail several relevant self-report questionnaires for the family to complete prior to the intake visit, then review these materials prior to meeting with the child. If it is apparent from these materials that comorbid depression or other anxiety problems besides OCD are prominent, we focus on these symptoms as well in the intake.

For surveying history of OCD symptoms and current symptom severity, we use the Children's Yale–Brown Obsessive Compulsive Scale (CY-BOCS) checklist and severity scale (Scahill et al., 1997). Before administering this scale, it is important to determine whether the child should be interviewed with or without the parent present. In our randomized controlled trial, we conduct a conjoint interview, directing questions to the child but soliciting parental feedback as well. Nonresearch settings offer more flexibility, and the decision to interview the child alone or with a parent present can be made by discussing these choices with the parent in advance or by observing the child's and family's behavior in the waiting area; it can even be made during the interview if necessary. For example, if it becomes clear that a patient is reluctant to discuss certain symptoms with a parent present (e.g., sexual obsessions), the therapist can skip that item on the CY-BOCS checklist and save some time at the end of the interview to revisit these potentially sensitive issues alone with the patient. Our mantra in the clinic is "get the information," meaning that if parental presence increases the validity of the assessment, then do that; if not, then interview the child alone.

Prior to administering the CY-BOCS, the therapist should explain the concepts of obsessions and compulsions, using examples if the child or parents have difficulty grasping the concepts. We also take this opportunity to tell children and adolescents about the prevalence, nature, and treatment of OCD, which may increase their willingness to disclose their specific symptoms. Children may be particularly vulnerable to feeling as if they are the only ones on earth with obsessive fears of hurting a loved one, so prefacing the examples with, "I once met a kid who . . . " can help to dispel this myth and minimize the accompanying sense of isolation. During the intake, it is also important to observe the child's behavior and ask whether certain behaviors (e.g., unusual movements, vocalizations) are compulsions designed to neutralize obsessions or to reduce distress. Tic disorders are commonly comorbid with OCD, and it is important to try to make a differential diagnosis, as compulsions and tics would be targeted by different treatment procedures. Furthermore, as mentioned previously, some children who are aware of their obsessional content may be fearful of talking about the fears. Surveying common obsessions with a checklist instead of asking the child to disclose the fears tends to help with this problem, as does encouragement on the part of the therapist (e.g., "Lots of the kids I see have a hard time talking about these kinds of fears"). We have found that flexibility in manner of disclosing the obsession is warranted. Thus, for example, we allow children to write down the fears or to nod their heads as the therapist describes examples of similar fears in order to help the children share their OCD problems. In this way we can convey to the child and family that we recognize the difficulty associated with disclosure. We also use examples from children we had evaluated in the past (e.g., "I remember a few months ago when a kid about your age told me she would be scared to touch her dog for fear she might lose control and hurt him"), although we let the children and families know we are careful not to violate confidentiality when citing such examples. Following are brief descriptions of other core assessments.

Conners–March Developmental Questionnaire

The Conners–March Developmental Questionnaire (CMDQ) is specially designed to save time in collecting valuable information that would otherwise have to be gathered during history taking (Conners & March, 1999). The CMDQ covers the following clinically useful information: description of problem(s), home environment, treatment history, birth history, early development and temperament, medical and psychiatric history, school behavior and performance, and a detailed history of the family and child.

Anxiety Disorders Interview Schedule for Children

The Anxiety Disorders Interview Schedule for Children (ADIS-C; Silverman & Albano, 1996) is a semistructured interview that can be used to examine comorbid problems in greater detail; we used the ADIS in our collaborative study examining the relative efficacy of CBT, sertraline, combined treatment, and pill placebo (Franklin, Foa, & March, 2003). The ADIS, which uses an interviewer–observer format, thereby allowing the clinician to draw information both from the interview and from clinical observations, shows excellent psychometric properties for internalizing conditions relative to other available instruments, such as the Diagnostic Interview Schedule for Children (DISC; Silverman & Albano, 1996). Scores are derived for specific diagnoses and for level of diagnosis-related interference. Adequate psychometric properties have been demonstrated.

Conners' Rating Scales – Revised

We use the Conners' Parent Rating Scale—Revised (CRPS-R) to provide a broad view of childhood and adolescent psychopathology and problem behavior in children and adolescents (ages 3–17 years), with particular attention to the assessment of attention-deficit/hyperactivity disorder (ADHD; Conners, 1997).

Children's OCD Impact Scale

We also obtain child and parent versions of the OCD Impact Scale, which shows preliminary evidence favoring psychometric adequacy and sensitivity to change (Piacentini, Jaffer, Bergman, McCracken, & Keller, 2001), for use in analyses of functional impairment from OCD. This instrument enables us to estimate whether the CY-BOCS improvements result in normalization as assessed by functional impairment. A new and shorter version of this scale has been developed recently, and the psychometric properties of this scale appear to be favorable (Piacentini et al., 2001).

Multidimensional Anxiety Scale for Children

The Multidimensional Anxiety Scale for Children (MASC) has four factors and six subfactors: Physical Anxiety (tense/restless, somatic/autonomic), Harm Avoidance (perfectionism, anxious coping), Social Anxiety (humiliation/rejection, performance anxiety), and Separation Anxiety. It is in use in a variety of treatment outcome studies. The MASC shows test–retest reliability in clinical (intraclass correlation coefficient [ICC] > .92) and school samples (ICC > .85); convergent–divergent validity is similarly superior (March, 1998; March & Sullivan, 1999).

Children's Depression Inventory

The Children's Depression Inventory (CDI; Kovacs, 1985) is a 27-item self-report scale that measures cognitive, affective, behavioral, and interpersonal symptoms of depression. Each item consists of three statements, of which the child is asked to select the one statement that best describes his or her current functioning. Items are scored from 0 to 2; therefore, scores on the CDI can range from 0 to 54. The CDI shows adequate reliability and validity (Kovacs, 1985). This scale is useful to assess for symptoms of depression, which helps in tailoring the treatment plan.

In brief, the aforementioned scales, interviews, and questionnaires may be useful to help generate relevant clinical information at pretreatment and in helping us to evaluate treatment gains once treatment has ended. In our research-oriented settings, this is part of routine clinical practice, and perhaps the development of an efficient packet for evaluating outcome may stimulate more interest in effectiveness research in real-world clinical settings. However, financial, time, and personnel constraints may limit general usefulness, especially of the structured interview component of the test battery.

Treatment

To date, the efficacy of cognitive-behavioral therapy and pharmacotherapy for pediatric OCD has been well established. Inspection of posttreatment outcomes, however, indicates that neither treatment administered alone is completely or universally effective for pediatric OCD, and the need to develop other treatments and to test combined treatment remains apparent (March, Frances, Kahn, & Carpenter, 1997). Concerns about relapse on discontinuation of SRIs in OCD (Leonard et al., 1991) and the unknown risks associated with long-term SRI pharmacotherapy (Leonard, March, Rickler, & Allen, 1997) have generated interest in the question of whether combining SRI pharmacotherapy with CBT, which appears to be a more durable treatment (March et al., 1994), may protect against loss of treatment gains when the medication is discontinued as, ideally, it should be once a patient is in sustained remission.

Cognitive-Behavioral Psychotherapy

A wide variety of dynamic, family, and supportive psychotherapies have been and continue to be inconsistently and, in light of current knowledge, inappropriately applied to children and adolescents with OCD. For the most part, insight-oriented psychotherapy, whether delivered individually or in the family setting, has proven disappointing in both youths (Hollingsworth, Tanguay, & Grossman, 1980) and adults (Esman, 1989). Conversely, effective, flexible, empirically supported cognitive-behavioral treatments are now available for many childhood mental illnesses, including OCD (March, Franklin, Nelson, & Foa, 2001).

In adults, the cognitive-behavioral treatment of OCD generally involves a three-stage approach consisting of information gathering; therapist-assisted exposure and response prevention (EX/RP), including homework assignments; and generalization training and relapse prevention. Both graded exposure and flooding procedures have garnered strong empirical and clinical support (Franklin, Rynn, March, & Foa, 2002). Component analyses suggest that both exposure and response prevention are active ingredients of treatment, with exposure reducing phobic anxiety and response prevention reducing rituals (Foa, Steketee, Grayson, Turner, & Latimer, 1984; Foa, Steketee, & Milby, 1980). Relaxation has been shown to be an inert component of behavioral treatment for OCD and has been used as an active placebo in brief (4–6 weeks) studies in adults (Marks, 1987). Similarly, cognitive interventions seem less potent than EX/RP in reducing OCD symptoms (van Oppen et al., 1995).

Although CBT is routinely described as the psychotherapeutic treatment of choice for children and adolescents with OCD (King, Leonard, & March, 1998), robust empirical support is only now emerging (March et al., 2001). In practice, treatment components, especially exposure and ritual prevention, that generally parallel the identical interventions in adults make up the typical CBT treatment package (Franklin et al., 1998, 2002; March & Mulle, 1998).

As applied to OCD, the exposure principle relies on the fact that anxiety usually attenuates after sufficient duration of contact with a feared stimulus (Foa & Kozak, 1985). Thus a child with a fear of germs must confront relevant feared situations until his or her anxiety decreases. Repeated exposure is associated with decreased anxiety across exposure trials, with anxiety reduction largely specific to the domain of exposure, until the child no longer fears contact with specifically targeted phobic stimuli (Franklin et al., 2001; March & Mulle, 1995; March et al., 1994). Adequate exposure depends on blocking the negative reinforcement effect of rituals or avoidance behavior, a process termed "response prevention." For example, a child with germ worries must not only touch "germy things" but must refrain from ritualized washing until his or her anxiety diminishes substantially. EX/RP is typically implemented in a gradual fashion (sometimes termed graded exposure), with exposure targets under patient or, less desirably, therapist control (March & Mulle, 1996; March et al., 1994).

However, intensive prescriptive approaches work equally well for children who subscribe in advance to this approach (Franklin et al., 1998). Intensive approaches may be especially useful with treatment-resistant OCD or with patients who desire a very rapid response.

A wide variety of cognitive interventions have been used to provide the child with a "tool kit" to facilitate compliance with EX/RP (Soechting & March, 2002). The goals of cognitive therapy, which may be more or less useful or necessary depending on the child and the nature of the OCD, typically include increasing a sense of personal efficacy, predictability, controllability, and self-attributed likelihood of a positive outcome within EX/RP tasks. Specific interventions include: (1) constructive self-talk (Kendall, Howard, & Epps, 1988), (2) cognitive restructuring (March et al., 1994; van Oppen & Arntz, 1994), and (3) cultivating nonattachment (Schwartz, 1996), or, stated differently, minimizing the obsessional aspects of thought suppression (Salkovskis, Westbrook, Davis, Jeavons, & Gledhill, 1997). Each must be individualized to match the specific OCD symptoms that afflict the child and must mesh with the child's cognitive abilities, developmental stage, and individual differences in preference among the three techniques.

Because blocking rituals or avoidance behaviors remove the negative reinforcement effect of the rituals or avoidance, response prevention technically is an extinction procedure. By convention, however, extinction is usually defined as the elimination of OCD-related behaviors through removal of parental positive reinforcement for rituals. For example, parents of a child with reassurance-seeking rituals may be asked to refrain from gratifying the child's reassurance seeking. Extinction frequently produces rapid effects, but it can be hard to implement when the child's behavior is bizarre or very frequent. In addition, nonconsensual extinction procedures often produce unmanageable distress on the part of the child, disrupt the therapeutic alliance, miss important EX/RP targets that are not amenable to extinction procedures, and, most important, fail to help the child internalize a strategy for resisting OCD. Hence, as with EX/RP, placing the extinction program under the child's control leads to increased compliance and improved outcomes (March & Mulle, 1998).

Modeling—whether overt (the child understands that the therapist is demonstrating more appropriate or adaptive coping behaviors) or covert (the therapist informally models a behavior)—may help improve compliance with in-session EX/RP and generalization to between-session EX/RP homework. Intended to increase motivation to comply with EX/RP, shaping involves positively reinforcing successive approximations to a desired target behavior. Modeling and shaping reduce anticipatory anxiety and provide an opportunity for practicing constructive self-talk before and during EX/RP (Thyer, 1991). Because EX/RP has not proven particularly helpful with obsessional slowness, modeling and shaping procedures are currently the behavioral treatment of choice for children with this OCD subtype (Ratnasuriya, Marks, Forshaw, & Hymas, 1991), although relapse often occurs when therapist-assisted shaping, limit setting, and temporal speeding procedures are withdrawn (Wolff & Rapoport, 1988).

Clinically, positive reinforcement seems not to directly alter OCD symptoms but rather helps to encourage compliance with EX/RP, and so produces a noticeable, if indirect, clinical benefit. In contrast, punishment (defined as imposition of an aversive event) and response–cost (defined as removal of a positive event) procedures have shown themselves to be un-helpful in the treatment of OCD (Harris & Wiebe, 1992). Most CBT pro-grams use liberal positive reinforcement for EX/RP and proscribe aversive contingency management procedures unless they are targeting disruptive behavior outside the domain of OCD (March & Mulle, 1996). Because OCD itself is a powerful tonic aversive stimulus, successful EX/RP breeds willingness to engage in further EX/RP via negative reinforcement (e.g., elimination of OCD symptoms boosts compliance with EX/RP) as mani-fested by unscheduled generalization to new EX/RP targets as treatment proceeds (March et al., 1994).

Finally, family psychopathology is neither necessary nor sufficient for the onset of OCD; nonetheless, families affect and are affected by the disor-der (Amir, Freshman, & Foa, 2000; Lenane, 1989). Hence, although empir-ical data is lacking, clinical observations suggest that a combination of indi-vidual and family sessions is best for most patients (March & Mulle, 1996).

A Typical CBT Protocol

The protocol used by Franklin and colleagues (2003) (discussed subse-quently), which is fairly typical of a gradual exposure regimen (March & Mulle, 1998), consists of 14 visits over 12 weeks spread across five phases: (1) psychoeducation, (2) cognitive training, (3) mapping OCD, (4) expo-sure and response prevention, and (5) relapse prevention and generalization training. As shown in Table 10.2, except for weeks 1 and 2, in which patients come twice weekly, all visits are administered on a once per week basis, last 1 hour, and include one between-visit 10-minute telephone contact scheduled during weeks 3–12. Psychoeducation, defining OCD as the identified problem, cognitive training, and development of a stimulus hierarchy (mapping OCD) take place during visits 1–4; EX/RP take up vis-its 5–12, with the last two sessions incorporating generalization training and relapse prevention. Each session includes a statement of goals, a review of the previous week, provision of new information, therapist-assisted practice, homework for the coming week, and monitoring procedures.

Parents are centrally involved at sessions 1, 7, and 11, with the latter

TABLE 10.2. CBT Treatment Protocol

Visit number	Goals	Targets
Weeks 1 and 2	Psychoeducation Cognitive training	Neurobehavioral model Labeling OCD as OCD
Week 2	Mapping OCD Cognitive training	Set up stimulus hierarchy Cognitive restructuring
Weeks 3–12	Exposure and response prevention	Imaginal and *in vivo* EX/RP
Weeks 11–12	Relapse prevention	Targets, relapse, follow-up plans
Visits 1, 7, and 9	Parent sessions	Decrease reinforcement of OCD Enlist parents as cotherapists

two sessions devoted to guiding the parents about their central role in helping their child to accomplish the homework assignments. Sessions 13 and 14 also require significant parental input. Parents check in with the therapist at each session, and the therapist provides feedback describing the goals of each session and the child's progress in treatment. The therapist works with parents to help them refrain from insisting on inappropriate EX/RP tasks, a common problem in pediatric OCD treatment. The therapist also encourages parents to praise the child for resisting OCD, while at the same time refocusing their attention on positive elements in the child's life, an intervention technically termed "differential reinforcement of other behavior" (DRO). In some cases, extensive family involvement in rituals or the developmental level of the child or both require that family members play a more central role in treatment. It is important to note that the CBT protocol provides sufficient flexibility to accommodate variations in family involvement dictated by the OCD symptom picture.

Crucial to the success of any CBT protocol is the ability to deliver protocol-driven treatments in a developmentally appropriate fashion (Clarke, 1995). In our hands, CBT has been shown effective in children as young as 5. We promote developmental appropriateness by allowing flexibility in CBT within the constraints of fixed session goals. More specifically, the therapist adjusts the level of discourse to the cognitive functioning, social maturity, and capacity for sustained attention of each patient. Younger patients require more redirection and activities in order to sustain attention and motivation. Adolescents are generally more sensitive to the effects of OCD on peer interactions, which in turn require more discussion. Cognitive interventions in particular require adjustment to the developmental level of the patient, so, for example, adolescents are less likely to appreciate giving OCD a "nasty" nickname than younger children are.

Developmentally appropriate metaphors relevant to the child's areas of interest and knowledge are also used to promote active involvement in the treatment process. For instance, an adolescent male football player treated with CBT was better able to grasp treatment concepts by casting them in terms of offensive and defensive strategies employed during football games (e.g., blitzing). Patients whose OCD symptoms entangle family members will require more attention to family involvement in treatment planning and implementation than those without as much family involvement. On the other hand, although the CBT manual includes a section on developmental sensitivity that is specific for each treatment session, the general format and goals of the treatment sessions will be the same for all children.

Medication Management

Until the mid-1980s, psychopharmacological interventions in OCD were thought to be largely ineffective. Positive effects were attributed to relief of depressive symptoms or to a reduction in overall anxiety. However, it is now clear that drug treatment can benefit the majority of pediatric patients with OCD.

Although today it is considered second, after the selective serotonin reuptake inhibitors (Leonard et al., 1997), clomipramine (Anafranil), was the first medication to be studied in treating OCD in children and adolescents (DeVeaugh-Geiss et al., 1992). Besides clomipramine, which is a nonselective tricyclic compound, the selective serotonin reuptake inhibitors (SSRIs) fluvoxamine (Luvox), sertraline (Zoloft), paroxetine (Paxil), fluoxetine (Prozac), and citalopram and escitalopram (Celexa and Lexapro) also are likely effective treatments for OCD in youths. Controlled studies now support the efficacy of all but citalopram and escitalopram in the treatment of pediatric OCD (Geller et al., 2001; March et al., 1998; Riddle et al., 2001). Based on large multicenter trials, fluvoxamine (for ages 8–18) and sertraline (for ages 6–18) alone among the selective agents currently hold FDA approval for pediatric OCD.

The following clinically relevant lessons originate from the multicenter trials: (1) In contrast to depressed patients treated with medications, there is little or no placebo effect in patients with OCD. (2) Clinical effects appear as early as 2 to 3 weeks and plateau at 10 to 12 weeks. (3) SSRIs produce about a 30% reduction in OCD symptoms, corresponding to a rating of moderately to markedly improved on a measure of patient satisfaction, which means that partial response is the rule rather than the exception. Side effects and magnitude of improvement in pediatric trials are comparable to those seen in adult trials. Given that most participants on average remain in the mildly to moderately ill range at the conclusion of an adequate trial, the SSRIs are not a panacea for all patients. The absence of typical tricyclic side effects, including cardiac toxicity (Wilens et al., 1999), give the SSRIs significant advantages over clomipramine, which is usually given only after two or three failed SSRI trials.

Although many patients will respond early to one of the serotonin uptake inhibitors, a substantial minority will not respond until 8 or even 12 weeks of treatment at therapeutic doses, and it often takes 3 to 4 weeks (the time–response window) for evidence of benefit (the dose–response effect) to emerge. Thus it is important to wait at least 3 weeks between dose increases and 6 to 8 weeks at therapeutic doses before changing agents or undertaking augmentation regimens. Parenthetically, fixed-dose studies suggest that dosing schedules for OCD are not dissimilar to those for depression; that is, 50 mg of sertraline or 20 mg of fluoxetine are as effective as higher doses (Greist et al., 1995). The "myth" that OCD requires higher doses likely resulted from (1) increasing the dose too early in the time–response window for a drug effect to emerge and (2) exclusion of exposure instructions, as exposure is necessary for reduction in OCD in the drug state just as it is in the nondrug state (Marks, 1990).

Approximately one-third of patients will fail to be helped by monotherapy with an SSRI. Patients who are partial responders will benefit from combination pharmacology—for example, with a neuroleptic such as risperidone—especially when comorbid schizotypal personality disorder or a tic-spectrum disorder is present. In general, however, much unnecessary suffering attends drug switching or augmentation trials that continue to produce partial response, when augmenting drug treatment with CBT to normalization of symptoms is the far better strategy. When pharmacological augmentation is appropriate, clonazepam, clomipramine, and L-tryptophan have been successfully used as augmenting agents, whereas lithium and buspirone seem not to be effective in controlled studies with adults and anecdotal experience with youths. Clinical evidence suggests that a successful augmenting response may depend in part on comorbidity. For example, augmentation with clonazepam may be particularly helpful when comorbid panic symptoms are present. When augmenting an SSRI, adding 25–50 mg of clomipramine to an SSRI may be the best choice. However, it is important to watch for p450 2D6 inhibition of clomipramine (CMI) by fluoxetine or paroxetine; sertraline and fluvoxamine are less likely to cause high CMI levels that may potentially lead to cardiac arrythmias or to seizures (Leonard et al., 1997). Fluvoxamine may be the best choice to augment with CMI because it inhibits p450 1A2, which is the enzyme that demethylates CMI to its inactive desmethyl metabolite, thereby keeping more of the active parent compound available.

Side effects of clomipramine—primarily anticholinergic, antihistaminic, and alpha-blocking effects—are comparable to (but typically milder than) those seen in the adult multicenter CMI trial (Katz, DeVeaugh, & Landau, 1990; Leonard et al., 1989). Although long-term clomipramine maintenance has not revealed any unexpected adverse reactions (DeVeaugh-Geiss et al., 1992; Leonard et al., 1991), tachycardia and slightly increased PR, QRS, and QT-corrected intervals on the electrocardiogram are common in children treated with both desipramine and clomipramine (Leonard et al., 1995). Given the potential for TCA-related cardiotoxic effects, pretreatment and periodic electrocardiographic and therapeutic drug monitoring is warranted (Elliott & Popper, 1991; Leonard, Swedo, March, & Rapoport, 1996; Schroeder et al., 1989). Because of greater potential for side effects, most expert psychiatrists begin with an SSRI, proceeding to a clomipramine trial after two or three failed SSRI trials (March et al., 1997).

Although comparisons are limited by the differences between studies in design and dosing regimen, the side effects for the SSRIs in the pediatric multicenter trials are generally comparable to the safety findings in previous placebo-controlled studies of SSRIs in adults with OCD. The most frequently occurring adverse events are: nausea and diarrhea, insomnia or somnolence, hyperstimulation, headache, and sexual side effects. Importantly, side-effect data from the fluvoxamine and sertraline multicenter trials do not support the need for a lower SSRI starting dose in children as compared with adolescents, irrespective of body weight, age, or gender.

PANDAS

As noted earlier, the term "pediatric autoimmune neuropsychiatric disorder associated with streptococcal infection" (PANDAS) has been used to identify a subset of children with infection-related obsessive–compulsive or tic disorders that meet the following five criteria: (1) presence of OCD, a tic disorder, or both; (2) prepubertal symptom onset; (3) episodic course of symptom severity; (4) association with group A ß-hemolytic streptococcal (GABHS) infection; and (5) association with neurological abnormalities (Swedo et al., 1998). Because an accurate diagnosis of PANDAS implies the need for acute and possibly prophylactic antibiotic treatment or even riskier immunomodulatory treatments, such as plasmapheresis, either alone or in addition to conventional treatments for OCD, it is critical to accurately establish the presence of PANDAS in order to prevent inappropriate application of immunomodulatory therapies (Giulino et al., 2002; Singer, 1999; see also *http://intramural.nimh.nih.gov/research/pdn/web.htm*).

Combined Treatment in a Stages-of-Treatment Framework

Evidence-based clinical practice guidelines that employ a stages-of-treatment model are assuming increasing importance in pediatric as in adult psychiatry. Most discussions of practice guidelines focus only on selection of initial treatment or management of treatment-refractory patients. However, maximum clinical utility requires a stages-of-treatment model that addresses selection of initial treatment, the management of partial response, maintenance treatment, treatment resistance, and comorbidity. We were instrumental in developing the only two practice guidelines that so far have been published for the treatment of OCD in youth: the Expert Consensus Guidelines (March et al., 1997) and the American Academy of Child and Adolescent Psychiatry Practice Parameters for OCD (King et al., 1998). Both recommend starting with CBT or CBT plus an SSRI, depending on severity and pattern of comorbidity; both recommend that patients started on SSRI monotherapy who are partial responders be augmented with CBT. Thus experts generally consider CBT a first-line augmentation strategy and medication augmentation a second-line option.

Modifiers of Treatment Outcome

The question of paramount interest to clinicians and to researchers attempting to refine and improve treatment outcome is, Which treatment for which child with what characteristics?

Conventional wisdom holds that patients with OCD who benefit from CBT and medication differ in important if ill-understood ways. However, other than comorbid schizotypy (Baer et al., 1992) and tic disorders (McDougle et al., 1993), which may represent treatment impediments and possible indications for neuroleptic augmentation, the meager empirical literature on moderators of treatment outcome in adults provides no clear support for any of the putative predictors proposed by Goodman and colleagues (1994) in their review of pharmacotherapy trial methodology in OCD. Conversely, predictors of a successful response to behavior therapy include the presence of rituals, the desire to eliminate symptoms, the ability to monitor and report symptoms, the absence of complicating comorbidities, the willingness to cooperate with treatment, and psychophysiological indicators (Foa & Emmelkamp, 1983; Steketee, 1994).

Although many have suggested that the presence of comorbidity—especially with the tic disorders—lack of motivation or insight, and the presence of family psychopathology might predict a poor outcome in children undergoing CBT, there is as yet little or no empirical basis on which to predict treatment outcome in children undergoing psychosocial treatment. In contrast, a rather extensive literature on prediction of outcome for drug treatment has failed to identify any predictor variables (March & Leonard, 1996). For example, in a recently published multicenter trial of sertraline and pill placebo in children and adolescents with OCD (March & Mulle, 1998), neither age, race, gender, body weight, baseline OCD score, baseline depression score, comorbidity, socioeconomic status, or plasma sertraline or desmethylsertraline level predicted the outcome of treatment.

In research studies, the answer to the question of which treatment is best for which child focuses on moderation and mediation of treatment response. In general, moderators are variables that change the size or direction of relationships between independent and dependent variables (Holmbeck, 1997). In clinical trials, moderators comprise those individual, familial, or wider systemic variables that exist prior to treatment assignment and that may be associated with differential response to intervention (Kraemer, 2000). Thus moderator analyses afford an understanding of which types of participants respond optimally to assigned interventions and under what circumstances treatments yield optimal effects. In pediatric studies, six groups of moderator variables that correspond to outcome domains prespecified by the National Institute of Mental Health consensus panel are typically evaluated: demographics, baseline OCD score, comorbidity, secondary adversities, family status (e.g., single parent), and functioning (e.g., family or academic functioning; Jensen, Hoagwood, & Petti, 1996). In contrast to moderator variables, which predate randomization, a mediator variable helps to explain the relationship between an independent and a dependent variable in such a manner that, when the mediator is accounted for, the relationship between the independent and dependent variables is attenuated or eliminated (Holmbeck, 1997). That is, inclusion of the mediator "explains" the relationship. For clinical trials, Kraemer, Wilson, Fairburn, and Agras (2002) defines a mediator as a variable that follows random assignment and that may help to explain a particular pattern of treatment results. With respect to mediational effects, two mediating variables are often examined: (1) compliance with treatment, defined as attendance at a prespecified percentage of the manualized treatment sessions, and (2) compliance with treatment, defined as compliance with EX/RP homework.

Given that the research literature is as yet undecided on which treatments—CBT, pharmacotherapy with an SSRI, or their combination—are best for which children with OCD, the candidate predictors summarized in Table 10.3, which we will test as potential moderators of treatment outcome in our current comparative treatment trial of CBT and medication alone and in combination, should be evaluated at least by history when structuring treatment plans for children and adolescents with OCD.

FUTURE DIRECTIONS

Despite the by-now routine recommendation of CBT alone or the combination of CBT and a serotonin reuptake inhibitor as the treatment of choice for OCD in the pediatric population (March et al., 1997), the relative efficacy of CBT and medication, alone and in combination, remains uncertain. Thus, as Kendall has clearly stated (Kendall & Lipman, 1991), well-

TABLE 10.3. Sets of Predictor Variables

Set	Variables evaluated
Demographics	Age, sex, race, socioeconomic status
Neurocognitive profile	Full-Scale, Verbal, and Performance IQs
Medical history	PANDAS, weight and height, and obstetrical history
OCD-specific factors	Symptom profile, initial severity, impact on functioning, insight, and treatment history
Treatment expectancy	Treatment expectancy
Comorbidity	Internalizing and externalizing disorders and symptoms, tic disorders
Parental psychopathology	General symptoms, depression, anxiety, OCD
Family functioning	Parental stress, expressed emotion, marital distress

designed comparative treatment outcome studies are necessary with both adults and children. Of particular importance, then, we will shortly complete a comparative treatment outcome study of initial treatments in OCD (Franklin et al., 2003). Using a volunteer sample of 120 (60 per site) youths ages 8–16 with a DSM-IV diagnosis of OCD, this 5-year treatment outcome study contrasts the degree and durability of improvement obtained across four treatment conditions: medication with sertraline (MED), OCD-specific cognitive behavior therapy (CBT), both MED and CBT (COMB), and two control conditions, placebo (PBO) and educational support (ES). The experimental design covers two phases. Phase 1 compares the outcome of MED, CBT, COMB, and control conditions. In Phase 2, responders advance to a 16-week discontinuation study to assess treatment durability. The primary outcome measure is the Yale–Brown Obsessive Compulsive Scale. Assessments blind to treatment status take place at week 0 (pretreatment); weeks 1, 4, 8, 12 (Phase 1 treatment); and weeks 16, 20, 24, and 28 (Phase 2 discontinuation). Besides addressing comparative efficacy and durability of the specified treatments, this study also examines time–action effects; differential effects of treatment on specific aspects of OCD, including functional impairment; and predictors of response to treatment. Once completed, this study will be followed by an augmentation trial of CBT versus an atypical neuroleptic in SSRI partial responders.

SUMMARY

Despite limitations in the research literature, it is now clear that OCD (with the exception of PANDAS) is similar to and continuous with the adult form of the disorder, though etiopathogenic factors may differ. Cognitive-behavioral psychotherapy, alone or in combination with pharmacotherapy, is the psychotherapeutic treatment of choice for OCD in children and adolescents. Ideally, young persons with OCD should first receive CBT that has been optimized for treating childhood-onset OCD and, if not rapidly responsive, either intensive CBT or concurrent pharmacotherapy with a serotonin reuptake inhibitor (Franklin et al., 1998; March et al., 1997). Moreover, because cognitive-behavioral psychotherapy, including booster treatments during medication discontinuation, may improve both short- and long-term outcome in drug-treated patients, all patients who receive medication also should receive concomitant CBT. In this regard, arguments advanced against CBT for OCD, such as symptom substitution, danger of interrupting rituals, uniformity of learned symptoms, and incompatibility with pharmacotherapy, have all proven unfounded. Perhaps the most insidious myth is that CBT is a simplistic treatment that ignores "real problems." We believe that the opposite is true. Helping patients make rapid and difficult behavior change over short time intervals takes both clinical savvy and focused treatment. Currently, state-of-the-art treatments for pediatric OCD are best delivered by a multidisciplinary team usually, but not always, located in a subspecialty clinic setting (March, Mulle, Stallings, Erhardt, & Conners, 1995). Translation of specialty practice to community settings is essential if demonstrably effective treatments, such as CBT, for OCD are to be made available to the children and adolescents suffering from this disorder (Kendall & Southam-Gerow, 1995).

ACKNOWLEDGMENTS

This work was supported by NIMH Grant Nos. 1 K24 MHO1557 (to John S. March) and 1 R10 MH55121 (to John S. March and Edna B. Foa) and by contributions from the Robert and Sarah Gorrell family and by the Lupin Family Foundation.

REFERENCES

Adams, G. B., Waas, G. A., March, J. S., & Smith, M. C. (1994). Obsessive compulsive disorder in children and adolescents: The role of the school psychologist in identification, assessment, and treatment. *School Psychology Quarterly, 94*(4), 274–294.

American Psychiatric Association. (1994). *Diagnostic and statistical manual of mental disorders* (4th ed.). Washington DC: Author.

Amir, N., Freshman, M., & Foa, E. B. (2000). Family distress and involvement in relatives of obsessive–compulsive disorder patients. *Journal of Anxiety Disorders, 14*(3), 209–217.

Baer, L., Jenike, M. A., Black, D. W., Treece, C., Rosenfeld, R., & Greist, J. (1992). Effect of axis II diagnoses on treatment outcome with clomipramine in 55 patients with obsessive–compulsive disorder. *Archives of General Psychiatry, 49*(11), 862–866.

Barr, L. C., Goodman, W. K., Price, L. H., McDougle, C. J., & Charney, D. S. (1992). The serotonin hypothesis of obsessive compulsive disorder: Implications of pharmacologic challenge studies. *Journal of Clinical Psychiatry, 53,* 17–28.

Baxter, L. R., Jr. (1992). Neuroimaging studies of obsessive compulsive disorder. *Psychiatric Clinics of North America, 15*(4), 871–884.

Clarke, G. N. (1995). Improving the transition from basic efficacy research to effectiveness studies: Methodological issues and procedures. *Journal of Consulting and Clinical Psychology, 63*(5), 718–725.

Cohen, D. J., & Leckman, J. F. (1994). Developmental psychopathology and neurobiology of Tourette's syndrome [Review]. *Journal of the American Academy of Child and Adolescent Psychiatry, 33*(1), 2–15.

Conners, C. (1997). *Conners' Rating Scales.* Toronto: Multi-Health Systems.

Conners, C., & March, J. (1999). *The Conners/March Developmental Questionnaire.* Toronto: Multi-Health Systems.

Cox, C., Fedio, P., & Rapoport, J. (1989). Neuropsychological testing of obsessive-compulsive adolescents. In J. Rapoport (Ed.), *Obsessive–compulsive disorder in children and adolescents* (pp. 73–86). Washington, DC: American Psychiatric Press.

Denckla, M. (1989). Neurological examination. In J. Rapoport (Ed.), *Obsessive–compulsive disorder in children and adolescents* (pp. 107–118). Washington, DC: American Psychiatric Press.

DeVeaugh-Geiss, J., Moroz, G., Biederman, J., Cantwell, D., Fontaine, R., Greist, J. H., Reichler, R., Katz, R., & Landau, P. (1992). Clomipramine hydrochloride in childhood and adolescent obsessive–compulsive disorder: A multicenter trial. *Journal of the American Academy of Child and Adolescent Psychiatry, 31*(1), 45–49.

Elliott, G., & Popper, C. (1991). Tricyclic antidepressants: The QT interval and other cardiovascular parameters. *Journal of Child and Adolescent Psychopharmacology, 1,* 187–191.

Esman, A. (1989). Psychoanalysis in general psychiatry: Obsessive–compulsive disorder as a paradigm. *Journal of the American Psychoanalytical Association, 37,* 319–336.

Flament, M. F., Whitaker, A., Rapoport, J. L., Davies, M., Berg, C. Z., Kalikow, K., Sceery, W., & Shaffer, D. (1988). Obsessive compulsive disorder in adolescence: an epidemiological study. *Journal of the American Academy of Child and Adolescent Psychiatry, 27*(6), 764–771.

Foa, E., & Emmelkamp, P. (1983). *Failures in behavior therapy.* New York: Wiley.

Foa, E., & Kozak, M. (1985). Emotional processing of fear: Exposure to corrective information. *Psychological Bulletin, 90,* 20–35.

Foa, E. B., Steketee, G., Grayson, B., Turner, M., & Latimer, P. (1984). Deliberate exposure and blocking of obsessive–compulsive rituals: Immediate and long-term effects. *Behavior Therapy, 15*(5), 450–472.

Foa, E. B., Steketee, G., & Milby, J. B. (1980). Differential effects of exposure and response prevention in obsessive–compulsive washers. *Journal of Consulting and Clinical Psychology, 48*(1), 71–79.

Franklin, M., Foa, E., & March, J. S. (2003). The Pediatric Obsessive–Compulsive Disorder Treatment Study (POTS): Rationale, design and methods. *Journal of Child and Adolescent Psychopharmacology, 13*(Suppl. 1), S39–S51.

Franklin, M. E., Kozak, M. J., Cashman, L. A., Coles, M. E., Rheingold, A. A., & Foa, E. B. (1998). Cognitive-behavioral treatment of pediatric obsessive–compulsive disorder: An open clinical trial. *Journal of the American Academy of Child and Adolescent Psychiatry, 37*(4), 412–419.

Franklin, M. E., Rynn, M., March, J. S., & Foa, E. B. (2002). Obsessive–compulsive disorder. In M. Hersen (Ed.), *Clinical behavior therapy: Adults and children* (pp. 276–303). New York: Wiley.

Franklin, M. E., Tolin, D. F., March, J. S., & Foa, E. B. (2001). Treatment of pediatric obsessive–compulsive disorder: A case example of intensive cognitive-behavioral therapy involving exposure and ritual prevention. *Cognitive and Behavioral Practice, 8*(4), 297–304.

Geller, D. A., Hoog, S. L., Heiligenstein, J. H., Ricardi, R. K., Tamura, R., Kluszynski, S., & Jacobson, J. G. (2001). Fluoxetine treatment for obsessive–compulsive disorder in children and adolescents: A placebo-controlled clinical trial. *Journal of the American Academy of Child and Adolescent Psychiatry, 40*(7), 773–779.

Giulino, L., Gammon, P., Sullivan, K., Franklin, M., Foa, E., Maid, R., & March, J. S. (2002). Is parental report of upper respiratory infection at the onset of obsessive–compulsive disorder suggestive of pediatric autoimmune neuropsychiatric disorder associated with streptococcal infection? *Journal of Child and Adolescent Psychopharmacology, 12*(2), 157–164.

Goodman, W., Rasmussen, S., Foa, E., & Price, L. (1994). Obsessive–compulsive disorder. In R. Prien & D. Robinson (Eds.), *Clinical evaluation of psychotropic drugs: Principles and guidelines* (pp. 431–466). New York: Raven Press.

Greist, J. H., Jefferson, J. W., Kobak, K. A., Chouinard, G., DuBoff, E., Halaris, A., Kim, S. W., Koran, L., Liebowtiz, M. R., Lydiard, B., et al. (1995). A 1 year double-blind placebo-controlled fixed dose study of sertraline in the treatment of obsessive–compulsive disorder. *International Clinical Psychopharmacology, 10*(2), 57–65.

Hamburger, S. D., Swedo, S., Whitaker, A., Davies, M., & Rapoport, J. L. (1989). Growth rate in adolescents with obsessive–compulsive disorder. *American Journal of Psychiatry, 146*(5), 652–655.

Harris, C. V., & Wiebe, D. J. (1992). An analysis of response prevention and flooding procedures in the treatment of adolescent obsessive–compulsive disorder. *Journal of Behavior Therapy and Experimental Psychiatry, 23*(2), 107–115.

Hollander, E., Schiffman, E., Cohen, B., Rivera, S. M., Rosen, W., Gorman, J. M., Fyer, A. J., Papp, L., & Liebowitz, M. R. (1990). Signs of central nervous system dysfunction in obsessive–compulsive disorder [Comment]. *Archives of General Psychiatry, 47*(1), 27–32.

Hollingsworth, C., Tanguay, P., & Grossman, L. (1980). Long-term outcome of obsessive–compulsive disorder in childhood. *Journal of the American Academy of Child Psychiatry, 19*, 134–144.

Holmbeck, G. N. (1997). Toward terminological, conceptual, and statistical clarity in the study of mediators and moderators: Examples from the child clinical and pediatric psychology literatures. *Journal of Consulting and Clinical Psychology,* 65(4), 599–610.

Jenike, M. A. (1989). Obsessive–compulsive and related disorders: A hidden epidemic [Editorial and comment]. *New England Journal of Medicine, 321*(8), 539–541.

Jensen, P. S., Hoagwood, K., & Petti, T. (1996). Outcomes of mental health care for children and adolescents: 2. Literature review and application of a comprehensive model. *Journal of the American Academy of Child and Adolescent Psychiatry, 35*(8), 1064–1077.

Katz, R. J., DeVeaugh, G. J., & Landau, P. (1990). Clomipramine in obsessive–compulsive disorder [Comment]. *Biological Psychiatry, 28*(5), 401–414.

Kendall, P. C., Howard, B. L., & Epps, J. (1988). The anxious child. Cognitive-behavioral treatment strategies. *Behavior Modification, 12*(2), 281–310.

Kendall, P. C., & Lipman, A. J. (1991). Psychological and pharmacological therapy: Methods and modes for comparative outcome research. *Journal of Consulting and Clinical Psychology, 59*(1), 78–87.

Kendall, P. C., & Southam-Gerow, M. A. (1995). Issues in the transportability of treatment: The case of anxiety disorders in youths. *Journal of Consulting and Clinical Psychology, 63*(5), 702–708.

King, R., Leonard, H., & March, J. (1998). Practice parameters for the assessment and treatment of children and adolescents with obsessive–compulsive disorder. *Journal of the American Academy of Child and Adolescent Psychiatry, 37*(10, Suppl), 27–45.

Kovacs, M. (1985). The Children's Depression Inventory (CDI). *Psychopharmacology Bulletin, 21,* 995–998.

Kraemer, H. C. (2000). Pitfalls of multisite randomized clinical trials of efficacy and effectiveness. *Schizophrenia Bulletin, 26*(3), 533–541.

Kraemer, H. C., Wilson, G. T., Fairburn, C. G., & Agras, W. S. (2002). Mediators and moderators of treatment effects in randomized clinical trials. *Archives of General Psychiatry, 59,* 877–883.

Lenane, M. (1989). Families in obsessive–compulsive disorder. In J. Rapoport (Ed.), *Obsessive–compulsive disorder in children and adolescents* (pp. 237–249). Washington, DC: American Psychiatric Press.

Leonard, H., Swedo, S., March, J. S., & Rapoport, J. (1996). Obsessive–compulsive disorder. In G. Gabbard (Ed.), *Synopsis of treatments of psychiatric disorders* (pp. 143–148). Washington, DC: American Psychiatric Press.

Leonard, H. L., Goldberger, E. L., Rapoport, J. L., Cheslow, D. L., & Swedo, S. E. (1990). Childhood rituals: Normal development or obsessive–compulsive symptoms? *Journal of the American Academy of Child and Adolescent Psychiatry, 29*(1), 17–23.

Leonard, H. L., Lenane, M. C., Swedo, S. E., Rettew, D. C., Gershon, E. S., & Rapoport, J. L. (1992). Tics and Tourette's disorder: A 2- to 7-year follow-up of 54 obsessive-compulsive children. *American Journal of Psychiatry, 149*(9), 1244–1251.

Leonard, H. L., March, J. S., Rickler, K. C., & Allen, A. J. (1997). Pharmacology of the selective serotonin reuptake inhibitors in children and adolescents. *Journal of the American Academy of Child and Adolescent Psychiatry, 36*(6), 725–736.

Leonard, H. L., Meyer, M. C., Swedo, S. E., Richter, D., Hamburger, S. D., Allen, A. J., Rapoport, J. L., & Tucker, E. (1995). Electrocardiographic changes during desipramine and clomipramine treatment in children and adolescents [Comment]. *Journal of the American Academy of Child and Adolescent Psychiatry, 34*(11), 1460–1468.

Leonard, H. L., & Rapoport, J. L. (1989). Pharmacotherapy of childhood obsessive–compulsive disorder. *Psychiatric Clinics of North America, 12*(4), 963–970.

Leonard, H. L., & Swedo, S. E. (2001). Paediatric autoimmune neuropsychiatric disorders associated with streptococcal infection (PANDAS). *International Journal of Neuropsychopharmacology, 4*(2), 191–198.

Leonard, H. L., Swedo, S. E., Lenane, M. C., Rettew, D. C., Cheslow, D. L., Hamburger, S. D., & Rapoport, J. L. (1991). A double-blind desipramine substitution during long-term clomipramine treatment in children and adolescents with obsessive–compulsive disorder. *Archives of General Psychiatry, 48*(10), 922–927.

Leonard, H. L., Swedo, S. E., Lenane, M. C., Rettew, D. C., Hamburger, S. D., Bartko, J. J., & Rapoport, J. L. (1993). A 2- to 7–year follow-up study of 54 obsessive–compulsive children and adolescents. *Archives of General Psychiatry, 50*(6), 429–439.

Leonard, H. L., Swedo, S. E., Rapoport, J. L., Koby, E. V., Lenane, M. C., Cheslow, D. L., & Hamburger, S. D. (1989). Treatment of obsessive–compulsive disorder with clomipramine and desipramine in children and adolescents. A double-blind crossover comparison. *Archives of General Psychiatry, 46*(12), 1088–1092.

March, J. S. (1998). *Manual for the Multidimensional Anxiety Scale for Children (MASC)*. Toronto: Multi-Health Systems.

March, J. S., Frances, A., Kahn, D., & Carpenter, D. (1997). Expert consensus guidelines: Treatment of obsessive–compulsive disorder. *Journal of Clinical Psychiatry, 58*(Suppl. 4), 1–72.

March, J. S., Johnston, H., Jefferson, J., Greist, J., Kobak, K., & Mazza, J. (1990). Do subtle neurological impairments predict treatment resistance in children and adolescents with obsessive–compulsive disorder. *Journal of Child and Adolescent Psychopharmacology, 1*, 133–140.

March, J. S., & Leonard, H. (1996). Obsessive–compulsive disorder in children and adolescents: A review of the past 10 years. *Journal of the American Academy of Child and Adolescent Psychiatry, 35*(10), 1265–1273.

March, J. S., & Leonard, H. (1998). Neuropsychiatry of pediatric obsessive–compulsive disorder. In E. Coffey & R. Brumback (Eds.), *Textbook of pediatric neuropsychiatry* (pp. 546–562). Washington, DC: American Psychiatric Association Press.

March, J. S., & Mulle, K. (1995). Manualized cognitive-behavioral psychotherapy for obsessive–compulsive disorder in childhood: A preliminary single-case study. *Journal of Anxiety Disorders, 9*(2), 175–184.

March, J. S., & Mulle, K. (1996). Banishing obsessive–compulsive disorder. In E. Hibbs & P. Jensen (Eds.), *Psychosocial treatments for child and adolescent disorders* (pp. 82–103). Washington, DC: American Psychological Press.

March, J. S., & Mulle, K. (1998). *OCD in children and adolescents: A cognitive-behavioral treatment manual*. New York: Guilford Press.

March, J. S., Mulle, K., Stallings, P., Erhardt, D., & Conners, C. K. (1995). Organizing an anxiety disorders clinic. In J. S. March (Ed.), *Anxiety disorders in children and adolescents* (pp. 420–435). New York: Guilford Press.

March, J. S., Biederman, J., Wolkow, R., Safferman, A., Mardekian, J., Cook, E. H., Cutler, N. R., Dominguez, R., Ferguson, J., Muller, B., Riesenberg, R., Rosenthal, M., Sallee, F. R., & Wagner, K. D. (1998). Sertraline in children and adolescents with obsessive–compulsive disorder: A multicenter randomized controlled trial [Comment]. *Journal of the American Medical Association, 280*(20), 1752–1756.

March, J. S., Franklin, M., Nelson, A., & Foa, E. (2001). Cognitive-behavioral psychotherapy for pediatric obsessive–compulsive disorder. *Journal of Clinical Child Psychology, 30*(1), 8–18.

March, J. S., Mulle, K., & Herbel, B. (1994). Behavioral psychotherapy for children and adolescents with obsessive–compulsive disorder: An open trial of a new protocol-driven treatment package. *Journal of the American Academy of Child and Adolescent Psychiatry, 33*(3), 333–341.

March, J. S., & Sullivan, K. (1999). Test–retest reliability of the Multidimensional Anxiety Scale for Children. *Journal of Anxiety Disorders, 13*(4), 349–358.

Marks, I. (1987). *Fears, phobias, and rituals.* New York: Oxford University Press.

Marks, I. M. (1990). Drug versus behavioral treatment of obsessive–compulsive disorder. *Biological Psychiatry, 28*(12), 1072–1073.

McDougle, C. J., Goodman, W. K., Leckman, J. F., Barr, L. C., Heninger, G. R., & Price, L. H. (1993). The efficacy of fluvoxamine in obsessive–compulsive disorder: Effects of comorbid chronic tic disorder. *Journal of Clinical Psychopharmacology, 13*(5), 354–358.

Pauls, D. L., Alsobrook, J. P., Goodman, W., Rasmussen, S., & Leckman, J. F. (1995). A family study of obsessive–compulsive disorder. *American Journal of Psychiatry, 152*(1), 76–84.

Pauls, D. L., Towbin, K., Leckman, J., Zahner, G., & Cohen, D. (1986). Gilles de la Tourette syndrome and obsessive–compulsive disorder: Evidence supporting a genetic relationship. *Archives of General Psychiatry, 43*, 1180–1182.

Perlmutter, S. J., Leitman, S. F., Garvey, M. A., Hamburger, S., Feldman, E., Leonard, H. L., & Swedo, S. E. (1999). Therapeutic plasma exchange and intravenous immunoglobulin for obsessive–compulsive disorder and tic disorders in childhood [Comment]. *Lancet, 354*(9185), 1153–1158.

Piacentini, J., Jaffer, M., Bergman, R. L., McCracken, J., & Keller, M. (2001, October). *Measuring impairment in childhood OCD: Psychometric properties of the COIS.* Paper presented at the annual meeting of the American Academy of Child and Adolescent Psychiatry, Honolulu, HI.

Rasmussen, S. A. (1994). Obsessive–compulsive spectrum disorders. *Journal of Clinical Psychiatry, 55*(3), 89–91.

Rasmussen, S. A., & Eisen, J. L. (1990). Epidemiology of obsessive–compulsive disorder. *Journal of Clinical Psychiatry, 53*(Suppl.), 10–13.

Ratnasuriya, R. H., Marks, I. M., Forshaw, D. M., & Hymas, N. F. (1991). Obsessive slowness revisited [Comment]. *British Journal of Psychiatry, 159*, 273–274.

Rettew, D. C., Swedo, S. E., Leonard, H. L., Lenane, M. C., & Rapoport, J. L. (1992). Obsessions and compulsions across time in 79 children and adolescents with obsessive–compulsive disorder. *Journal of the American Academy of Child and Adolescent Psychiatry, 31*(6), 1050–1056.

Riddle, M. A., Reeve, E. A., Yaryura-Tobias, J. A., Yang, H. M., Claghorn, J. L., Gaffney, G., Greist, J. H., Holland, D., McConville, B. J., Pigott, T., & Walkup, J. T. (2001). Fluvoxamine for children and adolescents with obsessive–compulsive disorder: A randomized, controlled, multicenter trial. *Journal of the American Academy of Child and Adolescent Psychiatry, 40*(2), 222–229.

Riddle, M. A., Scahill, L., King, R., Hardin, M. T., Towbin, K. E., Ort, S. I., Leckman, J. F., & Cohen, D. J. (1990). Obsessive–compulsive disorder in children and adolescents: Phenomenology and family history. *Journal of the American Academy of Child and Adolescent Psychiatry, 29*(5), 766–772.

Rosenberg, D. R., & Keshavan, M. S. (1998). A. E. Bennett Research Award: Toward a neurodevelopmental model of obsessive–compulsive disorder. *Biological Psychiatry, 43*(9), 623–640.

Rosenberg, D. R., MacMillan, S. N., & Moore, G. J. (2001). Brain anatomy and chemistry may predict treatment response in paediatric obsessive–compulsive disorder. *International Journal of Neuropsychopharmacology, 4*(2), 179–190.

Rutter, M., Tizard, J., & Whitmore, K. (1970). *Education, health, and behavior.* London: Longmans.

Salkovskis, P. M., Westbrook, D., Davis, J., Jeavons, A., & Gledhill, A. (1997). Effects of neutralizing on intrusive thoughts: An experiment investigating the etiology of obsessive–compulsive disorder. *Behavior Research and Therapy, 35*(3), 211–219.

Sallee, F. R., & March, J. S. (2001). Neuropsychiatry of paediatric anxiety disorders. In W. Silverman & P. Treffers (Eds.), *Anxiety disorders in children and adolescents: Research, assessment and intervention* (pp. 90–125). New York: Cambridge University Press.

Scahill, L., Riddle, M. A., McSwiggin-Hardin, M., Ort, S. I., King, R. A., Goodman, W. K., Cicchetti, D., & Leckman, J. F. (1997). Children's Yale–Brown Obsessive Compulsive Scale: Reliability and validity. *Journal of the American Academy of Child and Adolescent Psychiatry, 36*(6), 844–852.

Schroeder, J. S., Mullin, A. V., Elliott, G. R., Steiner, H., Nichols, M., Gordon, A., & Paulos, M. (1989). Cardiovascular effects of desipramine in children. *Journal of the American Academy of Child and Adolescent Psychiatry, 28*(3), 376–379.

Schwartz, J. (1996). *Brain lock.* New York: HarperCollins.

Silverman, W., & Albano, A. (1996). *The Anxiety Disorders Interview Schedule for DSM-IV, Child and Parent Versions.* San Antonio, TX: Psychological Corporation.

Singer, H. S. (1999). PANDAS and immunomodulatory therapy [Comment]. *Lancet, 354*(9185), 1137–1138.

Soechting, I., & March, J. (2002). Cognitive aspects of obsessive–compulsive disorder in children. In R. Frost & G. Steketee (Eds.), *Cognitive approaches to obsessions and compulsions: Theory, assessment, and treatment* (pp. 299–314). Amsterdam: Pergamon/Elsevier.

Staebler, C. R., Pollard, C. A., & Merkel, W. T. (1993). Sexual history and quality of current relationships in patients with obsessive–compulsive disorder: A comparison with two other psychiatric samples. *Journal of Sex and Marital Therapy, 19*(2), 147–153.

Steketee, G. (1994). Behavioral assessment and treatment planning with obsessive–compulsive disorder: A review emphasizing clinical application. *Behavior Therapy, 25*(4), 613–633.

Swedo, S. (1989). Rituals and releasers: An ethological model of obsessive–compulsive disorder. In J. Rapoport (Ed.), *Obsessive–compulsive disorder in children and adolescents* (pp. 269–288). Washington, DC: American Psychiatric Press.

Swedo, S., Leonard, H., & Rapoport, J. (1990). Childhood-onset obsessive–compulsive disorder. In M. Jenike, L. Baer, & W. Minichello (Eds.), *Obsessive–compulsive disorder.* Littleton, MA: PSG.

Swedo, S., & Rapoport, J. (1990). Neurochemical and neuroendocrine considerations of obsessive–compulsive disorder in childhood. In W. Deutsch, A. Weizman, & R. Weizman (Eds.), *Application of basic neuroscience to child psychiatry* (pp. 275–284). New York: Plenum Press.

Swedo, S. E., Leonard, H. L., Garvey, M., Mittleman, B., Allen, A. J., Perlmutter, S., Dow, S., Zamkoff, J., Dubbert, B. K., & Lougee, L. (1998). Pediatric autoimmune neuropsychiatric disorders associated with streptococcal infections: Clinical description of the first 50 cases. *American Journal of Psychiatry, 155*(2), 264–271.

Swedo, S. E., Rapoport, J. L., Leonard, H., Lenane, M., & Cheslow, D. (1989). Obsessive–compulsive disorder in children and adolescents: Clinical phenomenology of 70 consecutive cases. *Archives of General Psychiatry, 46*(4), 335–341.

Thyer, B. A. (1991). Diagnosis and treatment of child and adolescent anxiety disorders. *Behavior Modification, 15*(3), 310–325.

Valleni-Basile, L. A., Garrison, C. Z., Jackson, K. L., Waller, J. L., McKeown, R. E., Addy, C. L., & Cuffe, S. P. (1994). Frequency of obsessive–compulsive disorder in a community sample of young adolescents. *Journal of the American Academy of Child and Adolescent Psychiatry, 33*(6), 782–791.

Valleni-Basile, L. A., Garrison, C. Z., Waller, J. L., Addy, C. L., McKeown, R. E., Jackson, K. L., & Cuffe, S. P. (1996). Incidence of obsessive–compulsive disorder in a community sample of young adolescents. *Journal of the American Academy of Child and Adolescent Psychiatry, 35*(7), 898–906.

van Oppen, P., & Arntz, A. (1994). Cognitive therapy for obsessive–compulsive disorder. *Behavior Research and Therapy, 32*(1), 79–87.

van Oppen, P., de Haan, E., van Balkom, A. J., Spinhoven, P., Hoogduin, K., & van Dyck, R. (1995). Cognitive therapy and exposure in vivo in the treatment of obsessive–compulsive disorder. *Behavior Research and Therapy, 33*(4), 379–390.

Wilens, T. E., Biederman, J., March, J. S., Wolkow, R., Fine, C. S., Millstein, R. B., Faraone, S. V., Geller, D., & Spencer, T. J. (1999). Absence of cardiovascular adverse effects of sertraline in children and adolescents. *Journal of the American Academy of Child and Adolescent Psychiatry, 38*(5), 573–577.

Wolff, R., & Rapoport, J. (1988). Behavioral treatment of childhood obsessive–compulsive disorder. *Behavior Modification, 12*(2), 252–266.

Chapter 11

Posttraumatic Stress Disorder

CATHERINE D. MCKNIGHT
SCOTT N. COMPTON
JOHN S. MARCH

Since posttraumatic stress disorder (PTSD) entered the psychiatric lexicon with DSM-III (American Psychiatric Association, 1980), numerous investigations have confirmed that exposure to life-threatening stressors often leads to PTSD in young persons (March, Amaya-Jackson, & Pynoos, 1996) just as in adults (Davidson & March, 1996). In particular, child psychiatrists and psychologists have come to appreciate the extent to which children are exposed to traumatic situations, the severity of their acute distress, and the potential serious long-term psychiatric sequelae. A strong empirical investigation of traumatic events and their posttraumatic sequelae has ensued in an attempt to position PTSD within a sound developmental framework. This chapter reviews the epidemiology, diagnosis and assessment, and medication and psychosocial management of PTSD. Interested readers may wish to peruse more in-depth treatments of developmental approaches (Pynoos, Steinberg, & Piacentini, 1999), assessment (March, 1999), and treatment (Cohen, Berliner, & March, 2000b).

EPIDEMIOLOGY

Most experts agree that PTSD is not only underdiagnosed and undertreated but that it is also common, chronic, and associated with considerable morbidity and mortality. In adults, traumatic events are experienced by an estimated 70% of the population and are linked etiologically to the development of PTSD (Kessler, Sonnega, Bromet, Hughes, & Nelson, 1995). Exposure to high-magnitude trauma also occurs at alarmingly high rates in children. For example, in one study, 40% of adolescents in a community school sample experienced a PTSD-qualifying trauma by age 18 (Giaconia et al., 1995). Of more than 1,000 middle and high school students in Chicago, 35% had witnessed a stabbing, 39% had seen a shooting, and almost 25% had seen someone being killed (Jenkins & Bell, 1994). These images were particularly salient as nearly half of the victims were acquaintances, such as friends, family members, classmates, or neighbors. Additionally, 46% of the adolescent sample reported being direct victims of at least one highly violent crime, including armed robbery, rape, and shootings or stabbings.

Although the events that cause PTSD are common (Reiss, Richters, Radke-Yarrow, & Scharrf, 1993), there is an absence of epidemiological studies that look specifically at the general population incidence or prevalence of PTSD in young persons. It is clear, however, that PTSD is more common in youths exposed to life-threatening events, such as criminal assault (Pynoos & Nader, 1988), hostage taking (Schwarz & Kowalski, 1991), combat (Clarke, Sack, & Goff, 1993), bone marrow transplantation (Stuber et al., 1991), hospitalization following accidental injury (Daviss et al., 2000), severe burns (Stoddard, Norman, & Murphy, 1989), suicide (Brent, 1995), and naval disaster (Yule, Udwin, & Murdoch, 1990; Yule & Williams, 1990). Studies crossing a variety of industrial (March, Amaya-Jackson, Terry, & Costanzo, 1997) and natural disasters (Burke, Moccia, Borus, & Burns, 1986; McFarlane, 1987) also show elevated rates of posttraumatic stress in disaster victims relative to controls.

Although the range of environmental events capable of producing PTSD varies somewhat between children and adults, effects of the stressor remain primary within and across a variety of settings (McNally, 1993). For example, Pynoos and colleagues (1987) showed that exposure (physical proximity) was linearly related to the risk of PTSD symptoms and that children's memory disturbances, indicating distorted cognitive processing during the event, closely followed exposure. Saigh (1991) later showed that PTSD could result from direct, witnessed, or verbal exposure. However, stressor-specific factors tend to influence the resulting symptom picture (Famularo, Kinscherff, & Fenton, 1990; Kendall-Tackett, Williams, & Finkelhor, 1993; Nader, Stuber, & Pynoos, 1991). Specifically, chronic physical and sexual abuse in childhood often results in severe psychopathology that bears little relationship to the classic PTSD symptom picture (Kendall-Tackett et al., 1993). In this regard, Terr (1991) makes the clinically useful distinction between Type I traumas (sudden, unpredictable single-incident stressor that may be repeated) and Type II traumas (chronic expected repeated stressor, usually childhood physical and/or sexual abuse), with these two broad categories representing differing literatures and alternate treatment approaches (Cohen et al., 2000b).

DIAGNOSIS AND PHENOMENOLOGY

Four criteria must be satisfied to establish a DSM-IV diagnosis of PTSD in both adults and children: (1) exposure to a PTSD magnitude stressor; (2) subsequent reexperiencing of the event; (3) consequent avoidance or numbing of general responsiveness; and (4) persistent increased arousal (American Psychiatric Association, 1994).

Stressor

Unique in the requirement for an etiopathogenic agent with enduring sequelae (March, 1993), the stressor criterion defines the primary risk factor for PTSD, namely exposure to a life-threatening event; the three latter criteria groupings point to important clinical parameters in the phenomenology of the disorder. Such traumatic experiences inevitably involve intense perceptual experiences and internal moment-to-moment appraisals of the threat and hence meet the DSM-IV criterion requiring terror, horror, and helplessness (Eth & Pynoos, 1985; March, 1993).

Reexperiencing

Children and adolescents with PTSD typically reexperience the traumatic event in distressing intrusive thoughts or memories, dreams, and, less commonly, flashbacks. Reexperiencing may occur spontaneously or in response to environmental cues that are linked to traumatic components within the event itself. For example, recurrent intrusive and distressing images, sounds, smells, or impressions often act as cues to moments of extreme terror or vulnerability during the event. This may be particularly salient following more public traumas, such as the terrorist activity on September 11, 2001, as continuous media coverage may prolong reminders of the event. Furthermore, children's traumatic dreams include repetitions of aspects of the experience, depiction of other life-threatening dangers, or, over time, more general fearful dreams—for example, in young children, of being pursued by monsters.

Traumatic play and reenactment behaviors are not uncommon manifestations of reexperiencing in traumatized children and adolescents. Traumatic play refers to the retelling or repetitive dramatization in play of elements or themes of the event, for example, scenes of violence, plane crashes, or "earthquake" games (Terr, 1990). Children sometimes involve siblings or peers in their traumatic play, with incorporation of traumatic elements that impede the developmentally normative purpose of play (Pynoos & Nader, 1990). Oftentimes this disturbing play goes unnoticed by parents and teachers unless it is overtly distressing, dangerous, violent, suicidal, or sexually precocious. In contrast, reenactment behavior refers to unconscious replication of some aspect of the traumatic experience (Saylor, Swenson, & Powell, 1992; Terr, 1990). In younger children, the behavior may be an "action memory." For example, an abused preschool child who was locked in a closet repeatedly hid in small spaces, such as boxes or under desks, while consciously avoiding closets. Reenactment behavior in adolescents can be especially dangerous due to increased access to guns, automobiles, and drugs.

Avoidance and Numbing

Children with PTSD invariably make conscious attempts to avoid traumatic reminders—namely, thoughts, feelings, or activities that precipitate distressing recollections of the event (Pynoos et al., 1999). Technically, traumatic reminders are conditioned stimuli that provoke conditioned responses that are directly or indirectly related to the traumatic event itself, including the external circumstances of the event and the internal emotional and physical reactions of the child. Common reminders include the following: circumstances (e.g., anniversaries, location, preceding activity, clothes worn), precipitating conditions (e.g., high winds after a tornado, arguing, alcohol use), other signs of danger (e.g., staring eyes, alarms), unwanted results (e.g., fixed and dilated eyes, blood), endangering objects (e.g., trees, broken glass, weapons), and a sense of helplessness (e.g., cries for help, crying, fast heartbeat, a sinking feeling, ineffectualness, or moments of aloneness). Even normal school procedures and academic exercises may serve as reminders. For example, a fire drill may reevoke a sense of prior emergency, a balloon popping may rouse memories of a neighborhood shooting, or a civics class discussion of judicial proceedings may kindle fear and rage over the trial of a father's murderer.

Typically, traumatized children avoid specific thoughts, locations, concrete items, themes in their play, and human behaviors that remind them of the traumatic experience. They may discontinue pleasurable activities or unknown situations in order to avoid excitement or fear. Because avoidant behavior is likely to decease distress on a daily basis, these behaviors appear to increase over time (Laor et al., 1997). Traumatic avoidance may selectively restrict daily activity or generalize to more phobic behavior, impeding both academic development and positive social experiences. Diminished activity may represent a preoccupation with intrusive phenomena, a depressive reaction, avoidance of affect-laden states or of traumatic reminders, or an effort to reduce the risk of further trauma. Not surprisingly, children pay a high price for these survival strategies, which often spill over into other domains of functioning. For example, child survivors of trauma may show markedly diminished interest in usually significant activities or elevated somatic or autonomic symptoms (Nader & Fairbanks, 1994). The loss of previously acquired skills may leave a child less verbal or regressed to behaviors such as thumb sucking or enuresis. Rather than reporting feeling "numb," younger children report not wanting to know how they feel, tell of feeling alone with their subjective experience, or describe efforts to keep an emotion from emerging, for example, by going to sit alone. Although initial clinical attention suggested a relative absence of major amnesia in children, recent studies have demonstrated a variety of memory disturbances (Moradi, Doost, Taghavi, Yule, & Dalgleish, 1999), including microamnesias and temporal or spatial distortions, such as proximity, duration, or sequencing. Less commonly, dissociative memory disturbances also occur, especially in response to physical coercion, molestation, or abuse (Putnam & Trickett, 1993).

Hyperarousal

Sleep disturbances, irritability, neediness, difficulty concentrating, hypervigilance, exaggerated startle responses, and outbursts of aggression are evidence that the child is in a state of increased physiological arousal (Perry, 1994; Perry & Pate, 1994). Somatic symptoms of autonomic hyperactivity may be both tonic and phasic in nature, with the latter occurring more often when the child encounters traumatic reminders (Nader & Fairbanks, 1994). The child is "on alert," anticipating the environmental threat, and is continuously ready to respond (Ornitz & Pynoos, 1989). Especially in school-age children, physiological reactivity may include somatic symptoms as a form of reexperiencing (Pynoos, Steinberg, Ornitz, & Goenjian, 1997). Sleep disturbance may be severe and persistent; changes seen in sleep architecture have been noted in adult studies (Pitman, 1992). Sleepwalking and night terrors are not uncommon. These sleep problems can further decrease the child's ability to concentrate and attend to important tasks and thus may also adversely affect learning and behavior in school. Hypervigilance and exaggerated startle may alter a child's usual behavior by leading to chronic efforts to ensure personal security or the safety of others and continuous worry for their well-being (Ornitz & Pynoos, 1989;

Pynoos et al., 1997). Last, temporary or chronic difficulty in modulating aggression can increase irritability and reduce the child's threshold for anger in response to normal demands and slights of peers and family members, resulting in unusual acts of aggression or social withdrawal (Yule & Canterbury, 1994).

COMORBIDITY

As in adults (Davidson & March, 1996), children and adolescents with PTSD tend to exhibit higher rates of psychiatric comorbidity than those without PTSD. Depressive-spectrum conditions, ranging from simple demoralization through melancholic major depression, are among the most common secondary symptoms (Brent et al., 1995; Yule, 1994). Giaconia and colleagues (1995) reported that more than 41% of adolescents with PTSD met criteria for major depression by age 18, compared with 8% among their peers without PTSD, and that PTSD was associated with a significantly increased risk for social anxiety (33%), specific phobia (29%), alcohol dependence (46%), and drug dependence (25%). Moreover, for many, the onset of PTSD preceded or co-occurred with the onset of these disorders, suggesting that PTSD triggered their occurrence. In a study of children traumatized by an industrial fire, exposure (independent of posttraumatic stress symptoms) strongly predicted general anxiety, depression, and externalizing symptomatology (March et al., 1997). Finally, a variety of collateral symptoms important to functional outcomes also have been reported in traumatized children. For example, adolescents with PTSD are at substantially greater risk for suicidal thoughts and attempts, lower perceived health, greater numbers of sick days per month at school, lower high school grade point averages, and greater school-related problems (Giaconia et al., 1995; Saigh, Mroueh, & Bremner, 1997).

ASSESSMENT

As in all psychiatric disorders, the first step in setting up a program of treatment for PTSD is a careful assessment (March, 1999, Table 11.1). Drawing from a recent National Institute of Mental Health (NIMH) consensus conference on assessing PTSD, March (1999) recently summarized the variables thought essential in treatment-outcome and other studies of PTSD, including PTSD-specific factors, as well as non-PTSD outcomes, and risk and protective factors, noting that three types of instruments are available for assessing PTSD in youths. These include: (1) structured interviews that

TABLE 11.1. Assessment Requirements

Domain/subgroup	Population	Clinical	Treatment outcome
Criterion A	E	E	E
Core PTSD symptoms	E	E	E
Functioning	E	E	E
Loss/grief	R	R	R
Life events	R	R	O
Child intrinsic variables	E/R	E/R	E/R
Comorbidity	E/R	E/R	E/R
Social context	O	R	O
Parent psychopathology	O	E/R	O
Social cognition	O	E/R	O
Social skills	O	E/R	O
Biological	O	E/R	O
Outcome	NR	NR	E

Note. E, essential; R, recommended; O, optional.

include a PTSD module, (2) PTSD-specific interviews, and (3) self-report checklists (March, 1999).

Although semistructured interviews are *de rigeur* for assessing psychiatric disorders in children and adolescents, reliability and validity data regarding the PTSD modules for commonly employed instruments have only recently become available (Costello, Angold, March, & Fairbank, 1998; Silverman & Albano, 1996).

Among PTSD-specific instruments, the most commonly used measure, the Pynoos–Nader version of the Posttraumatic Stress Reaction Index (PTS-RI; Pynoos et al., 1987), shows modest empirical support as a semistructured interview, although it does not adequately capture the DSM-IV criteria; hence it is more widely used as a self-report measure of PTSD assessed dimensionally (Lonigan, Shannon, Finch, Daugherty, & Taylor, 1991). With the support of the National Center for PTSD, Nader, Blake, Kriegler, and Pynoos (1994) recently developed the Clinician-Administered PTSD Scale—Child and Adolescent Version (CAPS-C). Although detailed (and thus cumbersome to use in the clinic), the CAPS-C allows for reliable and valid current and lifetime diagnoses and dimensional assessment of DSM-IV PTSD symptoms.

In addition to its use as a structured interview, the Pynoos–Nader version of the Posttraumatic Stress Reaction Index has been the most common scalar measure for assessing PTSD used as a self-report measure in epidemiological studies, including studies of hurricanes (Shaw et al., 1995); earthquake (Bradburn, 1991; Goenjian et al., 1995), and war zone exposure (Nader et al., 1993). However, careful psychometric studies have not been completed of the PTS-RI, which also does not provide a stressor inventory or normative data. To address these problems, March (1999) and colleagues recently developed a normed self-report PTSD measure termed the Child and Adolescent Trauma Survey (CATS) and modeled on the Multidimensional Anxiety Scale for Children (MASC; March, Parker, Sullivan, Stallings, & Conners, 1997) and the DSM-IV PTSD criteria set (American Psychiatric Association, 1994). In addition to a change-sensitive PTSD symptom scale (March, Amaya-Jackson, Murray, & Schulte, 1998), the CATS alone among self-report measures includes stable indices of non-PTSD life events and PTSD qualifying stressors.

With the caveat that parents in general are better at evaluating children's externalizing than internalizing symptoms (Costello, 1989), a multimethod multitrait evaluation is preferable, including information from multiple sources (Amaya-Jackson & March, 1993). For example, parent–teacher measures, such as the Conners' Parent and Teacher Rating Scales (Conners, 1995), are efficient adjuncts for assessing collateral externalizing symptoms. Self-report measures, such as the Children's Depression Inventory (CDI; Kovacs, 1985) or the MASC (March, Parker, et al., 1997), can be used to assess internalizing comorbidities.

Last, very little is known about the role of moderating and mediating variables in either the development or treatment of PTSD in youths (Garbarino, Kostelny, & Dubrow, 1991; March & Amaya-Jackson, 1994). Demographic factors such as age (Green et al., 1991), gender (March, Amaya-Jackson, et al., 1997), race (March, Amaya-Jackson, et al., 1997), psychiatric comorbidity (Pynoos et al., 1987), other life events (Pynoos et al., 1987), negative cognitions (March, Amaya-Jackson, et al., 1997), and family functioning (Green et al., 1991) have been suggested as potential predictor variables, but empirical studies of these predictors in children are mostly lacking.

ACUTE STRESS DISORDER

After exposure, acute reactions (instantiated as acute stress disorder [ASD] in DSM-IV) presumably are the most important predictors of downstream psychopathology, including but not limited to PTSD. However, whereas the construct of ASD has received limited support in research with adults (Bryant & Harvey, 1997), ASD in youths has garnered little critical attention. Most reports tend to treat ASD as "provisional PTSD"—meaning that children evidence ASD on the way to a formal diagnosis of PTSD—while speculating on factors that might moderate or mediate the transformation of ASD into PTSD (Pynoos et al., 1999). Thus additional attention needs to be given to nosological validation of ASD as a diagnostic construct and to understanding how, from an experimental point of view, exposure to a traumatic stressor can lead to an acute stress response that then evolves into chronic PTSD. Within the general context of risk factor modeling (Kraemer, Stice, Kazdin, Offord, & Kupfer, 2001)—and, more specifically, modeling risk when the stressor is conceptualized as analogous to a treatment in a treatment outcome study (Kraemer, Wilson, Fairburn, & Agras, 2002)—March (2003) briefly reviewed the literature on ASD in youths in the context of outlining a testable multivariate model for understanding acute stress responses in youths.

DEVELOPMENT

PTSD is a multiply determined process initiated by a high-magnitude stressor with symptoms maintained by a variety of cognitive and environmental processes that may serve as either risk or protective factors. Thus the assessment of PTSD in children and adolescents necessarily must be embedded within the child's developmental and social matrices. Moreover, because posttraumatic sequelae vary with the nature of the stressor—witness the division in the field between abuse and sudden trauma research studies—and because many children experience multiple events in both categories, the ability to map the event or events onto important domains of outcome within a developmental framework is critical to developing an intelligent and efficacious treatment plan. To some extent, this renders the DSM-IV framework, which underemphasizes developmental differences and social contextual factors, less than adequate for evaluating childhood-onset PTSD. For example, some aspects of the PTSD symptom complex may be best reported by the affected child, others by parents, and still others by teachers or other observers, with these timing issues varying with the developmental stage of the child. Moreover, because the child's social matrix—neighborhood, family, peer, and school environments—may strongly condition the risk, characteristics, and course of PTSD and corollary symptoms, it is important to consider variables such as loss, secondary adversities, family functioning, and attachment-related symptoms, such as separation anxiety, when evaluating PTSD. For example, childhood victims of abuse and neglect demonstrate an increased risk of developing PTSD in young adulthood; however, prior abuse and neglect do not remain significant predictors after adjusting for behavior problems, marital disruption, and

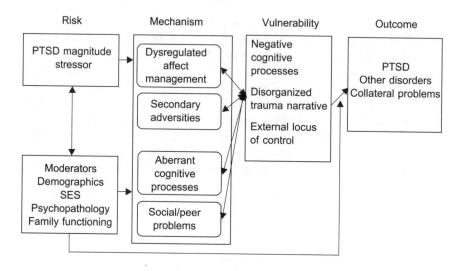

FIGURE 11.1. Developmental model.

alcohol or drug use. Useful primarily for heuristic purposes, Figure 11.1 presents a much-simplified developmental model for the genesis and maintenance of PTSD in youths, adapted from our previous work (Kendall, 1993; March, 1995; March et al., 1996), and, by analogy, from depression (Goodman & Gotlib, 1999).

TREATMENT

Although it is beyond the scope of this chapter to review the extensive (as contrasted, unfortunately, to the much smaller empirical) literature on the clinical treatment of pediatric PTSD, a wide variety of techniques have been found to be effective in clinical practice. (Fortunately, a review was recently conducted under the auspices of the International Society for Traumatic Stress Studies [Cohen, Berliner, & March, 2000a; Cohen et al., 2000b], to which the interested reader is referred.) Looked at from a broad vantage point, a prevention–intervention model—which incorporates triage for children exposed to stressor events, supporting and strengthening coping skills for anticipated grief and trauma responses, treating other disorders that may develop or exacerbate in the context of PTSD, and treatment for acute PTSD symptoms—is recommended (American Academy of Child and Adolescent Psychiatry, 1998). Although the horror of the trauma can never be undone and hence "cure" may not be the appropriate treatment goal, victims can become well-functioning survivors if appropriate treatment is given and facilitation of healing takes place.

From the standpoint of evidence-based practice, recommendations for treatment are more narrowly defined. In their comprehensive review, Cohen and colleagues (2000a) reached the following conclusions concerning the treatment of PTSD in youths:

> Children and adolescents with PTSD would likely benefit from treatment focused on PTSD symptomatology. Of the available treatments, CBT has the most empirical support and is therefore the initial treatment of choice. The particular format of CBT should be dictated by the nature of the trauma, with specific protocols focused on either abuse or sudden trauma. Because of their favorable side-effect profile and evidence supporting effectiveness in treating both depressive and anxiety disorders, SSRIs often are the first psychotropic medication chosen for treating pediatric PTSD, especially when dictated by a SSRI-responsive comorbidity. Clonidine may be helpful for some children and adolescents with prominent hyperarousal symptoms, especially elevated startle responses. (pp. 331–332)

Cognitive-Behavioral Psychotherapy

Although a wide variety of psychotherapeutic techniques have been employed (March et al., 1996), empirical support for psychosocial treatments of PTSD in children is strongest for cognitive-behavioral therapy (Cohen et al., 2000a, 2000b). Historically, behavioral therapy (the BT in CBT) evolved within the theoretical framework of classical and operant conditioning. The cognitive interventions (the C in CBT) have assumed a prominent role with the increasing recognition that cognitive processes mediate person–environment interactions. Behavioral therapists work with patients to change behaviors and thereby to reduce distressing thoughts and feelings. Cognitive therapists work to first change thoughts and feelings, with improvements in functional behavior following in turn. For the most part, these two main conceptual positions have been integrated within more recent approaches, such as information processing. Their clinical applications to treatment have also been subsumed within the broad umbrella of social learning theory (Hibbs & Jensen, 1996).

March and colleagues recently completed a pilot study of group school-based CBT for PTSD after single-incident trauma, which illustrates the general principles involved (March et al., 1998a) and draws significantly on earlier work with adults by Foa and colleagues (Foa, 1997). As shown in Table 11.2, treatment took place over 18 weekly sessions. Each

TABLE 11.2. Typical Treatment Outline

Session 1	Getting Started
Session 2	Naming and Mapping
Session 3	Anxiety Management Training 1
Session 4	Anxiety Management Training 2
Session 5	Grading Feelings
Session 6	Anger Coping 1
Session 7	Anger Coping 2
Session 8	Cognitive Training 1
Session 9	Cognitive Training 2
Session 10a	Introducing Exposure and Response Prevention
Session 10b	Pullout Session
Session 11	Trial Exposure
Session 12	Narrative Exposure 1
Session 13	Narrative Exposure 2
Session 14	Worst Moment Exposure 1
Session 15	Worst Moment Exposure 2
Session 16	Right Beliefs
Session 17	Relapse Prevention/Generalization
Session 18	Graduation Party

Note. Sessions 1 and 18 are 90 minutes; all others are 50–60 minutes.

session includes a statement of goals, a careful review of the preceding week, introduction of new information, therapist-assisted "nuts and bolts" practice, homework for the coming week, and monitoring procedures. Sessions 1 and 2 provide an overview of the treatment process, initiate information gathering, and introduce the concept of "bossing back PTS" by introducing a silly nickname for PTSD. Session 1 also defines rules for group process, including confidentiality, turn taking, plans for conflict resolution, and attendance procedures. Sessions 3–5 are devoted to anxiety management training. Session 3 introduces progressive, cue-controlled, and differential muscle relaxation. Session 4 extends relaxation training by teaching diaphragmatic breathing to relieve any "suffocation" symptoms associated with panic states. Session 5 introduces a distress scale in the form of an analog fear thermometer and then uses the fear thermometer to grade thoughts and feelings with respect to anxiety, anger, and PTS in response to traumatic reminders. Sessions 6 and 7 address anger and aggression by taking an interpersonal problem-solving approach to anger control (Lochman, Lampron, Gemmer, & Harris, 1987). Session 6 examines anger-producing self-statements and, building on techniques learned in anxiety management training (AMT), introduces "perspective taking" as a cognitive strategy for managing angry cognitions and aggressive behaviors. Session 7 builds on Session 6 by taking a role-playing approach to conflict resolution. Sessions 8 and 9 address cognitive training for "bossing back PTS" by adapting the approach used for AMT and anger coping more specifically to PTSD. Session 8 helps the child develop positive self-talk emphasizing personal efficacy, predictability, and controllability of the environment, realistic risk appraisal, and positive statements countering PTS intrusions. Session 9 continues cognitive training but more tightly couples cognitive training to PTSD. Session 10A provides an overview of exposure and response prevention and introduces the concept of the stimulus hierarchy. Session 10B is an individual session that has three goals: (1) using a moment-by-moment trauma replay procedure, constructing a stimulus hierarchy based on identification of conditioned stimuli (traumatic reminders within fear structures) that are referable to the child's trauma; (2) introducing narrative exposure; and (3) providing corrective information regarding trauma-specific misattributions and distortions. Sessions 11, 12, and 13 introduce narrative exposure, in which each child tells his or her story to the group so as to encourage habituation. As indicated, the therapist and group members introduce corrective information regarding spatial and temporal distortions, global attributions that reinforce lack of personal efficacy, normalization, and positive coping. These sessions also involve practicing imaginal exposure and introduce *in vivo* exposure as homework. For example, the child who avoids going outside might spend time playing in the front yard, assuming that it is safe to do so. Homework during this stage of treatment involves selecting *in vivo* exposure targets. Session 14 and 15 extend the approach used in sessions 12 and 13 to verbalize the "worst moment" for each child. Homework for these sessions involves practicing the techniques learned in groups for increasingly difficult *in vivo* exposure targets. In this context, the focus switches more to contrived exposure to traumatic reminders. Session 16 directly confronts PTSD-induced dysfunctional beliefs or schemas; homework is to practice substituting helpful beliefs for unskillful ones. Session 17 underscores that the children have learned how to "boss back PTS" across many situations and into the future. The goal for this session is to summarize, review, reinforce, and promote generalization of the techniques of AMT, anger coping, and exposure. Session 18 is a graduation party during which each child will receive a graduation certificate for "becoming the boss of PTS." During Sessions 17 and 18 the therapist gradually fades out therapist assistance and emphasizes independence.

Despite robust evidence favoring CBT as a treatment for PTSD across the age range, it is likely that most children do not receive state-of-the-art cognitive-behavioral interventions following life-threatening events (Kendall & Southam-Gerow, 1995). One reason is the lack of empirically supported manualized treatment protocols that can be exported to clinical settings (Clarke, 1995). Moreover, as Kendall and Southam-Gerow (1995) point out, controlled trials of protocol-driven treatments are clearly necessary before moving to effectiveness research protocols conducted in clinical populations. Thus it is encouraging that protocols for treating PTSD, stemming from both single-incident trauma (March et al., 1998) and sexual and physical abuse, are becoming more widely available (Cohen & Mannarino, 1996b; Deblinger, McLeer, & Henry, 1990).

Pharmacotherapy

Although PTSD has an exogenous origin and likely requires psychological treatment, the disorder is nevertheless, using Kardiner's (1941) term, a true physioneurosis (Perry, 1994), and psychotropic medication may, in selected cases, prove helpful in relieving PTSD and collateral symptoms (Davidson & March, 1996). Ideally, medications should decrease intrusions, avoidance, and anxious arousal; minimize impulsivity and improve sleep; treat secondary disorders; and facilitate cognitive-behavioral interventions. On the other hand, although a variety of psychopharmacological agents have been advocated or used—including propranolol (Famularo, Kinscherff, & Fenton, 1988), carbamezapine (Looff, Grimley, Kuller, Martin, & Shonfield, 1995), clonidine (Newcorn et al., 1998), and various antidepressants (Pfefferbaum, 1997)—relatively little data exist to guide medication of children and adolescents with these compounds (Donnelly, Amaya-Jackson, & March, 1999). Controlled trials with adults suggest that standard antidepressants may improve PTSD symptoms, with the SSRIs currently favored because of demonstrated efficacy and a more favorable side-effect profile (Davidson, 1997); a similar response has been seen clinically in children and adolescents (Donnelly et al., 1999). Clonidine has been shown to decrease startle responses in some children with PTSD (Ornitz & Pynoos, 1989), and Horrigan recently completed an open study in which a long-acting alpha-2 agonist, guanfacine, successfully reduced startle responses and nightmares in children with PTSD (Horrigan, personal communication), suggesting that the alpha-2 agonists may be helpful to some children with PTSD characterized by prominent hyperarousal symptoms.

Including Families

Parental emotional reaction to the traumatic event and parental support of the child are potentially powerful influences on the child's PTSD symptomatology. Hence, despite limited evidence to the contrary (King et al., 2000; March et al., 1998), most experts assert that inclusion of parents and supportive others in treatment is important for resolution of PTSD symptoms in children (March et al., 1996). At a minimum, including parents in treatment helps them monitor the child's symptomatology and learn appropriate behavioral management techniques, both in the intervals between treatment sessions and after therapy is terminated. In addition, helping parents resolve their emotional distress related to the trauma, to which the parent usually has had either direct or vicarious exposure, can help the parent be more perceptive of and responsive to the child's emotional needs (Burman & Allen-Meares, 1994). Not surprisingly, parent interventions are considered imperative in the child abuse literature, in which most authors recommend one or more parent-directed components (Cohen et al., 2000b; Cohen & Mannarino, 1996a; Deblinger et al., 1990).

Combined Treatment

It is widely recognized that assessment and treatment of PTSD must address a variety of symptoms or dysfunctions beyond those that make up or even are attributable to PTSD per se (March, 2002). However, there is little or no empirical evidence to support combining treatments within or across treatment modalities. In particular, there is no empirical evidence to support the common clinical belief that the combination of medication management and psychotherapy is superior to psychotherapy alone.

Duration of Treatment

Clinically, most children and adolescents with uncomplicated PTSD will make substantial improvement with 12–20 sessions of PTSD-specific CBT. A smaller number of children require long-term treatment. Exposure to massive violence, intrafamilial homicide or suicide, prolonged abuse, or exposure to repetitively distressing events suggests that brief trauma work may not be enough. The presence of preexisting psychopathology in the child or a parent, prior history of abuse, or ongoing exposure to a disruptive living situation also suggests a need for intensive longer term intervention. Long-term treatment can occur weekly or as "pulsed intervention" based on the child's developmental phase, capacity for response, and clinical issues. Pulsed intervention assumes that brief therapy is suspended (rather than terminated) until further treatment becomes necessary—such as during developmental transitions, changes in living situation, formation of intimate relationships, marriage, and so forth. "Pulsing" the treatment helps prevent ongoing helplessness by minimizing dependence on the therapist as "the only one who really understands." Unfortunately, severe PTSD requires arduous and critical dedication to treatment on the part of the patient and therapist. Longer term therapy also may be necessary when issues related to character formation and capacity to form meaningful relationships are present.

Future Directions

Recognizing the need for informed, evidence-based assessments, interventions, and treatments for children and adolescents who experience trauma, the National Child Traumatic Stress Network has coordinated a collaboration of 10 research development and evaluation sites and 26 community mental health centers across the United States. By integrating previously fragmented services, they aim to produce developmentally appropriate, evidence-based treatments that are informed by practice sites such as child advocacy groups, juvenile justice systems, school-based services, and medical centers. Under the umbrella of the National Network, interventions are being evaluated for the individualized needs of pediatric cancer patients, children who lost parents on September 11, 2001, refugee burn victims, and sufferers of sexual abuse. From training police and emergency room personnel who deal with the acute phase of trauma to developing manualized interventions for 0- to 5-year-old children, the joint expertise of the National Network will clarify what are both feasible and effective components of treatment for children and families who have experienced trauma.

CONCLUSION

Incontrovertible evidence reveals that PTSD occurs in children and adolescents in much the same form as in adults, though substantially colored by developmental and socioecological factors. Young persons with PTSD likely benefit from treatment focused on PTSD symptomatology. Of the available treatments, CBT has the most empirical support and is therefore the initial treatment of choice. The particular format of CBT should be dictated by the nature of the trauma, with specific protocols focused on either abuse or sudden trauma. Because of their favorable side-effect profile and evidence supporting effectiveness in treating both depressive and anxiety disorders, SSRIs often are the first psychotropic medication chosen for treating pediatric PTSD, especially when dictated by an SSRI-responsive comorbidity. Given early recognition and adequate treatment, many if not most children can be helped to resume a normal developmental trajectory.

ACKNOWLEDGMENTS

Supported by NIMH Grant No. 1 K24 MHO1557 to John S. March and by contributions from the Robert and Sarah Gorrell family.

REFERENCES

Amaya-Jackson, L., & March, J. (1993). Posttraumatic stress disorder in children and adolescents. In H. L. Leonard (Ed.), *Child psychiatric clinics of North America: Anxiety disorders* (Vol. 2, pp. 639–654). New York: Saunders.

American Academy of Child and Adolescent Psychiatry. (1998). Summary of the practice parameters for the assessment and treatment of children and adolescents with posttraumatic stress disorder. *Journal of the American Academy of Child and Adolescent Psychiatry, 37*(9), 997–1001.

American Psychiatric Association. (1980). *Diagnostic and statistical manual of mental disorders* (3rd ed.). Washington, DC: Author.

American Psychiatric Association. (1994). *Diagnostic and statistical manual of mental disorders* (4th ed.). Washington DC: Author.

Bradburn, I. S. (1991). After the earth shook: Children's stress symptoms 6–8 months after a disaster. *Advances in Behavior Research and Therapy, 13*(3), 173–179.

Brent, D. A. (1995). Risk factors for adolescent suicide and suicidal behavior: Mental and substance abuse disorders, family environmental factors, and life stress. *Suicide and Life-Threatening Behavior, 25*(Suppl.), 52–63.

Brent, D. A., Perper, J. A., Moritz, G., Liotus, L., Richardson, D., Canobbio, R., Schweers, J., & Roth, C. (1995). Posttraumatic stress disorder in peers of adolescent suicide victims: Predisposing factors and phenomenology. *Journal of the American Academy of Child and Adolescent Psychiatry, 34*(2), 209–215.

Bryant, R. A., & Harvey, A. G. (1997). Acute stress disorder: A critical review of diagnostic issues. *Clinical Psychology Review, 17*(7), 757–773.

Burke, J. D., Moccia, P., Borus, J. F., & Burns, B. J. (1986). Emotional distress in fifth-grade children ten months after a natural disaster. *Journal of the American Academy of Child Psychiatry, 25*(4), 536–541.

Burman, S., & Allen-Meares, P. (1994). Neglected victims of murder: Children's witness to parental homicide. *Social Work, 39*(1), 28–34.

Clarke, G., Sack, W. H., & Goff, B. (1993). Three forms of stress in Cambodian adolescent refugees. *Journal of Abnormal Child Psychology, 21*(1), 65–77.

Clarke, G. N. (1995). Improving the transition from basic efficacy research to effectiveness studies: Methodological issues and procedures. *Journal of Consulting and Clinical Psychology, 63*(5), 718–725.

Cohen, J. A., Berliner, L., & March, J. S. (2000a). Treatment of children and adolescents. In E. B. Foa, T. M. Keane, & M. J. Friedman (Eds.), *Effective treatments for PTSD* (pp. 330–332). New York: Guilford Press.

Cohen, J. A., Berliner, L., & March, J. (2000b). Treatment of children and adolescents. In E. B. Foa, T. M. Keane, & M. J. Friedman (Eds.), *Effective treatments for PTSD* (pp. 106–138). New York: Guilford Press.

Cohen, J. A., & Mannarino, A. P. (1996a). Factors that mediate treatment outcome of sexually abused preschool children. *Journal of the American Academy of Child and Adolescent Psychiatry, 35*(10), 1402–1410.

Cohen, J. A., & Mannarino, A. P. (1996b). A treatment outcome study for sexually abused preschool children: Initial findings. *Journal of the American Academy of Child and Adolescent Psychiatry, 35*(1), 42–50.

Conners, C. (1995). *Conners' Rating Scales.* Toronto: Multi-Health Systems.

Costello, E. (1989). Developments in child psychiatric epidemiology. *Journal of the American Academy of Child and Adolescent Psychiatry, 28*, 836–841.

Costello, E. J., Angold, A., March, J. S., & Fairbank, J. (1998). Life events and post-traumatic stress: The development of a new measure for children and adolescents. *Psychological Medicine, 28*(6), 1275–1288.

Davidson, J., & March, J. (1996). Traumatic stress disorders. In A. Tasman, J. Kay, & J. Lieberman (Eds.), *Psychiatry* (Vol. 2, pp. 1085–1098). Philadelphia: Saunders.

Davidson, J. R. (1997). Biological therapies for posttraumatic stress disorder: An overview. *Journal of Clinical Psychiatry, 58*(Suppl. 9), 29–32.

Daviss, W. B., Racusin, R., Fleischer, A., Mooney, D., Ford, J. D., & McHugo, G. J. (2000). Acute stress disorder symptomatology during hospitalization for pediatric injury. *Journal of the American Academy of Child and Adolescent Psychiatry, 39*(5), 569–575.

Deblinger, E., McLeer, S. V., & Henry, D. (1990). Cognitive behavioral treatment for sexually abused children suffering posttraumatic stress: Preliminary findings. *Journal of the American Academy of Child and Adolescent Psychiatry, 29*(5), 747–752.

Donnelly, C. L., Amaya-Jackson, L., & March, J. S. (1999). Psychopharmacology of pediatric posttraumatic stress disorder. *Journal of Child and Adolescent Psychopharmacology, 9*(3), 203–220.

Eth, S., & Pynoos, R. (1985). *Posttraumatic stress disorder in children.* Washington, DC: American Psychiatric Press.

Famularo, R., Kinscherff, R., & Fenton, T. (1988). Propranolol treatment for childhood posttraumatic stress disorder, acute type: A pilot study. *American Journal of Diseases of Children, 142*(11), 1244–1247.

Famularo, R., Kinscherff, R., & Fenton, T. (1990). Symptom differences in acute and chronic presentation of childhood posttraumatic stress disorder. *Child Abuse and Neglect, 14*(3), 439–444.

Foa, E. B. (1997). Psychological processes related to recovery from a trauma and an effective treatment for PTSD. *Annals of the New York Academy of Sciences, 821*, 410–424.

Garbarino, J., Kostelny, K., & Dubrow, N. (1991). What children can tell us about living in danger. *American Psychologist, 46*(4), 376–383.

Giaconia, R. M., Reinherz, H. Z., Silverman, A. B., Pakiz, B., Frost, A. K., & Cohen, E. (1995). Traumas and posttraumatic stress disorder in a community population of older adolescents. *Journal of the American Academy of Child and Adolescent Psychiatry, 34*(10), 1369–1380.

Goenjian, A. K., Pynoos, R. S., Steinberg, A. M., Najarian, L. M., Asarnow, J. R., Karayan, I., Ghurabi, M., & Fairbanks, L. A. (1995). Psychiatric comorbidity in children after the 1988 earthquake in Armenia. *Journal of the American Academy of Child and Adolescent Psychiatry, 34*(9), 1174–1184.

Goodman, S. H., & Gotlib, I. H. (1999). Risk for psychopathology in the children of depressed mothers: A developmental model for understanding mechanisms of transmission. *Psychological Review, 106*(3), 458–490.

Green, B. L., Korol, M., Grace, M. C., Vary, M. G., Leonard, A. C., Gleser, G. C., & Smitson-Cohen, S. (1991). Children and disaster: Age, gender, and parental effects on PTSD symptoms. *Journal of the American Academy of Child and Adolescent Psychiatry, 30*(6), 945–951.

Hibbs, E., & Jensen, P. (1996). *Psychosocial treatments for child and adolescent disorders.* Washington, DC: American Psychological Press.

Jenkins, E. J., & Bell, C. C. (1994). Violence among inner city high school students and posttraumatic stress disorder. In S. Friedman (Ed.), *Anxiety disorders in African Americans* (Vol. 246, pp. 76–88). New York: Springer.

Kardiner, A. (1941). *The traumatic neurosis of war.* New York: Hoeber.

Kendall, P. (1993). Guiding theory for therapy with children and adolescents. In P. C. Kendall (Ed.), *Child and adolescent therapy* (pp. 3–22). New York: Guilford Press.

Kendall, P. C., & Southam-Gerow, M. A. (1995). Issues in the transportability of treatment: The case of anxiety disorders in youths. *Journal of Consulting and Clinical Psychology, 63*(5), 702–708.

Kendall-Tackett, K. A., Williams, L. M., & Finkelhor, D. (1993). Impact of sexual abuse on children: A review and synthesis of recent empirical studies. *Psychological Bulletin, 113*(1), 164–180.

Kessler, R. C., Sonnega, A., Bromet, E., Hughes, M., & Nelson, C. B. (1995). Posttraumatic stress disorder in the National Comorbidity Survey. *Archives of General Psychiatry, 52*(12), 1048–1060.

King, N. J., Tonge, B. J., Mullen, P., Myerson, N., Heyne, D., Rollings, S., Martin, R., & Ollendick, T. H. (2000). Treating sexually abused children with posttraumatic stress symptoms: A randomized clinical trial. *Journal of the American Academy of Child and Adolescent Psychiatry, 39*(11), 1347–1355.

Kovacs, M. (1985). The Children's Depression Inventory (CDI). *Psychopharmacology Bulletin, 21,* 995–998.

Kraemer, H. C., Stice, E., Kazdin, A., Offord, D., & Kupfer, D. (2001). How do risk factors work together? Mediators, moderators, and independent, overlapping, and proxy risk factors. *American Journal of Psychiatry, 158*(6), 848–856.

Kraemer, H. C., Wilson, G. T., Fairburn, C. G., & Agras, W. S. (2002). Mediators and moderators of treatment effects in randomized clinical trials. *Archives of General Psychiatry, 59,* 877–883.

Laor, N., Wolmer, L., Mayes, L. C., Gershon, A., Weizman, R., & Cohen, D. J. (1997). Israeli preschool children under Scuds: A 30-month follow-up. *Journal of the American Academy of Child and Adolescent Psychiatry, 36*(3), 349–356.

Lochman, J., Lampron, L., Gemmer, T., & Harris, S. (1987). Anger coping intervention with aggressive children: A guide to implementation in school settings. In P.

Keller & S. Heyman (Eds.), *Innovations in clinical practice: A source book* (Vol. 6, pp. 339–356). Sarasota, FL: Professional Resource Exchange.

Lonigan, C. J., Shannon, M. P., Finch, A. J., Daugherty, T. K., & Taylor, C. M. (1991). Children's reactions to a natural disaster: Symptom severity and degree of exposure. *Advances in Behavior Research and Therapy, 13*(3), 135–154.

Looff, D., Grimley, P., Kuller, F., Martin, A., & Shonfield, L. (1995). Carbamazepine for PTSD [Letter]. *Journal of the American Academy of Child and Adolescent Psychiatry, 34*(6), 703–704.

March, J. S. (1993). What constitutes a stressor? The "Criterion A" issue. In J. Davidson & E. Foa (Eds.), *Posttraumatic stress disorder: DSM-IV and beyond* (pp. 37–54). Washington, DC: American Psychiatric Press.

March, J. S. (Ed.). (1995). *Anxiety disorders in children and adolescents.* New York: Guilford Press.

March, J. S. (1999). Assessment of pediatric posttraumatic stress disorder. In P. Saigh & D. Bremner (Eds.), *Post-traumatic stress disorder* (pp. 199–218). Washington, DC: American Psychological Press.

March, J. S. (2002). Combining medication and psychosocial treatments: An evidence-based medicine approach. *International Review of Psychiatry, 14*(2), 155–163.

March, J. S. (2003). Acute stress disorder in youth: A multivariate prediction model. *Biological Psychology, 53*(9), 809–816.

March, J. S., & Amaya-Jackson, L. (1994). Posttraumatic stress disorder in children and adolescents. *PTSD Research Quarterly, 4*(4), 1–7.

March, J. S., Amaya-Jackson, L., Murray, M. C., & Schulte, A. (1998). Cognitive-behavioral psychotherapy for children and adolescents with post-traumatic stress disorder following a single-incident stressor. *Journal of the American Academy of Child and Adolescent Psychiatry, 37*(6), 585–593.

March, J. S., Amaya-Jackson, L., & Pynoos, R. (1996). Pediatric posttraumatic stress disorder. In J. Weiner (Ed.), *Textbook of child and adolescent psychiatry* (2nd ed.). Washington, DC: American Psychiatric Press.

March, J. S., Amaya-Jackson, L., Terry, R., & Costanzo, P. (1997). Post-traumatic stress in children and adolescents after an industrial fire. *Journal of the American Academy of Child and Adolescent Psychiatry, 36*(8), 1080–1088.

March, J. S., Parker, J., Sullivan, K., Stallings, P., & Conners, C. (1997). The Multidimensional Anxiety Scale for Children (MASC): Factor structure, reliability and validity. *Journal of the American Academy of Child and Adolescent Psychiatry, 36*(4), 554–565.

McFarlane, A. (1987). Life events and psychiatric disorder: The role of a natural disaster. *British Journal of Psychiatry, 151,* 362–367.

McNally, R. J. (1993). Stressors that produce posttraumatic stress disorder in children. In J. R. T. Davidson & E. B. Foa (Eds.), *Posttraumatic stress disorder: DSM-IV and beyond* (pp. 57–74). Washington, DC: American Psychiatric Press.

Moradi, A. R., Doost, H. T., Taghavi, M. R., Yule, W., & Dalgleish, T. (1999). Everyday memory deficits in children and adolescents with PTSD: Performance on the Rivermead Behavioral Memory Test. *Journal of Child Psychology and Psychiatry, 40*(3), 357–361.

Nader, K., Blake, D., Kriegler, J., & Pynoos, R. (1994). *Clinician Administered PTSD*

Scale for Children (CAPS-C), Current and Lifetime Diagnosis Version, and Instruction Manual. Los Angeles: UCLA Neuropsychiatric Institute and National Center for PTSD.

Nader, K., Stuber, M., & Pynoos, R. S. (1991). Posttraumatic stress reactions in preschool children with catastrophic illness: Assessment needs. *Comprehensive Mental Health Care, 1*(3), 223–239.

Nader, K. O., & Fairbanks, L. A. (1994). The suppression of reexperiencing: Impulse control and somatic symptoms in children following traumatic exposure. *Anxiety, Stress and Coping: An International Journal, 7*(3), 229–239.

Nader, K. O., Pynoos, R. S., Fairbanks, L. A., al-Ajeel, M., & al-Asfour, A. (1993). A preliminary study of PTSD and grief among the children of Kuwait following the Gulf crisis. *British Journal of Clinical Psychology, 32*(Part 4), 407–416.

Newcorn, J. H., Schulz, K., Harrison, M., DeBellis, M. D., Udarbe, J. K., & Halperin, J. M. (1998). Alpha 2 adrenergic agonists: Neurochemistry, efficacy, and clinical guidelines for use in children. *Pediatric Clinics of North America, 45*(5), 1009–1022.

Ornitz, E., & Pynoos, R. (1989). Startle modulation in children with posttraumatic stress disorder. *American Journal of Psychiatry, 146*, 866–870.

Perry, B. D. (1994). *Neurobiological sequelae of childhood trauma: PTSD in children.* Washington, DC: American Psychiatric Press.

Perry, B. D., & Pate, J. E. (1994). *Neurodevelopment and the psychobiological roots of posttraumatic stress disorder.* Springfield: Thomas.

Pfefferbaum, B. (1997). Posttraumatic stress disorder in children: A review of the last ten years. *Journal of American Academy of Child and Adolescent Psychiatry, 36*(11), 1503–1511.

Pitman, R. (1992). Biological findings in posttraumatic stress disorder: Implications for DSM-IV classification. In J. Davidson & E. Foa (Eds.), *Posttraumatic stress disorder: DSM-IV and beyond* (pp. 173–189). Washington, DC: American Psychiatric Press.

Putnam, F. W., & Trickett, P. K. (1993). Child sexual abuse: A model of chronic trauma. *Psychiatry, 56*(1), 82–95.

Pynoos, R. S., Frederick, C., Nader, K., Arroyo, W., Steinberg, A., Eth, S., Nunez, F., & Fairbanks, L. (1987). Life threat and posttraumatic stress in school-age children. *Archives of General Psychiatry, 44*(12), 1057–1063.

Pynoos, R. S., & Nader, K. (1988). Children who witness the sexual assaults of their mothers. *Journal of the American Academy of Child and Adolescent Psychiatry, 27*(5), 567–572.

Pynoos, R. S., & Nader, K. (1990). Children's exposure to violence and traumatic death. *Psychiatric Annals, 20*(6), 334–344.

Pynoos, R. S., Steinberg, A. M., Ornitz, E. M., & Goenjian, A. K. (1997). Issues in the developmental neurobiology of traumatic stress. *Annals of the New York Academy of Sciences, 821*, 176–193.

Pynoos, R. S., Steinberg, A. M., & Piacentini, J. C. (1999). A developmental psychopathology model of childhood traumatic stress and intersection with anxiety disorders. *Biological Psychiatry, 46*(11), 1542–1554.

Reiss, D., Richters, J. E., Radke-Yarrow, M., & Scharrf, D. (Eds.). (1993). *Children and violence.* New York: Guilford Press.

Saigh, P. A. (1991). The development of posttraumatic stress disorder following four different types of traumatization. *Behaviour Research and Therapy, 29*(3), 213–216.

Saigh, P. A., Mroueh, M., & Bremner, J. D. (1997). Scholastic impairments among traumatized adolescents. *Behaviour Research and Therapy, 35*(5), 429–436.

Saylor, C. F., Swenson, C. C., & Powell, P. (1992). Hurricane Hugo blows down the broccoli: Preschoolers' post-disaster play and adjustment. *Child Psychiatry and Human Development, 22*(3), 139–149.

Schwarz, E. D., & Kowalski, J. M. (1991). Posttraumatic stress disorder after a school shooting: Effects of symptom threshold selection and diagnosis by DSM-III, DSM-III—R, or proposed DSM-IV. *American Journal of Psychiatry, 148*(5), 592–597.

Shaw, J. A., Applegate, B., Tanner, S., Perez, D., Rothe, E., Campo-Bowen, A. E., & Lahey, B. L. (1995). Psychological effects of Hurricane Andrew on an elementary school population. *Journal of the American Academy of Child and Adolescent Psychiatry, 34*(9), 1185–1192.

Silverman, W., & Albano, A. (1996). *The Anxiety Disorders Interview Schedule for DSM-IV, Child and Parent Versions.* San Antonio, TX: Psychological Corporation.

Stoddard, F. J., Norman, D. K., & Murphy, J. M. (1989). A diagnostic outcome study of children and adolescents with severe burns. *Journal of Trauma, 29*(4), 471–477.

Stuber, M. L., Nader, K., Yasuda, P., Pynoos, R. S., & Cohen, S. (1991). Stress responses after pediatric bone marrow transplantation: Preliminary results of a prospective longitudinal study. *Journal of the American Academy of Child and Adolescent Psychiatry, 30*(6), 952–957.

Terr, L. C. (1990). *Too scared to cry: Psychic trauma in childhood.* New York: Harper & Row.

Terr, L. C. (1991). Childhood traumas: An outline and overview. *American Journal of Psychiatry, 148*(1), 10–20.

Yule, W. (1994). Posttraumatic stress disorder. In T. H. Ollendick, W. Yule, & N. J. King (Eds.), *International handbook of phobic and anxiety disorders in children and adolescents: Vol. 496. Issues in clinical child psychology* (pp. 223–240). New York: Plenum Press.

Yule, W., & Canterbury, R. (1994). The treatment of posttraumatic stress disorder in children and adolescents. *International Review of Psychiatry, 6*(2–3), 141–151.

Yule, W., Udwin, O., & Murdoch, K. (1990). The "Jupiter" sinking: Effects on children's fears, depression and anxiety. *Journal of Child Psychology and Psychiatry and Allied Disciplines, 31*(7), 1051–1061.

Yule, W., & Williams, R. M. (1990). Posttraumatic stress reaction in children. *Journal of Traumatic Stress, 3*(2), 279–295.

Chapter 12

Specific Phobia

NEVILLE J. KING
PETER MURIS
THOMAS H. OLLENDICK

Children display a variety of fears during the normal course of development (Gullone, 2000; Ollendick, Hagopian, & King, 1997), Typically, children evince fear reactions to stimuli such as strangers, separation, loud noises, darkness, water, imaginary creatures, and small animals such as snakes and spiders, as well as other circumscribed or specific events or objects (King, Hamilton, & Ollendick, 1988). For the most part, these fears appear to result from day-to-day experiences of growing children and to reflect the children's emerging cognitive and representational abilities (Muris & Merckelbach, 2001). Such fears are short-lived, are adaptive, and do not cause distress. On the other hand, some children exhibit fear reactions that persist, are maladaptive and cause much distress for the child. Extreme fears of this nature are known as "phobias" (Barrios & Hartmann, 1997; Ollendick, King, & Muris, 2002; Ollendick, King, & Yule, 1994).

SYMPTOM PICTURE

Common examples of childhood phobias include excessive fears of animals, heights, water, thunderstorms, darkness, and medical or dental procedures. Following the tripartite model originally developed by Lang (1968, 1977), childhood fears and phobias can be conceptualized in terms of three response systems: cognitive, physiological, and overt-behavioral (Barrios & Hartmann, 1997; King, Ollendick & Murphy, 1997; Silverman & Ginsburg, 1995). In relation to the cognitive system, common responses include thoughts of being scared ("I feel afraid"), negative self-statements about coping ("I do not know what to do"), and the expectation that confrontation with a fear stimulus will result in personal harm or negative outcomes ("the dog will bite"). In terms of the physiological system, increased heart rate is frequently reported, as well as sweating, dryness of the mouth, upset stomach, and changes in respiration (Beidel, 1989). In relation to the overt-behavioral response system, phobic children frequently avoid or escape from what is feared. When escape or avoidance behavior is not possible, inappropriate fear-related behavior may be evident, such as tantrums, freezing or rigid posture, thumb sucking, clinging to parents, or crying. Severe phobias frequently manifest themselves in all three response systems, although the interrelationship between the response systems is complex (King, Hamilton & Ollendick, 1988; Silverman & Rabian, 1994).

In recognition of their seriousness and persistence, phobias are included in the two most widely accepted mental health diagnostic classification systems (American Psychiatric Association, 1994; World Health Organization, 1992). For example, the fourth edition of the *Diagnostic and Statistical Manual of Mental Disorders* (DSM-IV; American Psychiatric Association, 1994) specifies the following criteria for "specific" phobia: (1) marked and persistent fear that is excessive or unreasonable, cued by the presence or anticipation of a specific object or situation; (2) exposure to the phobic stimulus almost invariably provokes an immediate anxiety response or panic attack; (3) the person recognizes that the fear is excessive or unreasonable; (4) the phobic situation(s) is avoided or else endured with intense anxiety; (5) the phobia causes significant interference to functioning, or there is marked distress about having the phobia; (6) in individuals under 18 years, the duration is at least 6 months, and (7) the anxiety or phobic avoidance are not better accounted for by another disorder, such as obsessive–compulsive disorder or separation anxiety disorder. Five subtypes of specific phobia are differentiated: animal type (fear cued by snakes, spiders, dogs, or bees/insects), natural environment type (fear cued by storms, heights, or water), blood–injection–injury type (fear cued by seeing blood or an injury or by receiving an injection), situational type (fear cued by specific situations such as tunnels, bridges, elevators, flying, public transportation), and a miscellaneous "other" type (fear cued by stimuli such as costumed characters and loud noises).

The DSM-IV (American Psychiatric Association, 1994) recognizes that children may not view their fears as excessive or unreasonable, and, further, that children's fears may be expressed in "childhood" ways such as crying, tantrums, freezing, or clinging. These are important acknowledgments, as these criteria recognize the developmental nature of children and the developmental course of their fears (Ollendick & King, 1991a; King, Muris & Ollendick, in press). In addition, the DSM-IV specifies parameters for the duration of specific phobias in children (i.e., 6 months). In previous editions of the DSM, duration was not specified.

Consistent with our own clinical impressions, emerging evidence suggests that children with specific phobias frequently have comorbid internalizing or externalizing disorders (Last, Perrin, Hersen & Kazdin, 1992; Silverman et al, 1999). In a study of 80 clinic-referred children with specific phobias, Last and colleagues (1992) found that 75% of the children had a lifetime history of additional anxiety disorders (most commonly separation anxiety disorder), 32.5% had a lifetime history of any depressive disorder, and 22.5% had a lifetime history of any disruptive behavior disorder. Similarly, Silverman and colleagues (1999) reported that of 104 children referred to a phobia outpatient treatment program, a majority (72%) of had at least one comorbid diagnosis: 19% had an additional specific phobia, 16% had separation anxiety disorder, 14% had overanxious disorder, and 6% were diagnosed with attention-deficit/hyperactivity disorder. The remaining 17% of the 72% who had a comorbid diagnosis were distributed over eight additional diagnostic categories. Thus, contrary to simplistic views or assumptions commonly held about children with phobias, these findings suggest that such children have a complex and varied diagnostic profile involving marked comorbidity. An important caveat here is that this conclusion is based on studies with clinic-referred children. Although further investigation is necessary, it appears that community samples probably have greater diagnostic "purity" and less comorbidity (Costello & Angold, 1995).

EPIDEMIOLOGY AND NATURAL HISTORY

Findings on the prevalence of specific phobia in children vary considerably and reflect differences in the sample selected (community vs. clinic-referred), the source assessed (child, parent or both), the assessment method used (structured or unstructured, rating scales) and whether an impairment criterion was part of the definition of a case (Silverman & Rabian, 1994). In their recent review of epidemiological studies, Costello and Angold (1995) concluded that

OAD/GAD (overanxious disorder/generalized anxiety disorder), separation anxiety, and simple (i.e., specific) phobia are nearly always the most commonly diagnosed anxiety disorders, occurring in around 5% of children, while social phobia, agoraphobia, panic disorder, avoidant disorder, and obsessive–compulsive disorder are rare, with prevalence rates generally well below 2%. (p. 115)

Specific phobia is also more prevalent among girls than boys (e.g., Anderson et al., 1987; Essau, Conradt & Petermann, 2000; McGee et al., 1990; Milne et al., 1995). Whether prevalence rates vary with socioeconomic status, ethnicity, and age remains to be clarified.

Longitudinal investigations are lacking, but limited findings on natural history suggest that severe phobic symptoms can persist for some children for at least 1- to 2- years (Hampe et al., 1973) and possibly up to 5-years (Agras, Chapin & Oliveau, 1972; Ollendick, 1979). As further evidence for the persistence of specific phobia, it should also be noted that adult phobic sufferers frequently report a childhood onset (Öst, 1987). In fact, the DSM-IV points out that each type of specific phobia (natural environment, animal, blood–injection–injury, and situational) frequently develops during childhood and can persist into adulthood. Specific phobias that persist into adulthood remit only infrequently (around 20% of cases (APA, 1994). Clearly, the severe phobic reactions of children should not be dismissed as something that will naturally "weaken" over the course of time and, therefore, not require treatment (Ollendick & King, 1994).

ETIOLOGY

Childhood phobias have a complex and multidetermined etiology (Muris & Merckelbach, (2001). Genetic influences, temperamental predispositions, parental psychopathology, parenting practices, and individual conditioning histories all contribute to the development and maintenance of childhood phobias. Inasmuch as any one specific phobia is acquired and maintained through such complex processes, treatment approaches will likely need to address these dimensions before evidenced-based treatments can be fully realized (Ollendick & King, 1998, 2000).

Genetic/Biological and Familial Influences

Genetic influences play an important but limited role. Although no known studies of heritability exist for children with specific phobias, studies with adults suggest that specific phobias may be largely due to nongenetic factors (Carey, 1990; Kendler, Neale, Kessler, Heath, & Eaves, 1992). In discussing the role of genetics in specific phobias, social phobia, and agoraphobia, Kendler and colleagues (1992) propose that these subtypes of phobias can be placed along an etiological continuum: at the one end of the continuum lies agoraphobia, which has the latest age of onset, the highest heritability estimate, and the least specific environmental influences. At the other end of the continuum lie the specific phobias, which have the earliest age of onset, the lowest heritability estimates, and the highest specific environmental influences. These authors conclude: "The estimated heritability of liability of phobias . . . indicates that genetic factors play a significant but by no means overwhelming role in the etiology of phobias. Individual-specific environment appears to account for approximately twice as much variance in liability to phobias as do genetic factors" (p. 279). Overall, genetic factors appear to be associated with a general state or propensity toward fearfulness.

Constitutional (i.e., temperament) characteristics of the child may play a role in the onset and maintenance of specific phobias in children. Kagan and colleagues use the term "behavioral inhibition" (BI) to describe the temperament of infants who are predisposed to withdraw from unfamiliar people and situations (Kagan, 1989; Kagan, Reznick, & Gibbons, 1989; Kagan, Reznick, & Snidman, 1988). These researchers report BI to be prevalent in 10–15% of European American infants. Children identified as BI at 21 and 31 months of age maintained this temperament at later assessments at 4, 5, and 7½ years. Biederman and colleagues (1990) examined the children at 7 to 8 years of age. Mothers of the 22 inhibited and 19 uninhibited children were systematically interviewed using a structured diagnostic interview. Although a variety of measures were obtained in this study, only the results of diagnoses for common childhood anxiety disorders are presented here. Findings revealed that the rates of all anxiety disorders were higher in inhibited than in uninhibited children: overanxious disorder (13.6% vs. 10.5%), separation anxiety disorder (9.1% vs. 5.3%), avoidant disorder (9.1% vs. 0%), and phobic disorders (31.8% vs. 5.3%). Only differences for phobic disorders were statistically significant. Clearly, the inhibited group was found to be at risk for anxiety disorder, particularly phobic disorders. Such evidence suggests a link between BI in young children and the emergence of specific phobias. Although beyond the scope of this chapter, a number of methodological issues have been raised about the research on BI (see review by Turner, Beidel & Wolff, 1996).

Learning Factors

Learning-based theories of phobia onset have been presented in the literature for nearly 100 years. Watson and Rayner's (1920) early laboratory demonstration with "little Albert" has provided dramatic testimony of the power of traumatic experience in phobia acquisition (classical aversive conditioning). In this study a young infant developed a fear of a rat as a result of an aversive sound being associated with the sight of the animal. However, we should emphasize that replication of this work has not always been successful. Furthermore, classical aversive conditioning theory has come under criticism on several additional grounds as a comprehensive account of children's phobias (see Davey, 1992; King et al., 1988). Quite simply, traumatic experience is not always reported as a factor in the etiology of the child's phobic reaction. Thus Rachman (1976, 1977) proposed that there are three distinct, though frequently overlapping, pathways to the acquisition of fears and phobias: direct conditioning (e.g., child being attacked by a dog and then developing a phobia of dogs), modeling (e.g., child observing fearful behavior of parents in presence of dogs) and instruction or information (e.g., child hearing media reports of dog attacks).

Recently, a number of retrospective studies have attempted to empirically evaluate Rachman's theory of fear and phobia acquisition in children (see King, Gullone & Ollendick, 1998, for critique). In the first of these investigations, Ollendick & King (1991b) explored the pathways in 1,092 Australian and American children ages 9–14 years. In response to 10 commonly reported fears in children (King, Ollier, et al., 1989), the youths were asked to indicate on a self-report questionnaire their own levels of fear and then whether: (1) they remembered having a bad or frightening experience with the feared object (direct conditioning experience), (2) their parents, friends, or other acquaintances ever showed fear or avoidance of the feared object (vicarious conditioning), or (3) they had been told or heard stories regarding the feared object from either parents, teachers, friends, or other acquaintances (instruction or information pathway). Results indicated that the majority of the children attributed the onset of their fears to vicarious and instructional factors (56 and 39%, respectively), rather than to direct conditioning events (37%). For a minority of children and adolescents, these indirect sources alone were sufficient to evoke high levels of fear. More commonly, however, and depending on the specific fear, it was necessary for both of these indirect sources of fear to be present or for them to be combined with direct conditioning experiences. This finding suggests that the three pathways of fear may not be independent but, rather, interactive. Overall, findings supported Rachman's three-pathways theory of fear acquisition.

However, surprising findings sometimes occur in the study of the fear pathways in children. For example, in surveying the parents of 50 children with water phobia (mean age 5½ years), Menzies and Clarke (1993) found that only 2% of parents attributed their child's phobia onset to a direct conditioning episode and that none believed that information on adverse consequences accounted for the water phobia. Vicarious conditioning episodes were seen as being influential by 26% of parents. Moreover, a majority of the parents (56%) believed that their child's fear had been present from the child's very first contact with water. The remaining 16% of the parents were not able to offer any explanation of onset, recalling no traumatic experience but reporting nonetheless that their child had not always displayed a fear of water.

Overall, these findings suggest that not all phobias are acquired through individual-specific learning histories and that other factors may need to be considered. Among these other factors are those related to the heritability of phobias, biological-constitutional factors of the child, and parenting influences on the growing child. Early on, Darwin (1877, cited in Marks, 1987, p. 112) asked, "May we not suspect that . . . fears of children, which are quite independent of experience, are the inherited effects of real dangers . . . during savage times?" Basically, Darwin suggested that aversive experiences with certain stimuli were not necessary for the acquisition of fear; rather, some fears were "independent of experience" and were largely innate. Advancing this notion, Seligman (1971) hypothesized that associations between certain stimuli and fear responses were more likely to be formed than others (i.e., "prepared" and constituting noncognitive forms of associative learning). The status of this notion of "inherited phobia proneness" is certainly controversial and well beyond the scope of this chapter (see Davey, 1992; Marks, 1987; Menzies & Clarke, 1995; and Muris, Merckelbach, de Jong, & Ollendick, 2002, for discussion of issues related to these theories).

TREATMENT

Extensive reviews of research on the treatment of specific phobia in children can be found elsewhere (King & Ollendick, 1997; Ollendick & King, 1998). At the general level, we note a lack of well controlled treatment outcome studies, a dearth of research on clinical samples of phobic children, insufficient diagnostic evaluations, lack of multimethod or multi-informant assessment procedures, and lack of systematic follow-up evaluations. The most systematic work on the development and evaluation of therapies for phobic children has been from the behavioral or cognitive-behavioral perspective (Silverman & Carmichael, 1999).

Cognitive-Behavioral Therapy

Many behavioral and cognitive treatment strategies have been successfully employed in the treatment of childhood phobias (King, Muris & Ollendick, in press). Nearly three decades ago, Marks posited that exposure is the underlying mechanism: "an important mechanism shared by all of these methods is exposure of the frightened subject to a frightening situation until he acclimatises" (Marks, 1975, p. 67). We still find exposure to be a useful guiding principle in planning the treatment of childhood phobias. In fact, exposure is generally accepted as a key aspect of "best practice." Cognitive-behavior therapy programs are multicomponet and exposure based. We now outline the most frequently used procedures: desensitization, contingency management, modeling, and self-control procedures.

Developed by Wolpe (1958), the classic phobia reduction method for adults is "systematic desensitization." However, variants of the original desensitisation procedure are usually required in the treatment of phobic children. Clinicians typically employ a graded series of real-life exposures to what elicits fear, ranging from the least to the most anxiety provoking ("real-life desensitization"). In addition to real-life desensitization, emotive imagery affords a "story telling" means of helping the child overcome his or her phobia (King, Cranstoun, & Josephs, 1989; Lazarus & Abramovitz, 1962). This procedure involves narrative descriptions of the child teaming up with superhero figures (e.g., Batman), with phobic stimuli being gradually interwoven into the story (for review, see King et al., 1998). Desensitization procedures are now an important component of contemporary cognitive-behavior therapy programs for phobic children.

Capitalizing on the power of observational learning, another behavioral treatment approach is to have the child with a specific phobia observe another child display or model appropriate approach and coping behavior without adverse consequences (known as "modeling"; Ollendick & King, 1998). Phobic children sometimes display significant skills deficits, something we have especially observed in children with animal and water phobias (King et al., 1988). For children afraid of dogs, for example, it is possible through modeling to teach dog-handling skills and protective behaviors (MacDonald, 1975). The "models" can be symbolic (i.e., filmed) or live. Furthermore, the child with a phobia can be assisted in approaching the feared stimulus, as in participant modeling (Silverman & Ginsburg, 1995).

Based on operant conditioning principles, contingency management procedures attempt to alter phobic behaviors through manipulation of their consequences. Shaping, positive reinforcement, and extinction are the contingency management procedures most frequently used to reduce phobic behavior (Morris & Kratochwill, 1983). Caregivers typically play a key role in contingency management interventions designed for children with specific phobias (Glasscok & MacLean, 1990). A limited amount of research has confirmed the presence of maladaptive cognitions in anxious children. During testing situations, for example, anxious children report more off-task thoughts, more negative evaluations, amd fewer positive evaluations (e.g., Beidel & Turner, 1988; King, Mietz, Tinney, & Ollendick, 1995). Therefore, it can also be profitable to teach specific thinking styles that can be used during exposure to fear-eliciting stimuli. Illustratively, Silverman and Rabian (1994) recently used the STOP acronym to teach this skill: S stands for "Scared?", T for "Thoughts," O for "Other thoughts" or "Other things I can do," and P for "Praise." Children who lack the requisite cognitive and verbal skills, as in the case of the very young, would obviously not be suitable for self-control procedures.

We now consider empirical support for the use of cognitive and behavioral strategies in the treatment of children with specific phobias. In an early pioneering investigation, Graziano and Mooney (1980) examined the efficacy of cognitive-behavioral treatment program for children ages 6–13 years who had severe nighttime fears. Families were randomly assigned to either a treatment group or a waiting-list control group. Treatment involved teaching relaxation and verbal coping skills to the children to counter feelings of being afraid through the night. Over the 3-week program, the parents played an important role in monitoring home practice and rewarding children for their progress with "bravery tokens" (to be exchanged for a McDonald's party). Results attested to the efficacy of the intervention on multiple outcome measures of nighttime fear behavior and self-reported willingness to go to sleep. Maintenance of improvement was reported for nearly all children at a 2- to 3-year follow-up (Graziano & Mooney, 1982).

More recently, Silverman, Kurtines and Ginsburg (1999) compared the efficacy of an exposure-based self-control treatment and an exposure-based contingency management treatment condition relative to an education and support control group in the treatment of children ages 6–17 years with specific phobias. All children met criteria for a primary DSM-III-R diagnosis of phobic disorder (simple phobia, $N = 87$; social phobia, $N = 10$; agoraphobia, $N = 7$) as determined by the Anxiety Disorders Interview Schedule for Children (Silverman & Nelles, 1988). Seventy-two percent of the sample had at least one comorbid diagnosis, the more common additional diagnoses being simple phobia, separation anxiety disorder, and overanxious disorder. In each condition, participants underwent a 10-week manual-based treatment program in which children and parents were seen in separate treatment sessions with the therapist, followed by a brief conjoint meeting. Multi-informant outcome measures included diagnostic status, child-completed measures of emotional distress and negative cognitive errors, and parent-completed measures of emotional and behavioral impairment. Results indicated that all three conditions produced effective therapeutic change on the main outcome measures (child, parent, and clinician). The gains were maintained at 3-, 6-, and 12-month follow-ups. The finding that the education and support condition helped children overcome their specific phobias provides food for thought, as this condition was included as a nonexposure intervention to control for the nonspecific aspects of treatment.

Medication

A variety of pharmacological agents, such as anxiolytics, antidepressants, and antihistamines, have been used in the treatment of childhood anxiety and phobic disorders. However, as pointed out by Silverman and Carmichael (1999), much of the research on pharmacological agents predates DSM-IV, and ambiguous terms such as "neurosis," "phobic neurosis," or "school phobia" were used to describe the children, thus calling into question the current relevance of these studies. Recent literature reviews have concluded that, with the exception of clomipramine and fluoxetine for the treatment of obsessive–compulsive disorder and benzodiazepines for panic disorder, the efficacy of pharmacological treatments for phobic disorders in children is unclear (Silverman & Carmichael, 1999). Moreover, although some medications appear helpful, it is generally recommended that they be used in combination with other therapies, particularly cognitive and behavioral interventions (e.g., Kutcher, Reiter, & Gardner, 1995). In our opinion, medications do not generally have a role in the management of specific phobia in children. Exposure-based interventions should be the first treatment of choice for children with phobias.

Alternative Treatments

Recognizing the diversity of theoretical paradigms in the study of childhood psychopathology and its treatment, our literature search on evidence-based practice also incorporated other major psychotherapeutic modalities relevant to the treatment of childhood phobias (see also Ollendick & King, 2000). Although we found encouraging case reports that suggested the usefulness of therapies from an interpersonal perspective or family systems perspective, we failed to find any controlled good outcome studies in the published literature. Furthermore, no controlled outcome studies from a psychodynamic orientation were found. However, one uncontrolled outcome study conducted by Fonagy and Target (1994), using retrospective chart reviews of 196 children who met diagnostic criteria for anxiety disorders at the Anna Freud Centre in London, suggested that child psychoanalysis might be effective (but then only for younger children who receive treatment four or five times a week for an average of 2 years). Treatment outcome was assessed via clinician-determined diagnostic status and two measures of clinically significant change (improvement or return to normal functioning). Although the children were identified as meeting diagnostic criteria for anxiety disorders, it is not clear what proportion had a specific phobic disorder. Despite methodological limitations of this study (e.g., method and timing of assessments, lack of random assignment and control group), it represents an initial step in identifying the types of child problems that may improve with psychodynamic treatment (Silverman & Carmichael, 1999).

Stages of Treatment

Intervention with the child with specific phobia and his or her parents is usually implemented over several stages. For example, Silverman and Carmichael (1999) recommend a three-phase cognitive-behavioral program for children with specific phobias: an educational phase, an application phase, and a relapse prevention phase. The education phase incorporates an age-appropriate explanation of how phobias are acquired and an introduction to the key change-producing procedure, that is, exposure. Parents are trained in contingency management procedures such as reinforcement and extinction. Therapy sessions with the child focus on the development of self-control procedures, typically relaxation training, cognitive restructuring, action plans, and self-evaluation and self-reward. In the application phase, the child is encouraged to work through a graded hierarchy involving exposure to the fear-eliciting stimuli (both in session and out of session). We find it better to be on the conservative side of taking it slowly with the child, having him or her repeat exposures, and to try variations on the exposure theme. Such caution pays dividends in terms of consolidation of learning and generalization. The relapse prevention phase recognizes that the child may experience setbacks or relapses after a successful intervention plan. Good clinical practice therefore involves "an eye to the future" over the course of an intervention program with the child. Final therapy sessions are dedicated specifically to future anxiety-provoking events, such as school entry and school transitions, and how these might be approached using the strategies taught during the program. Finally, we note that treatment manuals have become a popular means of dissemination on evidence-based practice. Manuals set out the stages of intervention for therapists in considerable detail and facilitate replication of programs (for discussion of the merits and disadvantages of manuals, see Ollendick & King, 2000).

FUTURE DIRECTIONS

Promising advances have occurred in the cognitive-behavioral treatment of specific phobia in children. Intensive parental involvement appears to be important to the long-term success of these interventions. Parents are often regarded as "cotherapists" responsible for the implementation of the procedures developed by the therapist. However, it may be fruitful to also provide parents with treatment for their own phobias and anxiety problems.

Although not all parents of phobic children are highly anxious or phobic themselves, it is clear from much research that many parents are afflicted with these disorders (Kendall et al., 1992; Silverman, Cerny & Nelles, 1988; Windheuser, 1977). In helping them overcome their own phobias and anxiety, we hope that parents will feel less stressed and more confident to act as behavior-change agents. Furthermore, parents can provide a more appropriate coping model to their child during treatment. Therefore, we hypothesize that a family-oriented behavioral intervention will prove to be more effective than traditional child-focused behavioral strategies in the treatment of children's phobias (cf., Ginsburg, Silverman & Kurtines, 1995).

Unfortunately, there has been little systematic evaluation of behavioural family therapy in the treatment of children's phobias. More recently, the "transfer-of-control" model (Ginsburg et al., 1995) and the family anxiety management model (FAM; Dadds, Heard & Rapee, 1992) have stressed the critical role of parents during treatment. The transfer-of-control model emphasizes the gradual fading of control from therapist to parent and then to child. Both approaches involve training parents in contingency management strategies to deal with their child's fears and anxieties and to facilitate the child's exposure to the phobic situation. Self-control strategies involving self-instruction and relaxation are taught to children so that they can control and manage their own anxiety and exposure to the feared situation. These approaches explicitly recognize and target parental anxiety, problematic family relationships, parent–child communication problems, and parental problem-solving skills. In a controlled group study involving 79 children with anxiety disorders, FAM was found to be superior to a waiting-list control group and a cognitive-behavioral therapy group after treatment and at 1-year posttreatment (Barrett, Dadds & Rapee, 1996). However, its utility to phobic disorders remains to be determined. For the moment, behavioral family therapy has experimental status only in the treatment of childhood phobias.

CONCLUSIONS

Although childhood fears are a part of normal development, a significant minority of children evince fears that interfere with their functioning (referred to as "specific phobia" in the DSM-IV). Specific fears and phobias have cognitive, physiological, and overt-behavioral referents ("multichannel" response systems). The developers of the DSM-IV outline five subtypes of specific phobia: animal type, natural environment type, blood–injection–injury type, situational type, and a miscellaneous other type. Phobic children referred to treatment clinics frequently have comorbid internalizing disorders. Children's phobias have a complex etiology: Genetic influences, temperamental tendencies, parental psychopathology, and individual conditioning histories likely converge to occasion the development and maintenance of phobic reactions.

Most research over past decades on the treatment of children's phobias has been done from a behavioral or cognitive-behavioral perspective. Notwithstanding lively debates about underlying mechanisms in phobia reduction, we still see exposure as a useful conceptualization. Identifying what is responsible for therapeutic change remains a major challenge, especially in view of the findings from a recent well-controlled trial highlighting the significance of nonspecific factors in therapy outcome with children with specific phobias (Silverman et al., 1999). Future directions should investigate the usefulness of family-wide behavioral interventions. In addition to its intuitive clinical appeal, this research direction makes good sense in terms of what is now known about the role of parenting practices/psychopathology in the development and maintenance of children's phobias.

REFERENCES

Agras, W. S., Chapin, N. H., & Oliveau, D. C. (1972). The natural history of phobias: Course and prognosis. *Archives of General Psychiatry, 26*, 315–317.

American Psychiatric Association. (1994). *Diagnostic and statistical manual of mental disorders* (4th ed.). Washington, DC: Author.

Anderson, J. C., Williams, S., McGee, R., & Silva, P. A. (1987). DSM-III disorders in preadolescent children. *Archives of General Psychiatry, 44*, 69–76.

Barrett, P. M., Dadds, M. R., & Rapee, R. M. (1996). Family treatment of childhood anxiety: A controlled trial. *Journal of Consulting and Clinical Psychology, 64*, 333–342.

Barrios, B. A., & Hartmann, D. P. (1997). Fears and anxieties. In E. J. Mash & L. G. Terdal (Eds), *Assessment of childhood disorders* (3rd ed, pp. 230–327). New York: Guilford Press.

Beidel, D. C. (1989). Assessing anxious emotion: A review of psychophysiological assessment in children. *Clinical Psychology Review, 9*, 717–736.

Biederman, J., Rosenbaum, J. F., Hirshfeld, D. R., Faraone, V., Bolduc, E., Gersten, M., Meminger, S., & Reznick, S. (1990). Psychiatric correlates of behavioral inhibition in young children of parents with and without psychiatric disorders. *Archives of General Psychiatry, 47*, 21–26.

Carey, G. (1990). Genes, fears, phobias, and phobic disorders. *Journal of Counseling and Development, 68*, 628–632.

Costello, E. J., & Angold, A. (1995). Epidemiology. In J. S. March (Ed.), *Anxiety disorders in children and adolescents* (pp. 109–124). New York: Guilford Press.

Dadds, M. R., Heard, P. M., & Rapee, R. M. (1992). The role of family intervention in the treatment of child anxiety disorders: Some preliminary findings. *Behaviour Change, 9*, 171–177.

Davey, G. C. L. (1992). Classical conditioning and the acquisition of human fears and phobias: A review and synthesis of the literature. *Advances in Behavior Research and Therapy, 14,* 29–66.

Essau, C. A., Conradt, J., & Petermann, F. (2000). Frequency, comorbidity, and psychosocial impairment of specific phobia in adolescents. *Journal of Clinical Child Psychology, 29,* 221–231.

Fonagy, P., & Target, M. (1994). The efficacy of psycho-analysis for children with disruptive disorders. *Journal of the American Academy of Child and Adolescent Psychiatry, 33,* 45–55.

Glasscock, S. E., & MacLean, W. E., Jr. (1990). Use of contact desensitization and shaping in the treatment of dog phobia and generalized fear of the outdoors. *Journal of Clinical Child Psychology, 19,* 169–172.

Ginsburg, G. S., Silverman, W. K., & Kurtines, W. K. (1995). Family involvement in treating children with phobic and anxiety disorders: A look ahead. *Clinical Psychology Review, 15,* 457–473.

Graziano, A. M., & Mooney, K. C. (1980). Family self-control instruction for children's nighttime fear reduction. *Journal of Consulting and Clinical Psychology, 48,* 206–213.

Graziano, A. M., & Mooney, K. C. (1982). Behavioral treatment of "nightfears" in children: Maintenance of improvement at 2½- to 3–year follow-up. *Journal of Consulting Clinical Psychology, 50,* 598–599.

Gullone, E. (2000). The development of normal fear: A century of research. *Clinical Psychology Review, 20,* 429–451.

Hampe, E., Noble, H., Miller, L. C., & Barrett, C. L. (1973). Phobic children one and two years posttreatment. *Journal of Abnormal Psychology, 82,* 446–453.

Kagan, J. (1989). Temperamental contributions to social behavior. *American Psychologist, 44,* 668–674.

Kagan, J., Reznick, J. S., & Gibbons, J. (1989). Inhibited and uninhibited types of children. *Child Development, 60,* 838–845.

Kagan, J., Reznick, J. S., & Snidman, N. (1988). Biological bases of childhood shyness. *Science, 240,* 167–171.

Kashani, J. H., Beck, N. C., Hoeper, E. W., Fallahi, C., Corcoran, C. M., McAllister, J. A., Rosenberg, T. K., & Reid, J. C. (1987). Psychiatric disorders in a community sample of adolescents. *American Journal of Psychiatry, 144,* 584–549.

Kendall, P. C., Ellsas, T. E., Kane, M. T., Kim, R. S., Kortlander, E., Ronan, K. R., Sessa, F. M., & Siqueland, L. (1992). *Anxiety disorders in youth. Cognitive-behavioral interventions.* Boston: Allyn & Bacon.

Kendler, K. S., Neale, M. C., Kessler, R. C., Heath, A. C., & Eaves, L. J. (1992). The genetic epidemiology of phobias in women: The interrelationship of agoraphobia, social phobia, situational phobia, and simple phobia. *Archives of General Psychiatry, 49,* 273–281.

King, N. J., Cranstoun, F., & Josephs, A. (1989). Emotive imagery and children's nighttime fears: A multiple baseline design evaluation. *Journal of Behavior Therapy and Experimental Psychiatry, 20,* 125–135.

King, N. J., Gullone, E., & Ollendick, T. H. (1998). Etiology of childhood phobias: Current status of Rachman's three pathways theory. *Behaviour Research and Therapy, 36,* 297–309.

King, N. J., Hamilton, D. I., & Ollendick, T. H. (1988). *Children's phobias: A behavioural perspective.* Chichester, UK: Wiley.

King, N. J., Mietz, A., Tinney, L., & Ollendick, T. H. (1995). Psychopathology and cognition in adolescents experiencing severe test anxiety. *Journal of Clinical Child Psychology, 24,* 49–54.

King, N. J., Molloy, G., Murphy, G., & Ollendick, T. H. (1998). Emotive imagery treatment for childhood phobias: A credible and empirically validated intervention? *Behavioural and Cognitive Psychotherapy, 26,* 103–113.

King, N. J., Muris, P., & Ollendick, T. H. (in press) Fears and phobias in children: Assessment and treatment. *Child and Adolescent Mental Health.*

King, N. J., & Ollendick, T. H. (1989). Children's anxiety and phobic disorders in school settings: Classification, assessment and intervention issues. *Review of Educational Research, 59,* 431–470.

King, N. J., & Ollendick, T. H. (1997). Treatment of childhood phobias. *Journal of Child Psychology and Psychiatry, 38,* 389–400.

King, N. J., Ollendick, T. H., & Gullone, E. (1990). Desensitisation of childhood fears and phobias: Psychophysiological analyses. *Behaviour Change, 7,* 66–75.

King, N. J., Ollendick, T. H., & Murphy, G. (1997). Assessment of childhood phobias. *Clinical Psychology Review, 17,* 667–687.

King, N. J., Ollier, K., Icuone, R., Schuster, S., Gullone, E., Bays, K., & Ollendick, T. H. (1989). Fears of children and adolescents: A cross-sectional Australian study using the Revised-Fear Survey Schedule for Children. *Journal of Child Psychology and Psychiatry, 30,* 775–784.

Kutcher, S. P., Reiter, S., & Gardner, D. (1995). Pharmacotherapy: Approaches and applications. In J. S. March (Ed.), *Anxiety disorders in children and adolescents* (pp. 341–385). New York: Guilford Press.

Lang, P. J. (1968). Fear reduction and fear behavior: Problems in treating a construct. In J. M. Shlien (Ed.), *Research in psychotherapy.* Washington, DC: American Psychological Association.

Lang, P. J. (1977). Fear imagery: An information processing analysis. *Behavior Therapy, 8,* 862–886.

Lazarus, A. A., & Abramovitz, A. (1962). The use of emotive imagery in the treatment of children's phobias. *Journal of Mental Science, 198,* 191–195.

Last, G. C., Perrin, S., Hersen, M., Kazdin, A. E (1992). DSM-III-R anxiety disorders in children: Sociodemographic and clinical characteristics. *Journal of the American Academy of Child and Adolescent Psychiatry, 31,* 1070–1071.

MacDonald, A. (1975). Multiple impact behavior therapy in a child's dog phobia. *Journal of Behavior Therapy and Experimental Psychiatry, 6,* 317–322.

Marks, I. M. (1975). Behavioral treatments of phobic and obsessive–compulsive disorders: A critical appraisal. In M Hersen, R. M. Eisler, & P. M. Miller (Eds), *Progress in behavior modification* (Vol. 1, pp. 65–158). New York: Academic Press.

Marks, I. M. (1987). *Fears, phobias, and rituals.* New York: Oxford University Press.

Menzies, R. G., & Clarke, J. C. (1993). The etiology of childhood water phobia. *Behaviour Research and Therapy, 31,* 499–501.

Menzies, R. G., & Clarke, J. C. (1995). The etiology of phobias: A nonassociative account. *Clinical Psychology Review, 15,* 23–48.

McGee, R., Feehan, M., Williams, S., Partridge, F., Silva, P. A., & Kelly, J. (1990). DSM-III disorders in a large sample of adolescents. *Journal of the American Academy of Child and Adolescent Psychiatry, 29,* 611–619.

Milne, J. M., Garrison, C. Z., Addy, C. L., McKeown, R., Jackson, K. L., Cuffe, S. P., & Waller, J. L. (1995). Frequency of phobic disorder in a community sample of young adolescents. *Journal of the American Academy of Child and Adolescent Psychiatry, 34,* 1202–1211.

Muris, P., & Merckelbach, H. (2001). The etiology of childhood specific phobia: A multifactorial model. In M. W. Vasey & M. R. Dadds (Eds), *The developmental psychopathology of anxiety* (pp. 355–385). New York: Oxford University Press.

Muris, P., Merckelbach, H., de Jong, P., & Ollendick, T. H. (2002). The etiology of specific fears and phobias in children: A critique of the non-associative account. *Behaviour Research and Therapy, 40,* 185–195.

Ollendick, T. H. (1979). Fear reduction techniques with children. In M. Hersen, R. M. Eisler, & P. M. Miller (Eds), *Progress in behavior modification* (Vol. 8, pp. 127–168). New York: Academic Press.

Ollendick, T. H., Hagopian, L. P., & King, N. J. (1997). Specific phobias in children. In G. C. L. Davey (Ed.), *Phobias: A handbook of theory, research and treatment* (pp. 201–224). Chichester, UK: Wiley.

Ollendick, T. H., & King, N. J. (1998). Empirically supported treatments for children with phobic and anxiety disorders. *Journal of Clinical Child Psychology, 27,* 156–167.

Ollendick, T. H., & King, N. J. (2000). Empirically supported treatments for children and adolescents. In P. C. Kendall (Ed.), *Child and adolescent therapy: Cognitive-behavioral procedures* (2nd ed., pp. 386–425). New York: Guilford Press.

Ollendick, T. H., & King, N. J. (1991a). Fears and phobias of childhood. In M. Herbert (Ed.), *Clinical child psychology: Social learning, development and behavior* (pp. 309–329). Chichester, England: Wiley.

Ollendick, T. H., & King, N. J. (1991b). Origins of childhood fears: An evaluation of Rachman's theory of fear acquisition. *Behaviour Research and Therapy, 29,* 117–123.

Ollendick, T. H., & King, N. J. (1994). Diagnosis, assessment and treatment of internalizing problems in children: The role of longitudinal data. *Journal of Consulting and Clinical Psychology, 62,* 918–927.

Ollendick, T. H., & King, N. J. (2000). Empirically supported treatments for children and adolescents. In P. C. Kendall (Ed.), *Child and adolescent therapy: Cognitive-behavioral procedures* (2nd ed., pp. 386–425). New York: Guilford Press.

Ollendick, T. H., King, N. J., & Muris, P. (2002). Fears and phobias in children: Phenomenology, epidemiology and aetiology. *Child and Adolescent Mental Health, 7,* 98–106.

Ollendick, T. H., King, N. J., & Yule, W. (Eds.). (1994). *International handbook of phobic and anxiety disorders in children and adolescents.* New York: Plenum Press.

Öst, L. G. (1987). Age of onset in different phobias. *Journal of Abnormal Psychology, 96,* 223–229.

Rachman, S. (1976). The passing of the two-stage theory of fear and avoidance: Fresh possibilities. *Behaviour Research and Therapy, 14,* 125–134.

Rachman, S. (1977). The conditioning theory of fear acquisition: A critical examination. *Behaviour Research and Therapy, 15,* 375–387.

Seligman, M. E. P. (1971). Phobias and preparedness. *Behavior Therapy, 2,* 307–320.

Silverman, W. K., & Carmichael, W. K. (1999). Phobic disorders. In R. T. Ammerman, M. Hersen, & C. L. Last (Eds.), *Handbook of prescriptive treatments for children and adolescents* (2nd ed., pp. 172–192). Boston: Allyn & Bacon

Silverman, W. K., Cerny, J. A., & Nelles, W. B. (1988). The familial influence in anxiety disorders: Studies on the offspring of patients with anxiety disorders. In B. B. Lahey & A. E. Kazdin (Eds), *Advances in clinical child psychology* (Vol. 11, pp. 223–248). New York: Plenum Press.

Silverman, W. K., &, Ginsburg, G. (1995). Specific phobias and generalized anxiety disorder. In J. S. March (Ed.), *Anxiety disorders in children and adolescents* (pp. 151–180). New York: Guilford Press.

Silverman, W. K., Kurtines, W. M., Ginsburg, G. S., Weems, C. F., Rabian, B., & Serafini, L. T. (1999). Contingency management, self-control, and education support in the treatment of childhood phobic disorders: A randomized clinical trial. *Journal of Consulting and Clinical Psychology, 67,* 675–687.

Silverman, W. K., & Nelles, W. B. (1988). The anxiety disorders interview schedule for children. *Journal of the American Academy of Child and Adolescent Psychiatry, 27,* 772–778.

Silverman, W. K., & Rabian, B. (1994). Specific phobia. In T. H. Ollendick, N. J. King, & W. Yule (Eds), *International handbook of phobic and anxiety disorders in children and adolescents* (pp. 87–109). New York: Plenum Press.

Simeon, J. G., Ferguson, H. B., Knott, V., Roberts, N., Gauthier, B., Dubois, C., & Wiggins, D. (1992). Clinical, cognitive and neurophysiological effects of alprazolam in children and adolescents with overanxious and avoidant disorders. *Journal of the American Academy of Child and Adolescent Psychiatry, 31,* 29–33.

Turner, S. M., Beidel, D. C., & Wolff, P. L. (1996). Is behavioral inhibition related to anxiety disorders? *Clinical Psychology Review, 16,* 157–172.

Watson, J. B., & Rayner, R. (1920). Conditioned emotional reactions. *Journal of Experimental Psychology, 3,* 1–14.

Windheuser, H. J. (1977). Anxious mothers as models for coping with anxiety. *Behaviour Analysis and Modification, 2,* 39–58.

Wolpe, J. (1958). *Psychotherapy by reciprocal inhibition.* Stanford, CA: Stanford University Press.

World Health Organization. (1992). *International classification of mental and behavioral disorders, clinical descriptions and diagnostic guidelines* (10th ed.). Geneva, Switzerland: Author.

Chapter 13

Selective Mutism

JENNIFER B. FREEMAN
ABBE M. GARCIA
LAUREN M. MILLER
SARA P. DOW
HENRIETTA L. LEONARD

The inclusion of selective mutism in this volume on childhood anxiety disorders represents a change in understanding and studying this unusual and interesting phenomenon. Although selective mutism is classified under "other disorders of childhood" and not as an anxiety disorder in the fourth edition of the *Diagnostic and Statistical Manual of Mental Disorders* (American Psychiatric Association, 1994), current investigations are reevaluating this determination. With the increasing focus on both the biologically mediated temperamental components of selective mutism and the continuity of anxiety disorders from childhood to adulthood, this phenomenon deserves systematic reevaluation. This chapter reviews selective mutism in the context of both the early literature and future lines of study.

HISTORY, MODELS, AND ETIOLOGY

Elective, or selective, mutism was first identified by Kussmaul (1877) as "aphasia voluntaria," although it received little subsequent attention. The term "elective mutism" was used by Tramer (1934) to describe the behavior of children who spoke only in certain situations or only to certain people. Hesselman (1983) suggested that the term "selective mutism" was more descriptive, and this term replaced "elective mutism" in the change from DSM-III-R to DSM-IV (American Psychiatric Association, 1987, 1994).

In reviewing the past 100 years of literature, it appears that the diagnosis of elective mutism described a heterogeneous population. Historically, the disorder was attributed to a response to an early trauma, to a change of environment, or to a manifestation of intrapersonal and family dynamics (Wright, 1985). More recently, selective mutism has been seen as a manifestation of an anxiety disorder, and it is this conceptualization that is reflected in current literature.

The cause of selective mutism is unknown and probably is multifactorial and differs between individuals. Hayden (1980) described five different subtypes, and these serve to help understand both different approaches and possible etiologies. Only the subtype "biological mutism," in which mutism is a secondary consequence of another disorder (such as autism or deafness) would be excluded under current diagnostic criteria.

Hayden's (1980) first subtype, *symbiotic mutism*, suggested that the phenomenon could be explained by the nature of the relationship between the patient and the (enmeshed) mother, in which the child uses a "clinging, shy, and sensitive exterior" to manipulate and control his or her environment (p. 123). In the second subtype, *passive–aggressive mutism*, the child's "defiant refusal to speak" is a manifestation of his or her hostility (p. 126). Clearly, ideas of the older literature predominated—the *enmeshed mother,* the "oppositional child"—but such were the explanations for most childhood psychiatric symptoms at the time. The third subtype, *reactive mutism,* was felt to be the consequence of a traumatic event, such as starting school, emigration, hospitalization, severe or prolonged illness, and early psychological or physical traumatic experiences (which would include physical and sexual abuse). The fourth subtype, *speech-phobic mutism,* was characterized by the "active fear of hearing one's own voice" (p. 124); this is closest to our current understanding of social phobia.

The reconceptualization of selective mutism as an anxiety disorder stemmed from several lines of observation. Historically, many reports noted that electively mute children were shy and timid and that the mutism might be a manifestation of an "underlying anxiety state or depressive equivalent" (Wilkins, 1985, p. 202). More recent empirical evidence favors viewing anxious presentations as more likely, with oppositional features secondary if present at all (Black & Uhde, 1992, 1995; Dummit et al., 1997; Kratochwill, 1981; Leonard & Topol, 1993; Steinhausen & Juzi, 1996; Wright, Cuccaro, Leonhardt, Kendall, & Anderson, 1995). Shyness and reserve have been reported as characteristic of the families of children with selective mutism (Hayden, 1980; Kolvin & Fundudis, 1981; Wergeland, 1979; Wright, 1968), and systematic research has documented the familial transmission of other anxiety disorders (Silverman, Cerney, & Nelles, 1988; Silverman, Cerney, Nelles, & Burke, 1988; Weissman, Leckman, Merikangas, Gammon, & Prusoff, 1984).

Research on the biological components of temperament also merits specific attention. One model for childhood anxiety, behavioral inhibition to the unfamiliar, has identified children who are "inhibited" (Biederman et al., 1993). These children are identifiable between 2 and 3 years of age; they resist challenging or new situations, show a characteristic autonomic nervous system response to foreign (stressful) situations, and are at increased risk for subsequent anxiety disorders (Biederman et al., 1993). Whether selectively mute children are temperamentally inhibited has not yet been studied.

The hypothesis that there is a specific relationship between selective mutism and either social phobia or panic disorder was first posited by Crumley (1990). A 20-year follow-up case report of an electively mute child (who had not spoken at all in school until the sixth grade) reported that the patient continued to have great anxiety about facing people and avoided social settings. Crumley noted that it was "difficult to decide which was more the object of fear, the panic or the social scrutiny" and concluded that "future research may show it to be an uncommon manifestation of common familiar disorders" (p. 319). Later that year, Golwyn and Weinstock (1990) described the first successful pharmacological treatment of an electively mute child and reported a dramatic clinical response to phenelzine. The child had elective mutism and "associated shyness." Her father had panic disorder that responded to phenelzine. "Her response to pharmacologic treatment for social phobia, her family history of panic disorder, and the shyness and anxiety reported in the selective mutism literature raise nosologic questions about selective mutism and its relationship to social phobia and the anxiety disorders" (p. 385). Subsequently, many authors have investigated the efficacy of pharmacological agents used in the treatment of pediatric anxiety in selectively mute children.

Alternatively, selective mutism may perhaps be viewed as an obsessive–compulsive spectrum disorder: It is difficult to separate the concept of an obsessive fear of speaking from the anxiety involved in doing so. Hayden (1980) reported that some of his patients displayed ritualistic behavior that would invalidate the effects of speech and allow them to talk at certain times or about certain things, although he did not label the behavior as obsessive per se. Several of the selectively mute children evaluated by the authors of this chapter had a comorbid obsessive–compulsive disorder (OCD) diagnosis at evaluation, although comorbid selective mutism has not previously been diagnosed in children with primary OCD (Swedo, Rapoport, Leonard, Lenane, & Cheslow, 1989).

Some researchers believe that selective mutism should not continue to be a separate diagnostic category but rather that it is a symptom or subtype of social phobia (Anstendig, 1999; Black & Uhde, 1992, 1995; Dow, Sonies, Scheib, Moss, & Leonard, 1995; Dummit et al., 1997; Leonard & Topol, 1993). Others take broader views. For example, Steinhausen and Juzi (1996) suggest that the anxious behaviors of selectively mute children are not only indicative of social phobia but may also represent a more general personality feature, such as shyness. In another vein, Kristensen (2000) hypothesizes that although selective mutism may be regarded as a symptom of anxiety, the cause of the anxiety may include underlying neurodevelopmental vulnerabilities that might be ignored if selectively mute children were simply lumped in with all other children with anxiety disorders. Regardless of its official classification in the DSM, understanding selective mutism as a variant of anxiety will be beneficial for the treatment of these children.

In conclusion, selective mutism is under systematic study at several sites around the world, and from these studies a better understanding of the neurobiology, etiology, and diagnostic classification should emerge.

PHENOMENOLOGY

Parents of a selectively mute child typically report that the child speaks loudly and freely at home but "doesn't say one word at school." The extent to which a selectively mute child speaks varies greatly. Characteristically, the selectively mute child converses freely at home, and some speak in very specific and familiar social situations. Selectively mute children usually do not speak out loud in public, where either strangers or less well-known people might hear; thus they will not order food at a restaurant or speak with a clerk in a store. However, some will speak to strangers in stores and restaurants but persistently do not speak at school or to people who know them. Some children are able to have long conversations with people on the telephone with whom they do not converse in person. There is usually a distinct hierarchy of people to whom the child does and does not speak.

Some individuals who have recovered from selective mutism recall that they were afraid to speak in public or to have others hear their voices. It is not unusual for a child to speak to a best friend in one of their homes but not at school, where others might hear his or her voice. Usually parents report that their child "has always been this way" but that they thought the child would outgrow the behavior. Thus most selectively mute children are not clinically identified until they start either preschool or kindergarten.

Only three systematic reports have compared selectively mute children with contrasting populations. Kolvin and Fundudis (1981) compared 24 electively mute children with a group of speech-retarded children (N = 84) and their matched control group (N = 102). Wilkins (1985) compared the case notes of 24 children with selective mutism to 24 matched controls with diagnoses of "emotional disorders." Kristensen (2000) compared 54 selectively mute children to a matched control group (N = 108). The largest case descriptions have included sample sizes of 68 (Hayden, 1980), 100 (Steinhausen & Juzi, 1996), 54 (Kristensen, 2000), and 50 (Dummit et al., 1997). The most common finding in these studies is the association with comorbid anxiety disorders. Several comprehensive reviews of selective mutism are available, including papers by Anstendig (1998) and Black (1996).

DIFFERENTIAL DIAGNOSIS

Selective mutism is currently classified in DSM-IV (American Psychiatric Association, 1994) under "Disorders Usually First Diagnosed in Infancy, Childhood, or Adolescence." Whether systematic research will ultimately recommend that the disorder be classified as an anxiety disorder remains to be determined.

Selective mutism is characterized in DSM-IV by the "consistent failure to speak in specific social situations (in which there is an expectation for speaking, e.g., at school) despite speaking in other situations" (American Psychiatric Association, 1994, p. 115). The disorder must interfere with educational or occupational functioning or with social communication. The symptoms must have been present for at least a month and cannot be limited to the first month of school.

Generally speaking, in diagnosing selective mutism, one would want to distinguish between selective mutism and a developmental disorder or another psychiatric disorder in which mutism is a secondary condition, such as autism, schizophrenia, deafness, and aphonia. In mental retardation, pervasive developmental disorder, and other developmental disorders (including severe expressive language disorder), the child may have physical but not psychological difficulty in speaking.

The DSM-IV diagnostic criteria state that the symptoms must not be able to be "better accounted for by a Communication Disorder (e.g. Stuttering)" (American Psychiatric Association, 1994, p. 115). It is not known what the rate of either expressive or receptive language disorders is in the selectively mute population, but one would want to rule out any significant difficulty that might secondarily contribute to the child's difficulty and/or self-consciousness about speaking. An expressive or receptive language disability can be diagnosed in addition to the selective mutism, if both are present.

Assigning the diagnosis is more complicated in children from immigrant families who may not wish to speak in the new language or who have had some difficulty in learning two languages early in life. In these cases, the mutism may be due to a lack of knowledge rather than a fear of speaking. According to DSM-IV, the selective mutism diagnosis should not be assigned if there is a "lack of knowledge of, or comfort with, the spoken language required in the social situation" (American Psychiatric Association, 1994, p. 114).

Excessive shyness or timidity may be mistaken for selective mutism; distinguishing between them is difficult, because selectively mute children are characteristically shy. Comorbid anxiety disorders (social phobia, generalized anxiety disorder, OCD) may be diagnosed if those diagnostic criteria are met.

RELATED FEATURES

Whereas the majority of children with selective mutism are described as excessively shy, other clinical correlates of the disorder are heterogeneous. Children with selective mutism are also described as inhibited, withdrawn, anxious, and sometimes passive–aggressive, stubborn, disobedient, angry, manipulative, controlling, and oppositional. In the past, these features were used to classify children with selective mutism into two distinct subgroups: (1) withholding speech as a result of extreme anxiety and (2) withholding speech in an attempt to be manipulative or controlling. From a clinical standpoint, it is our opinion that these children are indeed "particularly sensitive, shy, afraid of everything strange or new" (Wergeland, 1979, p. 219). They appear unable to speak in the specific social setting, with anxiety rather than an oppositional stance inhibiting their ability to speak.

Empirical evidence also suggests that anxious presentations are more likely and that oppositional features, if present, are secondary aspects of the disorder (Black & Uhde, 1992, 1995; Dummit et al., 1997; Kratochwill, 1981; Leonard & Topol, 1993; Steinhausen & Juzi, 1996; Wright et al., 1995). Steinhausen and Juzi (1996) assessed 100 selectively mute children. The authors reported that 85% of their sample were characterized as shy, 66% were described as anxious, 21% were described as oppositional, and 17% as hyperactive. Kumpulainen, Rasanen, Raaska, and Somppi (1998) reported that, in their sample of selectively mute children, teachers described 63% of the sample as shy, 63% as withdrawn, 58% as serious, and, in contrast, only 13% as aggressive or hyperactive.

Comorbidity between selective mutism and other disorders has been systematically assessed in several studies. Three studies have reported high rates of comorbidity with anxiety disorders, including social phobia, avoidant disorder, and separation anxiety disorder (74–100% of samples with selective mutism met criteria for an anxiety disorder; Black & Uhde, 1995; Dummit et al., 1997; Kristensen, 2000). High rates of anxiety disorders and selective mutism also appear in the first-degree relatives of patients with selective mutism. In one study, 70% of patients had a first-degree relative with social phobia or avoidant disorder, and 37% had a first-degree relative with selective mutism (Black & Uhde, 1995).

Some researchers report comorbid obsessive–compulsive behaviors in patients with selective mutism (Hayden, 1980; Kolvin & Fundudis, 1981). Hayden (1980) reported that 18% (12 of 68) of the children in his study had obsessive–compulsive behaviors such as "having things just so" and "lining all the papers up a certain way" (p. 124). Wergeland (1979) noted "clear tendencies toward compulsion-neurosis in six" (p. 221) of 11 children, whereas Kolvin and Fundudis (1981) noted that 2 of 24 (8%) were "seriously obsessional" (p. 226). Whether some of these children have an obsessive fear of hearing their own voices or embarrassing themselves remains to be determined and merits further study.

In contrast, rates of externalizing disorders, in particular oppositional defiant disorder, were very low (1 in 50, Dummit et al., 1997; 3 in 30, Black & Uhde, 1995). Interestingly, elimination disorders appear to occur more frequently among children with selective mutism than in the general population (Kristensen, 2000; Steinhausen & Juzi, 1996).

The association between developmental delays, particularly language disorders, and selective mutism is unclear. Whereas some studies have reported no evidence of difficulties with speech and language functioning (Black & Uhde, 1995), others have reported that rates of language disorder or delays range from 11–65% in this population (Dummit et al., 1997; Kristensen, 1997, 2000; Kumpulainen et al., 1998; Steinhausen & Juzi, 1996). Steinhausen and Juzi (1996) reported that articulation and expressive language disorders were more common than receptive language problems or stuttering in their sample. Rates of motor delays have been reported to range from 18–65% (Kristensen, 1997).

The association between selective mutism and autistic spectrum disorders is controversial because of differing interpretations of the DSM-IV diagnostic criteria. DSM-IV states that selective mutism must not occur exclusively during the course of a pervasive developmental disorder (American Psychiatric Association, 1994). However, some have argued that, to the extent that being selectively mute can be an essential feature of a child's presentation that would not necessarily be captured by a developmental disorder (e.g., Asperger's disorder), then one should be able to assign both diagnoses when warranted. Based on this argument, a few research groups have looked at rates of comorbidity between selective mutism and Asperger's disorder. In one study 7.4% of the sample with selective mutism met criteria for Asperger's disorder (Kristensen, 2000), and in another study 1 of 5 children with selective mutism met all the criteria except one for Asperger's disorder (Kopp & Gillberg, 1997).

EPIDEMIOLOGY, DEMOGRAPHICS, AND NATURAL HISTORY

Recent evidence suggests that the age of onset of selective mutism usually ranges from 2 to 4 years (Black & Uhde, 1995; Dummit et al., 1997; Kristensen, 2000; Steinhausen & Juzi, 1996). Despite the early age of onset, children are most often referred for diagnosis and treatment upon entry to school. Boys in Hayden's (1980) study were referred an average of 2.3 years earlier than girls, a finding the author attributed to the greater tolerance of reticent behavior in females. Selective mutism is generally thought, however, to be more common in girls than in boys, with estimates ranging from 2.6:1 to 1.5:1 (females to males; Dummit et al., 1997; Kopp & Gillberg, 1997; Kristensen, 2000; Kumpulainen et al., 1998; Steinhausen & Juzi, 1996).

Although selective mutism is considered to be a rare disorder, it may actually be more prevalent, as most cases do not come to medical attention and do resolve with age. In one of the few epidemiological studies (Fundudis, Kolvin, & Garside, 1979), only 2 (.08%) selectively mute children were identified in a total city cohort of 3,300 7-year-old children. Brown and Lloyd (1975) reported that only .7% (42 of 6,072) of the 5-year-olds they studied were not speaking 8 weeks after starting first grade. More recently, two studies from Scandinavia reported prevalence rates for slightly older groups of children: 2% (38 of 2,010) among second graders in Finland (Kumpulainen et al., 1998) and .18% (5 of 2,793) among school-age children (ages 7–15) in Sweden (Kopp & Gillberg, 1997). These findings suggest that selective mutism in the young child entering school may be transient and resolve on its own. However, in a small percentage, the diagnosis and disability is ongoing.

The majority of cases "outgrow" the disorder, although it is not known whether remnants of shyness or anxiety persist. Certainly, most parents can be reassured that the child will outgrow it, although it is not uncommon for the disorder to persist for several years in elementary school. Because some treatments for this disorder appear to be effective, one could argue that interventions might shorten its course.

With the natural course of the illness characterized by spontaneous remissions, it is difficult to assess follow-up reports. Friedman and Karagan (1973) asserted that long-term improvement occurs despite lack of apparent immediate gains. Wright (1968) reported that at 6-month to 7-year follow-ups for 19 of an initial 24 children, all of the children were talking;

21% (N = 4) were evaluated as having had excellent response, 58% (N = 11) as good, 16% (N = 3) as fair, and 5% (N = 1) as poor (Wright, 1968). Others have reported less optimistic outcomes. Kolvin and Fundudis's (1981) 5- to 10-year follow-up of 24 selectively mute children suggested a poor outcome; only 46% (11 of 24) of the sample showed improvement. They concluded that those who fail to improve by 10 years of age are suffering from a more intractable form of selective mutism.

As a clinician, one might reassure the families of selectively mute children that in the majority of cases the symptoms resolve. However, children with symptoms lasting more than 6 months should be evaluated and treated. Most clinicians would suggest that the best prognosis is most likely with early diagnosis and treatment.

ASSESSMENT

Any child with selective mutism should have had a medical history and a physical examination completed. The assessor should ask about a history of recurrent ear infections and perform a hearing screening. Neurological examination should note any "soft signs" or motor delays. A developmental history of motor, language, cognitive, and social milestones should be obtained, which includes the prenatal and perinatal periods. Questions about the child's speech should assess articulation, comprehension, and fluency and find out whether the child stutters or repeats sounds.

A psychiatric assessment for comorbid diagnoses should be completed. Issues of temperament, including quality of inhibition and social interactions, are important to explore. Is the child interested in social relationships? Does the child have friends to whom he or she speaks? Often, the child will have several friends whom he or she speaks with at home but not in school. Does the child still socially interact, and is the child part of the group in school, even if he or she does not speak?

Cognitive and academic skills should also be assessed; typically, psychological testing is indicated to formally evaluate these skills. Formal speech and language assessments should also be completed. Parents can tape-record the child's voice at home for use by the speech therapist in assessing expressive skills. Receptive (comprehension), expressive, verbal, and nonverbal language and oral–motor performance should be noted.

Although there have been occasional reports of selective mutism following an early hospitalization or trauma, evaluations of the patients in our clinic have not suggested that selective mutism is caused by trauma. Certainly, a careful history should be taken, but parents of selectively mute children should not be assumed to be abusing their children. Parents have related stories about how mental health and school systems have confronted them about "presumed abuse." These unfortunate accusations appear to stem from the paucity of available information and the misunderstandings about selective mutism in both the general and the psychiatric communities.

TREATMENT

Historically, treatment for selective mutism has included a variety of behavioral, pharmacological, and individual and/or family psychodynamic psychotherapy approaches. However, the empirical treatment literature remains quite limited, with a small number of controlled group studies, some single-case experimental designs, and numerous uncontrolled case reports. For further reading, see several excellent reviews of the treatment literature (Anstendig, 1998; Kratochwill, 1981; Kratochwill, Brody, & Piersel, 1979; Wright, 1985).

Although selective mutism may be difficult to treat (Kolvin & Fundudis, 1981), early intervention has been hypothesized to prevent secondary problems with socializing and learning (Wright, 1968). Wright (1985) recommended that all children with a history of selective mutism longer than 6 months be referred for treatment. Generally, the literature has suggested that a behavioral approach, either with or without family intervention, is more effective than more traditional dynamic interventions (Kratochwill, 1981; Wright, 1985). Currently, a multidisciplinary approach is often considered, and pharmacotherapy may be indicated.

Behavioral Therapy

Behavioral therapy is generally the first and primary intervention for selective mutism, although it is time-consuming and requires the full cooperation of parents, teachers, and other school professionals. Although this type of treatment is the norm in clinical practice, the empirical literature is in fact quite limited. Studies to date include a number of uncontrolled case reports, a few single-case experimental designs, and only one small controlled group study (Anstendig, 1998; Cunningham, Cataldo, Mallion, & Keyes, 1984; Labbe & Williamson, 1984). The primary behavioral techniques that have been studied to date include contingency management, exposure-based techniques, and self-modeling.

Contingency management involves the use of positive or negative consequences in order to increase the frequency of speech and decrease the frequency of failure to talk. This type of approach can be executed in many ways. For example, the child may be rewarded for speaking, or reinforcement may be withheld if the child does not speak. Alternatively, an aversive consequence may be taken away when the child speaks or introduced when the child does not speak. The technique of shaping is often used, by which the child receives reinforcement for small, manageable, incremental goals toward speech (e.g., raising one's hand, whispering to a teacher, speaking in an audible voice). Stimulus fading strategies are also used, in which children are reinforced for gradual changes in the environment in which they speak (e.g., speaking alone with a therapist, speaking with the same therapist in another setting, speaking with the therapist and another new person). It is a mistake to expect a child to speak loudly in front of others in the beginning of the behavioral plan; the child is likely to be overwhelmed and fail.

Contingency management has received more empirical attention than other behavioral interventions in the treatment of selective mutism (Calhoun & Koenig, 1973; Cunningham et al., 1984; Griffith, Schnelle, McBNees, Bissinger, & Huff, 1975). Cunningham and colleagues (1984) noted that the six controlled single-case design studies and the one group study in the literature all used the technique of reinforcement, with or without stimulus fading. The authors report that for children with limited speech at baseline, reinforcement alone may be a strong enough intervention. However, for children with no baseline speech, reinforcement plus stimulus fading is the more common approach. Negative or aversive consequences, in which the child must speak to avoid an unpleasant consequence, have been reported in some case studies (e.g., Griffith et al., 1975; Krohn, Weckstein, & Wright, 1992; Matson, Esveldt-Dawson, & O'Donnell, 1979; Wulbert, Nyman, Snow, & Owen, 1977); however, use of these strategies alone is not considered effective (Crema & Kerr, 1978).

Exposure-based treatment approaches are built around the concept that for the child, anxiety about talking in itself inhibits speaking (negatively reinforces the behavior) and that not speaking reduces the anxiety. Given the connections that have been posited between selective mutism and anxiety, it makes sense to consider desensitization and the use of alternative coping strategies (e.g., relaxation, deep breathing, presence of a trusted adult). Children are encouraged to move gradually up a hierarchy of situations, ranked from least to most anxiety provoking, while using appropriate coping techniques. These strategies have not been well studied in the treatment of selective mutism, with only some case studies (e.g., Croghan & Craven, 1982; Rye & Ullman, 1999; Scott, 1977) and a few single-case designs (Cunningham et al., 1984; Sanok & Striefel, 1979; Wulbert et al., 1977) described in the literature. However, these techniques are often successful and deserve further experimental study.

A few studies have used self-modeling techniques to treat selective mutism (Holmbeck & Lavigne, 1992; Kehle, Owens, & Cressy, 1990; Pigott & Gonzales, 1987). In these interventions, children are first videotaped or audiotaped in a situation in which they speak comfortably (usually with a parent). The tape is then edited so that it appears as if the child is talking in other situations (e.g., at school or with a peer). The child then watches the tape of him- or herself modeling verbal behavior in target situations. The techniques are based on principles of observational learning and the belief that the child will increase his or her speech after watching his or her own verbal behavior displayed and reinforced.

Although the long-term outcome of behavioral treatment of selective mutism is not well studied, single-case studies certainly provide preliminary evidence for the effectiveness of these strategies. Specifically, behavioral strategies such as contingency management, exposure-based techniques, and self-modeling (often in combination) appear to hold the most promise. It is also important that the family be involved in the treatment. The reader is directed to some excellent reviews of the literature on behavioral therapy for further details (Anstendig, 1998; Cunningham et al., 1984; Labbe & Williamson, 1984).

Psychosocial Interventions

Psychosocial interventions are important components of the treatment plan. In general, efforts to coerce the child to speak are unsuccessful and may make the situation worse, as they further increase the child's anxiety. Successful efforts focus on involving the child in peer-group activities, emphasizing verbal skills when the child does talk, and encouraging home visits by relatives and friends. Parents should identify several friends who can be regular playmates and should arrange after-school play dates. An increasing number of social interactions and relationships with classmates may indirectly decrease stresses in the classroom. Additionally, the child should be encouraged to partake in nonverbal relationships with adults, to answer questions that require merely a one-word answer, and to participate in nonthreatening activities with strangers.

Of specific note, selectively mute children should remain in a regular classroom and should not be placed in emotionally disturbed or special education classrooms. An individualized behavioral treatment plan can be implemented in a regular classroom setting without great difficulty. Practically, the behavior modification program could be designed by the teacher, speech therapist, and school psychologist. A speech therapist can play an ongoing and unique role in providing a full speech and language workup and implementing treatment in school that might include pragmatically based small-group interactions.

Psychodynamic Psychotherapy

Psychodynamic theories have been based on the hypothesis that the symptom is a manifestation of intrapsychic conflict. Thus the disorder might represent a regression to a preverbal stage of development, a behavior that would compromise separation and individuation, or a manifestation of angry or manipulative affect (Browne, Wilson, & Laybourne, 1963). Psychodynamic treatments have focused on identifying the underlying conflict, and typically play therapy and sometimes art therapy were utilized because they enabled the child to express feelings nonverbally. The therapist might also try to involve other family members in the therapeutic process, and family psychotherapy may be needed in specific cases.

Browne and colleagues (1963) and Wergeland (1979) described 10 and 11 cases, respectively, of electively mute children treated with a psychodynamic approach, and they concluded that the treatment was lengthy and the outcome poor. The psychodynamic treatment literature relies predominantly on retrospective case reports, which limit systematic evaluation of treatment outcome. Additionally, information about the child's mutism, as well as information about the specific intervention techniques employed, is frequently omitted, thus making it difficult to generalize the use of these treatment modalities to other children with selective mutism. Psychodynamic therapy would not typically be recommended as the major intervention for the primary symptom, as there is no empirical evidence of its effectiveness; however, the modality may provide a supportive role in understanding and encouraging social interaction and addressing any family issues unique to that child.

Psychopharmacology

The systematic treatment literature on pharmacotherapy for the treatment of selective mutism remains limited at this point, despite the fact that medications are frequently used. In general, a behavioral treatment plan should be initiated first. If the child does not make sufficient progress, then adjunctive medication with ongoing behavioral treatment is sometimes considered. The bulk of the literature has been single-case studies, initially focusing on monoamine oxidase inhibitors (MAOIs) and then the use of selective serotonin reuptake inhibitors (SSRIs; Black & Uhde, 1992; Carlson, Kratochwill, & Johnston, 1994; Golwyn & Sevlie, 1999; Golwyn & Weinstock, 1990; Harvey & Milne, 1998; Thomsen, Rasmussen, & Andersson, 1999; Wright et al., 1995). There are no studies using a benzodiazepine or buspirone.

One open-treatment trial (Dummit, Klein, Tancer, Asche, & Martin, 1996) and one small, double-blind placebo-controlled trial (Black & Uhde, 1994) have been conducted, both with fluoxetine in children with selective mutism. The response of selectively mute children to pharmacological agents for social phobia and other anxiety disorders has led to discussions concerning the nosology of selective mutism. Obviously, a similar positive response to an agent does not allow conclusions about diagnoses.

Several cases report a positive response to the MAOI phenelzine. Golwyn and Sevlie (1999) reported four children, ages 5 to 7 years of age, who had a positive treatment response with phenelzine. Despite this case report, it would be extremely unusual to use an MAOI with a child, given the concerns of a hypertensive crisis or a serotonin syndrome when combined with certain medications or foods.

The largest literature on pharmacotherapy exists for the SSRIs. Fluoxetine, citalopram, and sertraline have all been anecdotally reported to be helpful (Carlson, Kratochwill, & Johnston, 1999; Harvey & Milne, 1998; Thomsen et al., 1999). Dummit and colleagues (1996) reported on 21 children, ages 5–14, who had a comorbid anxiety disorder and selective mutism. All children had to have had at least 4 weeks of behavioral psychotherapy prior to enrollment in the open drug trial. Interestingly, no child had shown enough improvement in the initial behavioral treatment to exclude him or her from entering into the open fluoxetine trial. Fluoxetine was administered in an open fashion for 9 weeks. Graduated doses (range 10–60 mg per day) were used—1.25 mg per day for the first week, 2.5 mg per day for the second week, 5 mg per day for the third week, and 10 mg per day in the fourth week. The mean dose at the end of treatment was 28.1 mg per day (1.1 mg per kg per day), with two children ending at 60 mg, four at 40 mg, and 15 at 20 mg per day. Two children were dropped from the study due to behavioral disinhibition. Clinical response was considered to be positive, with 76% (of 21 children) showing "clinical improvement" (defined by dichotomized Clinical Global Improvement scores) after 9 weeks of treatment. All measures indicated marked improvement in their symptoms for the group, but 5 of the 21 did not reach "improved" CGI (of 3 or less) at the end of treatment. Younger children showed a better response than did older children. The authors noted that complete remission of the symptoms required more than the 9-week trial (Dummit et al., 1996).

The only randomized double-blind study was completed by Black and Uhde (1994) using fluoxetine. Sixteen children started the single-blind placebo lead-in, and 15 of those children were subsequently randomly assigned to double-blind treatment for 12 weeks with fluoxetine ($N = 6$) or placebo ($N = 9$). The initial dose of fluoxetine was 0.2 mg per kg per day and was titrated up to a target dose of 0.6 mg per kg per day. The mean maximum dose was 21.4 mg per day (range 12 to 27 mg per day, 0.60 to 0.62 mg per kg per day). All of the 15 patients in the double-blind treatment completed the 12-week trial. The fluoxetine-treated patients were significantly more improved on parent ratings of mutism change and global change. The groups did not differ on the clinician and the teacher ratings. The authors speculated that this may be due in part to the difference in baseline severity (the fluoxetine group was more severe) and the small N enrolled. The authors concluded that, although some improvement was seen, both groups remained very symptomatic at the end of the study (Black & Uhde, 1994).

One single-case research trial with a double-blind placebo-controlled trial of sertraline with a multiple-baseline across-participants design ($N = 2$; $N = 3$) is included for completeness (Carlson et al., 1999). The study lasted 16 weeks. At the end of the study, there were no group changes in mutism, anxiousness, or shyness, although some individuals experienced some improvement. All parents chose to continue their children on sertraline (100 mg per day) at the end of the study. On a case-by-case basis, two children did not meet criteria for selective mutism after 10 weeks of sertraline treatment, and another was asymptomatic 20 weeks after the trial was completed. The reader may be interested in reviewing the authors' "ladder-like" paradigm for treating children with selective mutism when developing treatment plans (Carlson et al., 1999).

Although the literature is very limited, selective mutism is often treated as an anxiety disorder. If a medication were to be chosen, then an SSRI would be the likely choice. Interestingly, the systematic literature on the treatment of childhood anxiety disorder continues to grow. Fluvoxamine was shown to be superior to placebo in children with social phobia, separation anxiety, or generalized anxiety disorder (Walkup et al., 2001). Other reports on the safety of the SSRIs in children are derived from the pediatric OCD literature (March et al., 1998; Riddle et al., 2001) and depression literature (Emslie et al., 1997; Keller et al., 2001).

Despite the absence of large systematic treatment trials with children with selective mutism, some clinical observations have come from treating these children. It is preferable to treat the selectively mute child earlier and more intensively than previously thought, or often done. Several researchers have noted that it is much more difficult to treat the older child who has been symptomatic for a very long period of time (Black & Uhde, 1994; Dummit et al., 1996). The more anxious and inhibited children with selective mutism appear to respond better to medication than do the less anxious children. Children with selective mutism may take longer to respond to pharmacotherapy, sometimes 12 to 16 weeks, so a longer trial is usually recommended.

In conclusion, pharmacotherapy (usually with an SSRI) may be indicated in the overall treatment plan when the symptoms of selective mutism have not responded to a behavioral treatment plan or when the symptoms are long-standing and cause significant impairment. Pharmacotherapy may be used adjunctively with other treatments and should not be used as the sole intervention. Clearly, systematic trials are needed in this important area.

Combined Treatments

Wright and colleagues (1995) described the successful treatment of selective mutism in a preschool-age child using a multifaceted treatment approach. The intervention included fluoxetine, as well as family therapy, behavioral therapy, and play therapy. According to the authors, the components of the intervention reflect a conceptualization of selective mutism that views anxiety as a key feature but also focuses on associated features, particularly oppositional behaviors. Although this study has all of the limitations associated with a single-case design, it is included as an example of the comprehensive treatment approach that is often necessary for most children with selective mutism.

Intuitively, a combined multimodal treatment approach has clinical appeal, particularly in the treatment-refractory case or in the older child. Unfortunately, the limited systemic study of psychosocial or pharmacological treatments leaves the field with a paucity of evidence-based medicine. Certainly, combined treatments are often required for the child with a more severe symptom picture or with multiple comorbidities.

CASE EXAMPLE

K. M. is 5 years and 10 months old, in kindergarten, and was brought to us by her parents for evaluation because she did not speak at school to teachers or to peers and had not done so during her 2 previous years in preschool. Two years ago, K. M. had difficulties being left at preschool, and it took about 2 months before she could be left without crying. Although she does not talk to the other children, she interacts with them and participates in school activities. She has several friends whom she seems to like and whom she talks about at home. She has two friends in the neighborhood whom she speaks to. She speaks openly to all family members at home but does not speak to them in public if others might hear her.

K. M. says that she does not know why she does not talk, but she has told her mother that she feels "scared." Her mother describes her as shy and as a "worrier." She sometimes is afraid to go into another room by herself, and she is petrified of storms. No specific traumatic or abusive events in K. M.'s life could be identified. Her parents note that she internalizes her worries. They report that the shyness interferes with her making friends, although she has always had one or two special friends.

Developmental history was remarkable for a series of middle-ear infections that required tube placement. She did not consistently speak words until 2 years of age, but when her mother brought this to the pediatrician's attention, a tympanogram done at the time was normal. K. M.'s parents report that she speaks clearly with normal volume and fluency and without articulation difficulties. Her mother is not aware of any specific comprehension difficulties.

On evaluation, K. M. was alert and paid close attention to the questions. She appeared uncomfortable and did not smile at all. She would on occasion shake her head (yes or no) in response to a question, and she clung closely to her parents for most of the examination. Her mood appeared anxious. On psychological testing on the Leiter Performance Scale, she scored at the 6-year 9-month age level when she was chronologically 5 years and 10 months old. On the Peabody Picture Vocabulary Test—Revised she scored at the 4-year 8-month age level. A detailed speech and language evaluation reported a 6- to 12-month receptive language delay.

Diagnostic impressions included selective mutism, history of separation anxiety disorder, overanxious disorder, and receptive language delay. Recommendations included speech and language therapy within the school system and the development of a behavior modification program to be used at school and at home. No recommendations were made for pharmacotherapy until the response to ongoing assessment and a behavior modification program could be assessed.

RESEARCH ISSUES

Systematic phenomenological studies are needed to reconsider selective mutism in the light of new developments in the study of childhood anxiety disorders. Recent clinical experience suggests that most children with selective mutism are not "refusing" to talk (which implies a willful oppositional state) but that they feel unable to do so. Studies of the phenomenology, neurobiology, familial psychopathology, and treatment would provide information to determine whether selective mutism might be well classified as an anxiety disorder. Studies are needed to determine effective treatments, and more work is needed to clarify the efficacy of medications, although they appear promising at this point.

NOTE ON PATIENT ADVOCACY GROUPS

The Selective Mutism Foundation, a nonprofit national organization, provides support to those who are dealing with children with this disorder and information on the disorder. Organized by two mothers of children with selective mutism, the organization has encouraged research around the country in order to reassess old misconceptions about the disorder. Some areas of the country have local patient and family chapters of the national organization. For information on the national organization, contact the cofounders and codirectors: Mrs. Sue Leszcyk or Mrs. Carolyn Miller, Selective Mutism Foundation, P.O. Box 13133, Sissonville, WV 25360, or visit the foundation website at *http://www.orgsites.com/fl/selectivemutismfoundation.*

REFERENCES

American Psychiatric Association. (1987). *Diagnostic and statistical manual of mental disorders* (3rd ed., rev.). Washington, DC: Author.

American Psychiatric Association. (1994). *Diagnostic and statistical manual of mental disorders* (4th ed.). Washington, DC: Author.

Anstendig, K. (1998). Selective mutism: A review of the treatment literature by modality from 1980–1996. *Psychotherapy, 35*(3), 381–391.

Anstendig, K. D. (1999). Is selective mutism an anxiety disorder? Rethinking its DSM-IV classification. *Journal of Anxiety Disorders, 13*(4), 417–434.

Biederman, J., Rosenbaum, J. F., Bolduc-Murphy, E. A., Faraone, S. V., Chaloff, J., Hirshfeld, D. R., & Kagan, J. (1993). Behavioral inhibition as a temperamental risk factor for anxiety disorders. *Child and Adolescent Psychiatric Clinics of North America, 2*(4), 667–683.

Black, B. (1996). Social anxiety and selective mutism. In L. J. Dickstein, M. B. Riba, & J. M. Oldham (Eds.), *Review of psychiatry* (Vol. 15, pp. 469–495). Washington, DC: American Psychiatric Press.

Black, B., & Uhde, T. W. (1992). Elective mutism as a variant of social phobia. *Journal of the American Academy of Child and Adolescent Psychiatry, 31*(6), 1090–1094.

Black, B., & Uhde, T. W. (1994). Treatment of elective mutism with fluoxetine: A double-blind, placebo-controlled study. *Journal of the American Academy of Child and Adolescent Psychiatry, 33*(7), 1000–1006.

Black, B., & Uhde, T. W. (1995). Psychiatric characteristics of children with selective mutism: A pilot study. *Journal of the American Academy of Child and Adolescent Psychiatry, 34*(7), 847–856.

Brown, J. B., & Lloyd, H. (1975). A controlled study of children not speaking at school. *Association of Workers for Maladjusted Children, 3*, 49–63.

Browne, E., Wilson, V., & Laybourne, P. C. (1963). Diagnosis and treatment of elective mutism in children. *Journal of the American Academy of Child and Adolescent Psychiatry, 2*, 605–617.

Calhoun, J., & Koenig, K. P. (1973). Classroom modification of elective mutism. *Behavior Therapy, 4*, 700–702.

Carlson, J. S., Kratochwill, T. R., & Johnston, H. (1994). Prevalence and treatment of selective mutism in clinical practice: A survey of child and adolescent psychiatrists. *Journal of Child and Adolescent Psychopharmacology, 4*(4), 281–291.

Carlson, J. S., Kratochwill, T. R., & Johnston, H. F. (1999). Sertraline treatment of 5 children diagnosed with selective mutism: A single-case research trial. *Journal of Child and Adolescent Psychopharmacology, 9*(4), 293–306.

Crema, J. E., & Kerr, J. M. (1978). Elective mutism: A child care case study. *Child Care Quarterly, 1*, 215–226.

Croghan, L. M., & Craven, R. (1982). Elective mutism: Learning from the analysis of a successful case history. *Journal of Pediatric Psychology, 7*(1), 85–93.

Crumley, F. E. (1990). The masquerade of mutism. *Journal of the American Academy of Child and Adolescent Psychiatry, 29*, 318–319.

Cunningham, C. E., Cataldo, M. F., Mallion, C., & Keyes, J. B. (1984). A review and controlled single case evaluation of behavioral approaches to the management of elective mutism. *Child and Family Behavior Therapy, 5*(4), 25–49.

Dow, S. P., Sonies, B. C., Scheib, D., Moss, S. E., & Leonard, H. L. (1995). Practical guidelines for the assessment and treatment of selective mutism. *Journal of the American Academy of Child and Adolescent Psychiatry, 34*(7), 836–846.

Dummit, E. S., Klein, R. G., Tancer, N. K., Asche, B., & Martin, J. (1996). Fluoxetine treatment of children with selective mutism: An open trial. *Journal of the American Academy of Child and Adolescent Psychiatry, 35*(5), 615–621.

Dummit, E. S., Klein, R. G., Tancer, N. K., Asche, B., Martin, J., & Fairbanks, J. A. (1997). Systematic assessment of 50 children with selective mutism. *Journal of the American Academy of Child and Adolescent Psychiatry, 36*(5), 653–660.

Emslie, G. J., Rush, J., Weinberg, W. A., Kowatch, R. A., Hughes, C. W., Carmody, T., & Rintelmann, J. (1997). A double-blind, randomized, placebo-controlled trial of fluoxetine in children and adolescents with depression. *Archives of General Psychiatry, 54*(11), 1031–1037.

Friedman, R., & Karagan, N. (1973). Characteristics and management of elective mutism in children. *Psychology in the Schools, 10*, 249–254.

Fundudis, T., Kolvin, I., & Garside, R. (1979). *Speech retarded and deaf children: Their psychological development.* London: Academic Press.

Golwyn, D. H., & Sevlie, C. P. (1999). Phenelzine treatment of selective mutism in four prepubertal children. *Journal of Child and Adolescent Psychopharmacology, 9*(2), 109–113.

Golwyn, D. H., & Weinstock, R. C. (1990). Phenelzine treatment of elective mutism: A case report. *Journal of Clinical Psychiatry, 51*(9), 384–385.

Griffith, E. E., Schnelle, J. F., McBNees, M. P., Bissinger, C., & Huff, T. M. (1975). Elective mutism in a first grader: The remediation of a complex behavioral problem. *Journal of Abnormal Child Psychology, 3*, 127–134.

Harvey, B. H., & Milne, M. (1998). Pharmacotherapy of selective mutism: Two case studies of severe entrenched mutism responsive to adjunctive treatment with fluoxetine. *South African Journal of Child and Adolescent Mental Health, 10*(1), 59–66.

Hayden, T. L. (1980). Classification of elective mutism. *Journal of the American Academy of Child and Adolescent Psychiatry, 19*, 118–133.

Hesselman, S. (1983). Elective mutism in children 1877–1981. *Acta Paedopsychiatrica, 49*, 297–310.

Holmbeck, G., & Lavigne, J. (1992). Combining self-modeling and stimulus fading in the treatment of an electively mute child. *Psychotherapy, 29*(4), 661–667.

Kehle, T., Owens, S., & Cressy, E. (1990). The use of self-modeling as an intervention in school psychology: A case study of an elective mute. *School Psychology Review, 19*, 115–121.

Keller, M. B., Ryan, N. D., Strober, M., Klein, R. G., Kutcher, S. P., Birmaher, B., Hagino, O. R., Koplewicz, H., Carlson, G. A., Clarke, G. N., Emslie, G. J., Feinberg, D., Geller, B., Kusumakar, V., Papatheodorou, G., Sack, W. H., Sweeney, M., Wagner, K. D., Weller, E. B., Winters, N. C., Oakes, R., & McCafferty, J. P. (2001). Efficacy of paroxetine in the treatment of adolescent major depression: A randomized, controlled trial. *Journal of the American Academy of Child and Adolescent Psychiatry, 40*(7), 762–772.

Kolvin, I., & Fundudis, T. (1981). Elective mute children: Psychological, development, and background factors. *Journal of Child Psychology and Psychiatry, 22*, 219–232.

Kopp, S., & Gillberg, C. (1997). Selective mutism: A population-based study: A research note. *Journal of Child Psychology and Psychiatry, 38*(2), 257–262.

Kratochwill, T. R. (1981). *Selective mutism: Implications for research and treatment.* Hillsdale, NJ: Erlbaum.

Kratochwill, T. R., Brody, G. H., & Piersel, W. C. (1979). Elective mutism in children. *Advances in Clinical Child Psychology, 2*, 194–240.

Kristensen, H. (1997). Elective mutism—associated with developmental disorder/delay: Two case studies. *European Child and Adolescent Psychiatry, 7*, 234–239.

Kristensen, H. (2000). Selective mutism and comorbidity with developmental disorder/delay, anxiety disorder, and elimination disorder. *Journal of the American Academy of Child and Adolescent Psychiatry, 39*(2), 249–256.

Krohn, D. D., Weckstein, S. M., & Wright, H. L. (1992). A study of the effectiveness of a specific treatment for elective mutism. *Journal of the American Academy of Child and Adolescent Psychiatry, 31*(4), 711–718.

Kumpulainen, K., Rasanen, E., Raaska, H., & Somppi, V. (1998). Selective mutism among second-graders in elementary school. *European Child and Adolescent Psychiatry, 7*, 24–29.

Kussmaul, A. (1877). *Die Störungen der Sprache.* Leipzig, Germany: FCW Vogel.

Labbe, E. E., & Williamson, D. A. (1984). Behavioral treatment of elective mutism: A review of the literature. *Clinical Psychology Review, 4*, 273–292.

Leonard, H. L., & Topol, D. A. (1993). Elective mutism. *Child and Adolescent Psychiatric Clinics of North America, 2*, 695–707.

March, J. S., Biederman, J., Wolkow, R., Safferman, A., Mardekian, J., Cook, E. H., Cutler, N. R., Dominguez, R., Ferguson, J., Muller, B., Riesenberg, R., Rosenthal, M., Sallee, F. R., & Wagner, K. D. (1998). Sertraline in children and adolescents with obsessive–compulsive disorder: A multicenter randomized controlled trial. *Journal of the American Medical Association, 280*(20), 1752–1756.

Matson, J. L., Esveldt-Dawson, K., & O'Donnell, D. (1979). Overcorrection, modeling, and reinforcement procedures for reinstating speech in a mute boy. *Child Behavior Therapy, 1*, 363–371.

Pigott, H. E., & Gonzales, F. P. (1987). Efficacy of videotape self-monitoring in treating an electively mute child. *Journal of Clinical Child Psychology, 16*(2), 106–110.

Riddle, M. A., Reeve, E. A., Yaryura-Tobias, J. A., Yang, H. M., Claghorn, J. L., Gaffney, G., Greist, J. H., Holland, D., McConville, B. J., Pigott, T., & Walkup, J. T. (2001). Fluvoxamine for children and adolescents with obsessive–compulsive disorder: A randomized, controlled, multicenter trial. *Journal of the American Academy of Child & Adolescent Psychiatry, 40*(2), 222–229.

Rye, M. S., & Ullman, D. (1999). The successful treatment of long-term selective mutism: A case study. *Journal of Behavior Therapy and Experimental Psychiatry, 30*, 313–323.

Sanok, R., & Striefel, S. (1979). Elective mutism: Generalization of verbal responding across people and settings. *Behavior Therapy, 10*, 357–371.

Scott, E. (1977). A desensitization programme for the treatment of mutism in a 7–year-old girl: A case report. *Journal of Child Psychology and Psychiatry, 18*, 263–270.

Silverman, W., Cerney, J. A., & Nelles, W. B. (1988). The familial influence in anxiety disorders: Studies on the offspring of patients with anxiety disorders. In B. B. Lahey & A. E. Kazdin (Eds.), *Advances in clinical child psychology* (Vol. 11, pp. 223–247). New York: Plenum Press.

Silverman, W. K., Cerney, J. A., Nelles, W. B., & Burke, A. (1988). Behavior problems in children of parents with anxiety disorders. *Journal of the American Academy of Child and Adolescent Psychiatry, 27*, 779–784.

Steinhausen, H.-C., & Juzi, C. (1996). Elective mutism: An analysis of 100 cases. *Journal of the American Academy of Child and Adolescent Psychiatry, 35*(5), 606–614.

Swedo, S. E., Rapoport, J. L., Leonard, H. L., Lenane, M., & Cheslow, D. (1989). Obsessive–compulsive disorders in children and adolescents: Clinical phenomenology of 70 consecutive cases. *Archives of General Psychiatry, 46*, 335–343.

Thomsen, P. H., Rasmussen, G., & Andersson, C. B. (1999). Elective mutism: A 17–year-old girl treated successfully with citalopram. *Nordic Journal of Psychiatry, 53*(6), 427–429.

Tramer, M. (1934). Elective mutism in children. *Journal of Child Psychiatry, 1*, 30–35.

Walkup, J. T., Labellarte, M. J., Riddle, M. A., Pine, D. S., Greenhill, L., Klein, R., Davies, M., Sweeney, M., Abikoff, H., Hack, S., Klee, B., McCracken, J., Bergman, L., Piacentini, J., March, J., Compton, S., Robinson, J., O'Hara, T., Baker, S., Vitiello, B., Ritz, L. A., & Roper, M. (2001). Fluvoxamine for the treatment of anxiety disorders in children and adolescents. *New England Journal of Medicine, 344*(17), 1279–1285.

Weissman, M. M., Leckman, J. F., Merikangas, K. R., Gammon, G. D., & Prusoff, B. A. (1984). Depression and anxiety disorders in parents and children. *Archives of General Psychiatry, 41*, 845–852.

Wergeland, H. (1979). Elective mutism. *Acta Psychiatrica Scandanavica, 59*, 218–228.

Wilkins, R. (1985). A comparison of elective mutism and emotional disorders in children. *British Journal of Psychiatry, 146*, 198–203.

Wright, H. H. (1968). A clinical study of children who refuse to talk in school. *Journal of the American Academy of Child and Adolescent Psychiatry, 7*, 603–617.

Wright, H. H. (1985). Early identification and intervention with children who refuse to speak. *Journal of the American Academy of Child and Adolescent Psychiatry, 24*, 739–746.

Wright, H. H., Cuccaro, M. L., Leonhardt, T. V., Kendall, D. F., & Anderson, J. H. (1995). Case study: Fluoxetine in the multimodal treatment of a preschool child with selective mutism. *Journal of the American Academy of Child and Adolescent Psychiatry, 34*(7), 857–862.

Wulbert, M., Nyman, B. A., Snow, D., & Owen, Y. (1977). The efficacy of stimulus fading and contingency management in the treatment of elective mutism: A case study. *Journal of Applied Behavior Analysis, 6*, 435–441.

Part III

TREATMENT

Chapter 14

Cognitive-Behavioral Psychotherapy

KRISTEN SCHOFF D'ERAMO
GRETA FRANCIS

During the past decade, cognitive-behavioral treatments for childhood anxiety disorders have gained increasing recognition and support. The term "cognitive-behavioral" is meant to represent an integration of cognitive, behavioral, affective, and social strategies for change (Kendall et al., 1992). The cognitive-behavioral model emphasizes the learning process and the influence of contingencies and models in the individual's environment on the learning process (Kendall, Panichelli-Mindel, Sugarman, & Callahan, 1997).

The behavioral treatment of childhood anxiety has illustrious roots. Jones (1924) was among the first to demonstrate the application of learning theory to the treatment of childhood anxiety in her classic study of the deconditioning of a fear in "Little Peter." However, according to Ollendick and Cerny (1981), behavioral treatment of childhood disorders did not begin to gain popularity until the 1960s.

Although the past 40 years have been characterized by intense interest in behavioral therapy for childhood disorders, treatments for childhood internalizing disorders have only recently been a focus for development and testing by the scientific community (Kazdin & Weisz, 1998). During the past decade, significant progress has been made in the development and evaluation of empirically based treatments for childhood anxiety and phobic disorders.

As noted, the common link among all cognitive-behavioral treatment strategies is that they are based on models of learning. Principles of classical conditioning, operant conditioning, cognitive learning theory, and social learning theory are the underpinnings of cognitive-behavioral strategies used to treat childhood anxiety. In this chapter, we highlight a number of studies that exemplify the application of behavioral and cognitive-behavioral therapy to the treatment of childhood anxiety disorders. Applications of exposure-based strategies, contingency contracting, modeling, and cognitive procedures are illustrated, and an overview of Kendall and colleagues' (1992) integrated cognitive-behavioral treatment package is provided.

EXPOSURE-BASED STRATEGIES

Exposure-based treatments are based on principles of classical conditioning. Fears are classically conditioned responses that can be unlearned through counterconditioning. Counterconditioning requires that the child approach the anxiety-provoking situation in order to unlearn the fear response, thereby reducing anxiety. Exposure can be conducted imaginally or *in vivo*. We review several variants of exposure therapy with demonstrated efficacy for the treatment of childhood anxiety disorders.

Graduated Exposure

In graduated exposure, the child and the therapist generate a list of feared situations in a hierarchy, from least to most anxiety provoking. The child then approaches each situation sequentially, moving up the hierarchy as his or her anxiety level permits. It is important to start with situations that produce only minimal anxiety so as to facilitate success.

The literature includes a number of examples of the use of graduated exposure to treat childhood anxiety. Francis and Ollendick (1990) described a case study of the use of graduated *in vivo* exposure to treat an adolescent with generalized social phobia. The 16-year-old girl had a long history of school refusal and avoidance of most social situations. She reported intense social-evaluative fears. Treatment was conducted over a 3-month period. First, a fear hierarchy was developed, which ranged from least (going to a shopping mall with someone) to most (going to school alone and staying all day) anxiety provoking. Items from the hierarchy were used as homework assignments to be practiced between therapy sessions. Tasks were completed in a gradual fashion, with repeated practice for each one. For example, the client practiced riding the bus, going to a shopping mall alone, and going to a movie early and waiting in a crowded line. Although she was unable to return to her regular high school, she attended an alternative school program, obtained her GED, and enrolled in a local community college. By the end of treatment, although she still found some social situations anxiety provoking, she no longer engaged in avoidance behaviors.

Recently, Öst and colleagues have begun to apply one-session graduated exposure treatments designed for adults to the treatment of children's specific phobias. In a recent randomized trial, Öst, Svensson, Hellström, and Lindwall (2001) tested the efficacy of the single-session treatment in a group of 60 children ages 7–17 presenting with a variety of specific phobias. Children were randomly assigned to a one-session exposure alone, a one-session exposure with a parent present, or a wait-list control condition. Both exposure treatments lasted a maximum of 3 hours, were conducted *in vivo*, and were adjusted to the developmental level of the child. For example, with children ages 7–10 many playful activities were used, whereas children ages 15–17 were treated very much like adults. Children progressed through the exposure hierarchy at their own pace, moving on to subsequent steps in their hierarchy once they experienced at least a 50% drop in their subjective anxiety level. The specific steps of the hierarchy were determined by the child's specific phobia. For example, children with snake phobias progressed through interactions with snakes of varying sizes (e.g., a corn snake, a python, and a boa constrictor). Both treatment conditions produced significant improvements on multiple measures at posttreatment, and the effects were maintained at the 1-year follow-up. Interestingly, not only did the treatment positively affect the presenting specific phobia, but trends also suggested improvements in comorbid internalizing disorders following treatment.

Systematic Desensitization

Systematic desensitization involves pairing the feared situation or stimulus with a state that is antagonistic to anxiety (e.g., relaxation). Systematic desensitization consists of three steps: relaxation training, construction of the anxiety hierarchy, and pairing of relaxation with graduated exposure to anxiety-provoking situations (Wolpe, 1958). Relaxation training can include the use of progressive muscle relaxation (PMR), diaphragmatic breathing, and imagery. Koeppen (1974) produced a script for children that teaches PMR by using imagery. For example, a child is taught to tense and relax muscles in the hands by imagining that he or she is squeezing the juice from a lemon and to tense and relax muscles in the feet and legs by imagining that he or she is stepping into a big gooey mud puddle. PMR scripts for children differ from those suggested for adults. They are shorter in length and offer fewer distinctions among the muscle groups. Such modifications appear necessary to ensure attentiveness to the procedure, thereby increasing the likelihood of its effectiveness. Alternative strategies for inducing the anxiety-antagonistic state in children include feeding, storytelling, game playing, parental contact, therapist contact, and anger induction. Exposure to anxiety-provoking situations may involve imagining the feared situation while in a relaxed state, seeing pictures of feared stimuli, and *in vivo* exposure.

A large body of literature supports the use of systematic desensitization in the treatment of childhood fears and anxiety. Barrios and O'Dell (1998) reviewed 44 studies (66% of which were case studies) investigating the efficacy of systematic desensitization and its variants from 1924 through 1989 in more than 600 children treated for more than 16 different types of fear and anxiety reactions. Across studies, systematic desensitization produced positive effects on the targeted fear and anxiety reaction. Imaginal and *in vivo* variants of systematic desensitization were recently classified as "probably efficacious" for the treatment of fears and phobias (Ollendick & King, 1998). Emotive imagery, a variant of systematic desensitization that involves invoking support for the child from a favorite superhero, has some support for treating darkness phobias in children (Cornwall, Spence, & Schotte, 1996) and was recently labeled an experimental procedure in the treatment of childhood phobic and anxiety disorders (Ollendick & King, 1998).

Flooding

Flooding involves repeated and prolonged exposure to the feared stimulus with the goal of extinguishing the anxiety response. Such exposure can be conducted imaginally or *in vivo*. Throughout the flooding process, the child is asked to provide anxiety ratings and remains in the presence of the anxiety-provoking stimulus until his or her self-reported anxiety level diminishes. Although there are a few examples of the use of flooding to treat phobic conditions (Blagg & Yule, 1984; Harris & Goetsch, 1990) and posttraumatic fear (Saigh, 1986, 1987a, 1987b, 1987c), flooding has been used primarily to treat obsessive–compulsive disorder. For the treatment of obsessive–compulsive disorder, flooding is typically used in conjunction with response prevention, which requires that the child not engage in avoidance responses. Flooding and response prevention create more distress than some of the other interventions, at least in the initial stages. Therefore, it is important that the child clearly understand the treatment rationale, which may limit its applicability with younger children.

Francis and Gragg (1996) described the use of flooding and response prevention to treat an adolescent with very severe obsessive–compulsive disorder. The 15-year-old boy was admitted to an inpatient unit because of complete incapacitation due to his need to repeat behaviors and an expressed desire to commit suicide to alleviate associated distress. Assessment revealed that the boy experienced nearly constant obsessions about dying if he did not perform rituals to make amends to God for a broken promise. His rituals were varied (e.g., avoidance of preferred foods, compulsive checking, repetitive touching, lining up objects, hoarding objects) and typically involved repetition until they were performed "just right." At the time of his admission, he was having difficulty accomplishing even simple daily activities because he would become "stuck" repeating behaviors. For example, the boy required 20 minutes to leave his bedroom on the unit because he kept returning to touch a specific spot on the baseboard.

Treatment involved both medication management and behavioral intervention. A flooding approach to exposure and response prevention (EX/RP) was implemented. Because the adolescent felt incapable of preventing his ritualized behavior independently, unit staff were instructed to provide constant directions, such as issuing firm commands (e.g., "Come directly to me without touching anything") and providing strict time limits within which he was required to complete routine activities (e.g., 10 minutes to shower). By the 10th day of behavior therapy, the adolescent was getting stuck less often, performing tasks more quickly, and self-directing his avoidance of rituals more often. He was then gradually transferred to increasingly less restrictive settings, with ongoing outpatient therapy, and his parents and school staff were instructed in the implementation of EX/RP. Although the adolescent initially became more symptomatic during transitions, he was able to recover previous gains fairly quickly and continue to make new gains. After 4 weeks of outpatient therapy, the adolescent's symptomatology had improved significantly, but functional impairment was still noted, and ongoing behavioral and pharmacological treatment was recommended to further reduce impairment.

CONTINGENCY MANAGEMENT

Contingency management procedures are used to modify antecedents and consequent events that may influence the acquisition and/or maintenance of fearful or anxious behavior. Operant strategies such as positive reinforcement, shaping, extinction, and punishment fall under the rubric of contingency management. For example, a child may receive a reward for interacting with a feared stimulus or have a reward rescinded for refusing to interact with a feared stimulus. Contingency management is often combined with graduated exposure. For example, in reinforced practice, children are rewarded for progressing through the steps of the anxiety hierarchy. Contingency management can also be used to shape behavior by dispensing and rescinding rewards for making, or failing to make, progressively bolder steps toward the feared stimulus. Contingency management can be used in the context of a therapy session, and it also can be taught to parents for implementation in the home. At times, parents of anxious children require extensive teaching of operant strategies in order to successfully implement contingency management procedures. The involvement of parents or teachers in administering treatment in the home or school can be vital in facilitating generalization and maintenance of therapeutic gains.

Barrios and O'Dell (1998) reviewed 19 studies from 1936 to 1987 using contingency management procedures to treat 10 different types of anxiety and fear (most commonly related to school and social situations) in more than 59 children. Approximately half of these studies were controlled, and almost all reported success. In a recent comparison of the efficacy of contingency management, cognitive self-control, and psychoeducation for the treatment of childhood phobic disorders, Silverman, Kurtines, Ginsburg, Weems, Rabian, and colleagues (1999) described a 10-session contingency management protocol. Each of the 10 sessions was divided into 40 minutes spent with the child alone, 25 minutes spent with the parent alone, and 15 minutes spent with the parent and child together. The first 3 sessions were spent teaching parents behavioral strategies to facilitate child exposure (positive reinforcement, shaping, extinction, contingency contracting, following through, and consistency), devising the fear hierarchy, and creating a "reward list." The next 6 sessions were designed to facilitate a total of 11 exposures (6 in session and 5 out of session). Therapists assisted in the creation of parent–child contracts specifying the details of the exposure task and the reward to be administered upon successful completion of the exposure. Results suggested that contingency management was generally as effective as both cognitive self-control and psychoeducation. Upon completion of treatment, 55% of the 41 children in the contingency management condition no longer met diagnostic criteria for their initial phobia diagnosis. Ollendick and King (1998) rated reinforced practice a "well-established" treatment for fears and phobias, citing evidence that it is superior to verbal coping skills and live modeling.

MODELING

Social learning theory tells us that children learn an enormous amount by watching others (Bandura, 1977). An anxious child can benefit from observing a model approach and cope with a feared situation. Variants of modeling include covert, symbolic (e.g., filmed), live, and participant modeling. In covert modeling, the anxious child imagines a child or adult inter-acting appropriately with the feared stimulus, and in filmed modeling, the anxious child watches a videotape of the model. In live modeling, the model is in the presence of the anxious child, and in participant modeling, the live model interacts with the anxious child and guides his or her ap-proach to the feared stimulus.

Barrios and O'Dell (1998) reviewed 34 studies from 1924 to 1991 ex-amining the efficacy of modeling in more than 1,300 children presenting with 11 different types of fears and anxieties (most commonly phobias about small animals, dental procedures, and medical procedures). Fifty per-cent of the studies involved symbolic modeling, 20% involved participant modeling, and 30% involved two or more variants of modeling. Virtually all studies employed experimental designs, and virtually all found modeling to be effective. Studies suggested that participant modeling was more effec-tive than live, symbolic, or covert modeling. Furthermore, their review sug-gested that the more closely the anxious child resembled the model in terms of age, fear level, and previous experience with the feared stimulus, the greater the probability of a positive treatment outcome. Participant model-ing has been designated a "well-established treatment" for childhood fears and phobias, with studies showing that it is superior to imaginal systematic desensitization, as well as live and filmed modeling. Both live and filmed modeling are considered "probably efficacious" treatments for fears and phobias (Ollendick & King, 1998).

COGNITIVE STRATEGIES

Although pure behavioral techniques are effective for treating simple fears and specific phobias, they may be less effective in treating more complex anxiety disorders (Piacentini & Bergman, 2001). For such disorders, cogni-tive strategies may enhance the efficacy of treatment.

Cognitive procedures include a variety of techniques, such as self-instruction training and altering maladaptive self-talk. These strategies typically are taught using modeling, exposure, and behavioral rehearsal. Self-instruction training (Meichenbaum & Goodman, 1971) for anxious children was described by Hagopian and Ollendick (1993) as incorporating the following steps: (1) the therapist approaches the feared stimulus while talking aloud about coping, (2) the child approaches the feared stimulus and verbalizes coping statements at the direction of the therapist, (3) the child approaches the feared stimulus while saying coping statements aloud, (4) the child approaches the feared stimulus while whispering coping state-ments, (5) the child approaches the feared stimulus while thinking the cop-ing statement. Self-instruction training was recently classified as a "probably efficacious" treatment for childhood fears and phobias (Ollendick & King, 1998).

Maladaptive self-talk is the result of cognitive distortions. "Cognitive distortions involve active information processing that is faulty or misguided, resulting in misperceptions of oneself and/or the environment . . . [and] are a part of the psychology of children with internalizing difficulties" (Kendall, Panichelli-Mindel, et al., 1997, p. 30). To modify maladaptive self-talk, the child must first learn to identify and monitor self-statements associated with anxiety and avoidance behaviors. Once maladaptive self-talk is identified, the child works with the therapist to generate alternative self-statements that serve to decrease anxiety, facilitate approach behaviors, and improve coping (Kendall et al., 1992).

In their comparison of cognitive self-control therapy with contingency management and psychoeducation among children presenting with phobic disorders, Silverman, Kurtines, Ginsburg, Weems, Rabian, and colleagues (1999) found that all three treatments were efficacious. However, the cognitive self-control treatment did show a treatment advantage on two of the multiple treatment-outcome measures assessed. Specifically, children in the self-control condition were less likely to meet diagnostic criteria posttreatment (88%) relative to the other two conditions (55–56%), and they reported lower levels of subjective distress. The cognitive self-control condition involved ten 80-minute sessions divided into 40 minutes spent with the child alone, 25 minutes spent with the parent alone, and 15 minutes spent with the child and parent together. The first three sessions focused on instructing children in cognitive strategies of self-observation, self-talk, self-evaluation, and self-reward, helping parents understand treatment rationale and encouraging parental support for the anxious child, as well as creating the fear hierarchy. The next six sessions involved facilitation of six in-session and five out-of-session exposure tasks. Each exposure task was outlined for the child, and the child was instructed in the specific self-control strategies to be used during the task.

Unlike in the literature on adult anxiety disorders, cognitive strategies have rarely been studied as the sole treatment intervention for childhood anxiety disorders but have almost always been implemented in combination with behavioral techniques. This may be due, in part, to several cognitive limitations common among preadolescent children. Piacentini and Bergman (2001) suggest that therapists need to consider the developmental limitations of children when using cognitive strategies therapeutically. These limitations include an inability to engage in abstract or metacognitive thought, limited ability to identify and understand different emotion states, and a tendency to be more present oriented and less able to take the perspective that tasks that may be difficult now will be beneficial in the future (e.g., anxiety-provoking exposure treatments). These considerations have guided the development of cognitive treatment procedures for children. For example, in Kendall's Coping Cat treatment (an integrated cognitive-behavioral technique described in the next section), children are taught to identify distorted cognitions and the link between such cognitions and maladaptive behaviors through the use of cartoons with "thought bubbles." Developmental considerations also suggest that cognitive strategies may have little utility in children age 6 and under.

INTEGRATED COGNITIVE-BEHAVIORAL APPROACH

Over the past decade, a number of integrated cognitive-behavioral treatments have been developed and tested for childhood anxiety disorders (e.g., Barrett, Dadds, & Rapee, 1996; Kendall, 1994; Silverman, Kurtines, Ginsburg, Weems, Rabian, et al., 1999). The first to be developed, the Coping Cat program, has been promoted by Kendall and colleagues (1992). They outlined three goals of this treatment approach: (1) the child learns to recognize, experience, and cope with anxiety; (2) the child learns to reduce his or her level of anxiety; (3) the child learns to master developmentally appropriate, challenging, and difficult tasks.

The integrated cognitive-behavioral program, called the "Coping Cat" program, consists of 16–20 sessions and is divided into two segments, an 8-session skills training phase followed by an 8- to 12-session practice phase. In the skills acquisition phase, the child is taught (1) to recognize the physiological symptoms of anxiety, (2) to challenge and modify anxious self-talk, (3) to develop a plan to cope with the situation, and (4) to evaluate his or her performance and utilize self-reinforcement. Children are taught to remember these steps with the acronym FEAR: Feeling frightened? Expecting bad things to happen? Actions and attitudes that can help, Results and rewards. During the practice phase of treatment, the child applies acquired coping skills during a variety of individually tailored in vivo exposures. Other aspects of the program include the incorporation of behavioral training strategies (e.g., modeling, role play, relaxation training, and contingency management) and the application of coping skills to a variety of situations to promote generalization (Kendall et al., 1992). An accompanying Coping Cat workbook (Kendall, 1990) is available for children participating in the treatment.

Kendall and colleagues have demonstrated the efficacy of the Coping Cat program in several trials with children ages 9–13 who met criteria for generalized anxiety disorder (formerly overanxious disorder), separation anxiety disorder, or social phobia (formerly avoidant disorder). In two separate randomized clinical trials, 53–64% of children receiving 16 sessions of treatment no longer met diagnostic criteria, compared with only 5–6%

of children in the wait-list control group. Treatment gains were maintained at 1-year and at 3- to 5-year follow-ups (Kendall, 1994; Kendall, Flannery-Schroeder, et al., 1997; Kendall & Southam-Gerow, 1996). The treatment has been proven equally effective for both boys and girls and for African American and European American children (Treadwell, Flannery-Schroeder, & Kendall, 1995). Barrett and colleagues (1996) modified the treatment and essentially replicated the positive findings in an Australian sample of children, suggesting that the treatment is "probably efficacious" for the treatment of nonsimple phobia anxiety disorders in children (Kendall, Flannery-Schroeder, et al., 1997; Ollendick & King, 1998). The modified Australian "Coping Koala" version has also been used with children exhibiting anxiety symptoms who did not meet criteria for a diagnosed anxiety disorder. The program reduced the likelihood of children developing an anxiety disorder 6 months posttreatment (Dadds, Spence, Holland, Barrett, & Laurens, 1997). Although the effects faded at 12 months, they re-emerged at 24 months (Dadds et al., 1999), suggesting that integrated cognitive-behavioral treatments may be effective in preventing the development of anxiety disorders among children exhibiting subclinical levels of anxiety.

Kendall's Coping Cat program has been adapted for group use (Flannery-Schroeder & Kendall, 1996), and the individual and group formats have been compared (Flannery-Schroeder & Kendall, 2000). At posttreatment, 73% of children in the individual format and 50% in the group format no longer met diagnostic criteria for their primary anxiety disorder, compared with only 8% in the wait-list control condition (Flannery-Schroeder & Kendall, 2000). Other researchers have also found support for the efficacy of integrated cognitive-behavioral treatments administered in group formats. In two separate randomized clinical trials, researchers found that 64–75% of children in group cognitive-behavioral treatment no longer met criteria for an anxiety disorder, compared with only 13–25% of children in the wait-list control condition, and that treatment effects were maintained at 12-month follow-ups (Barrett, 1998; Silverman, Kurtines, Ginsburg, Weems, Lumpkin, et al., 1999). Overall, results from multiple studies support the efficacy of both individual and group CBT and suggest that the addition of a family treatment component may enhance individual treatments (Barrett et al., 1996).

APPLICATIONS TO SPECIFIC DISORDERS

Posttraumatic Stress Disorder

Practice parameters developed by the American Academy of Child and Adolescent Psychiatry advocate the use of trauma-focused cognitive-behavioral therapy in the treatment of childhood PTSD (Cohen & the Work Group on Quality Issues, 1998). CBT has been shown to be superior to no treatment (Goenjian et al., 1997), to community treatment (Deblinger, Lippman, & Steer, 1996; Deblinger, Steer, & Lippman, 1999), and to supportive therapy (Cohen & Mannarino, 1996) in the treatment of childhood PTSD. Cohen and the Work Group (1998) recommend that therapists instruct clients in stress management techniques, such as PMR, diaphragmatic breathing, thought stopping, and positive imagery, which can then be utilized during exposure sessions. Although Cohen and colleagues (1998) generally recommend that exposure take place through direct exploration of the trauma (i.e., asking the child what happened and what it meant to them), they acknowledge that some researchers and clinicians recommend more gradual exposure to trauma and that in some instances, such as those in which the child is not currently distressed by the trauma or is particularly resistant or embarrassed, direct exploration may be contraindicated. Cohen and the Work Group also recommend that therapists challenge cognitive distortions, such as "it's all my fault" and "nothing is safe," during therapy.

Cognitive-behavioral treatment programs developed for adults are sometimes useful in adolescent populations. These include manualized treatments targeting a broad range of PTSD symptoms (Foa & Rothbaum, 1998), as well as more focused treatments. For example, Shipherd, Beck, Hamblen, and Freeman (2000) have developed a 12-session manualized treatment for adolescents and adults with PTSD resulting from motor vehicle accidents. There are also cognitive-behavioral treatment programs designed specifically for children. Deblinger and Heflin (1996) developed a manualized treatment for children ages 3–13 with a history of sexual abuse and resulting PTSD or functional impairment. The treatment consists of therapy sessions with the child alone, the nonoffending parent alone, and the parent and child together that focus on (1) coping skills in emotional expression, relaxation, and cognitive techniques, (2) graduated exposure with cognitive-affective processing, (3) behavior management for parents, and (4) education about healthy sexual behavior and safety. John March and colleagues report promising results from a cognitive-behavioral group intervention they are developing for children and adolescents diagnosed with PTSD following a single-incident trauma (March, Amaya-Jackson, Murray, & Schulte, 1998).

Social Anxiety Disorder

Although there is extensive support for cognitive-behavioral treatments of social anxiety disorder in adults, the treatment-outcome literature with children is limited (King, Murphy, & Heyne, 1997). Several studies that demonstrate the efficacy of cognitive-behavioral therapy for childhood anxiety disorders have included children with social anxiety disorder, along with children diagnosed with other anxiety disorders (Barrett et al., 1996; Flannery-Schroeder & Kendall, 2000; Kendall, 1994; Kendall, Flannery-Schroeder, et al., 1997; Silverman, Kurtines, Ginsburg, Weems, Lumpkin, et al., 1999; Silverman, Kurtines, Ginsburg, Weems, Rabian, et al., 1999). Without treatment-outcome studies targeting childhood social anxiety disorder specifically, however, one must be cautious in inferring the utility of cognitive-behavioral therapy with this population.

Two recently developed cognitive-behavioral programs designed specifically for childhood social anxiety disorder show promise. Both are modeled after existing treatments for adults with social anxiety disorder. Key similarities between the programs are that both are conducted in a group format and both include innovative social skills training components. Cognitive Behavioral Group Therapy for Adolescents (CBGT-A; Albano, 2000) is designed for socially anxious adolescents ages 13–17. Group sessions initially focus on psychoeducation and skill building (e.g., social skills, problem solving, assertiveness) and then involve contrived exposure sessions. Cognitive restructuring is a critical component of treatment incorporated before, during, and after exposure sessions. One unique component of the treatment is a scheduled snack break designed to provide exposure to eating in public and opportunities for practicing social skills. Initial findings with five adolescents demonstrated improvements at 3- and 12-month follow-ups (Albano, Marten, Holt, Heimberg, & Barlow, 1995). Findings from the first randomized pilot test demonstrated significant improvement in clinician-rated interference and reduction in symptoms at posttreatment but no significant differences between treatment and control participants at the 12-month follow-up (Hayward et al., 2000).

Social effectiveness therapy for children (SET-C; Beidel, Turner, & Morris, 2000) is designed for socially phobic preadolescent children ages 7–13. One unique feature of the program is the recruitment of socially skilled peers to participate in group activities. This "peer generalization programming" encourages skills development through modeling. Results from a large controlled treatment trial reveal advantages for SET-C over an alternative, empirically supported treatment for test anxiety. Specifically, 67% of participants in SET-C no longer met criteria for social anxiety disorder at posttreatment, compared with only 5% in the alternative treatment. Treatment gains for the SET-C group increased at 6-month follow-up, with 85% no longer meeting criteria (Beidel et al., 2000).

Obsessive–Compulsive Disorder

Reviews of the literature on cognitive-behavioral treatments for OCD in children and adolescents provide some support for the use of behavioral techniques (i.e., extinction, modeling, and operant techniques) and cognitive techniques (i.e., thought stopping, cognitive restructuring, and satiation) but suggest that cognitive-behavioral treatments that incorporate exposure and response prevention (EX/RP) are most effective (Geffken, Pincus, & Zelikovsky, 1999; March, 1995; Piacentini, 1999). This finding is supported by the American Academy of Child and Adolescent Psychiatry (1998; King, Leonard, & March, 1998). Results from a recent randomized clinical trial indicated that exposure and response prevention were the key therapeutic components of OCD treatment and that outcomes did not improve with the addition of anxiety management therapy or medication (Franklin et al., 1998). A manualized treatment for childhood OCD is available (March & Mulle, 1998).

Panic Disorder

Only one systematic, controlled treatment for panic disorder has been empirically evaluated in adolescents (Ollendick, 1995). This study involved a multiple-baseline design with four adolescents. The cognitive-behavioral treatment was based on protocols designed by Barlow, Craske, Cerny, and Klosko (1989) and Öst, Westling, and Hellström (1993) for treating panic disorder in adults and included psychoeducation about panic disorder and anxiety, instruction in relaxation techniques (PMR, diaphragmatic breathing, cue-controlled relaxation, and applied relaxation), cognitive coping strategies (positive self-statements, coping procedures, and self-instruction strategies), and *in vivo* exposure. Treatment length varied depending on participants' response to treatment. The cognitive-behavioral treatment produced improvements in all four adolescents. Specifically, the treatment eliminated panic attacks, reduced avoidance, enhanced self-efficacy about their own ability to cope with future attacks, and brought levels of anxiety sensitivity, trait anxiety, fear, and depression to normative levels. Further research is needed to determine whether empirically validated treatments for panic disorder in adults are appropriate for children and adolescents. Based on their assessment of panic disorder presentations in adolescents, Kearney, Albano, Eisen, Allan, and Barlow (1997) have recommended addressing negative affectivity and adding cognitive therapy to techniques commonly used with adults.

School Refusal

Behavioral and cognitive-behavioral treatments are widely accepted as the preferred method for treating school refusal (Elliott, 1999; King, Tonge, Heyne, & Ollendick, 2000). However, because of relatively few empirical studies, cognitive-behavioral therapy does not yet meet the criteria for designation as a "well-established" treatment for school refusal (King et al., 2000). In the only two existing randomized clinical trials, cognitive-behavioral therapy was found to be superior to no treatment (N. J. King et al., 1998) but not to an attention-placebo control condition (Last, Hansen, & Franco, 1998). The specific strategies reported in the literature vary and include the full range of behavioral and cognitive techniques presented in this chapter. For example, some behavioral programs emphasize *in vivo* flooding (i.e., forced return), whereas others utilize a graduated exposure approach (Elliott, 1999). Perhaps the variability in treatment methods is reflective of the tremendous heterogeneity found among the population of school refusers. Possible reasons for school avoidance include, but are not limited to, specific phobias, social anxiety, separation anxiety, oppositionality, and the desire to engage in more pleasurable activities at home. The treatment of choice may depend on the individual child's particular presentation (Elliott, 1999). Preliminary support for the utility of prescriptive treatments for school refusal is found in Kearney and Silverman's (1990) innovative open clinical trial. The authors assigned each of seven children to one of four treatment conditions depending on whether they: (1) had a specific phobia or were generally overanxious, (2) were socially anxious, (3) were seeking attention or were having separation anxiety issues, or (4) were staying home to engage in more pleasurable activities. Each condition received a different treatment (e.g., relaxation training and systematic desensitization for the specific phobia/overanxious group and shaping and differential reinforcement for the attention-seeking group). Six of the seven children returned to school full time; the seventh child did not return to school but began working instead. Following is a case example of a cognitive-behavioral treatment for a school-refusing adolescent with a complex clinical picture.

CASE EXAMPLE

Lydia was a 14-year-old female who was referred to a therapeutic day treatment program by her school department because of anxiety and school avoidance. Prior to the manifestation of anxiety in school and subsequent school avoidance, her academic and social functioning in school was reportedly average. Lydia was an only child who lived with her biological mother and had relatively little contact with her biological father. Lydia and her mother reported having a close relationship, which was strained by Lydia's recent refusal to attend classes.

Lydia was evaluated during the first week of her placement in the day treatment program. The evaluation included clinical interviews with Lydia and her mother, administration of self-report questionnaires, and observations of Lydia's behavior in the day treatment program. Lydia presented with a lifelong history of excessive worrying about a variety of issues and a tendency to experience social-evaluative anxiety. These anxious tendencies had increased substantially during the previous several months, concurrent with the onset of school avoidance.

Lydia's problems with school avoidance began approximately 4 months prior to her admission to the treatment program. At that time, she reportedly developed a medical problem with urinary frequency. Despite successful pharmacological treatment of this medical condition, Lydia's anxiety about urinary frequency did not subside. She subsequently developed an acute onset of panic disorder. Lydia reported that her panic attacks came on quickly and that they were almost always triggered by fear that she would need to urinate and would not have immediate access to a bathroom. Lydia had experienced panic attacks in one of her classrooms, in several stores, on the bus, and while riding in the car. She endorsed multiple physical symptoms during her panic attacks, including breathlessness, sweaty palms, shaking, derealization, heart palpitations, nausea, and feeling faint. Lydia reported a high level of anticipatory anxiety about having another panic attack, and she engaged in avoidance behaviors related to situations in which she was fearful of having a panic attack. Her avoidance of the school bus and her classrooms were of primary concern to the school department and her mother.

Lydia was diagnosed with panic disorder with agoraphobia, social phobia, and generalized anxiety disorder. She and her mother were given feedback about her diagnostic formulation and about the proposed treatment. Lydia agreed to participate in individual cognitive-behavioral therapy several times weekly, and she and her mother agreed to participate in weekly family sessions with a separate family therapist. The primary focus of the family therapy sessions was to encourage Lydia's mother's support of treatment, which included psychoeducation and development of a contingency contract.

Lydia's individual treatment initially focused on psychoeducation. The functional nature of anxiety was emphasized, and the goal of treatment was described as being to regain control of, rather than to eliminate, anxiety. The behavioral, cognitive, and physiological components of anxiety were discussed, and distinctions were drawn between "worry" and panic attacks. Lydia was assigned readings on the physiology of anxiety to complete for homework, and her questions were answered during therapy sessions. Lydia seemed to benefit from the psychoeducational work, describing an increased sense of control over anxiety resulting from her understanding of anxiety as a natural process. Throughout the remainder of treatment, Lydia often referred back to her early readings about anxiety as a means to reestablish control in challenging situations.

Once Lydia had a basic understanding of the nature of anxiety and its components, we began to work on strategies for managing anxiety. Lydia reported that she had tried several relaxation strategies in the past, but it was clear that she had not done so in a systematic way. Lydia was first instructed in diaphragmatic breathing. We discussed diaphragmatic breathing as a "muscle memory skill" that needs to be practiced repeatedly so that it eventually becomes second nature and can be implemented in an anxiety-provoking situation. Lydia was asked to practice diaphragmatic breathing for 5 minutes twice daily during periods of low anxiety. During the course of therapy, Lydia's breathing assignments were altered to gradually increase the similarities between practice sessions and situations that Lydia found anxiety provoking. For example, she initially practiced in a quiet room away from the classrooms, then she practiced during silent reading periods in the classroom, and finally she practiced during active class periods. Over the course of treatment, Lydia was also instructed in other relaxation techniques (i.e., PMR and imagery).

We also worked on cognitive techniques for anxiety management. Lydia was able to generate lists of distorted cognitions that contributed to her anxiety in different situations. She was very good at evaluating the evidence for these cognitions and generating alternative thoughts that reduced her anxiety. Lydia reported that her use of relaxation techniques and cognitive strategies was helpful in reducing panic attacks and panic-like symptoms (she did not experience a full-blown panic attack after the second week of treatment). However, she reported no change in her tendency to worry about multiple topics at inopportune times (e.g., on the bus and in the classroom). Lydia described feeling the need to worry about "stuff" and said that she had become accustomed to worrying at specific times. To reduce the frequency of her worrying, we asked Lydia to designate a daily "worry time." Lydia estimated that she would need approximately 30 minutes each day to adequately worry about her problems. She was instructed to choose a 30-minute period in the afternoon or evening each day during which she did nothing but worry. Lydia chose to worry after dinner, and she designated her laundry room as the location for her worry time because she did not normally spend time in the laundry room. Within a week of daily worry time, Lydia reported extreme boredom during worry time. Within 2 weeks, she was reporting reductions in the amount of time spent worrying outside of her designated worry time. As the amount of unscheduled worry time decreased, we slowly reduced her scheduled worry time by 5-minute intervals.

After laying the foundation for treatment through psychoeducation and instruction in specific techniques for mastering her anxiety, we began to discuss transition back to high school during the fourth week of placement. Lydia worked with the therapist to identify her fears about entering the high school and to establish a hierarchy for exposure. During the fifth week of her placement, the hierarchy was clarified, and her family and individual therapists worked closely with key high school personnel (e.g., teachers, principal) to assess the feasibility of implementation. As the plan for transition was solidified, Lydia expressed increasing anxiety about the transition. Her anxiety initially manifested in specific statements about her fear that she would be unable to manage the transition. When it became clear to Lydia that the transition would still take place, she began to express a multitude of somatic complaints and other problems. These complaints were conceptualized as a manifestation of anxiety, and Lydia was informed that her transition would take place as scheduled. Lydia was assigned cognitive work sheets to help her work through some of her anxiety-producing automatic thoughts.

Lydia began *in vivo* exposure during the sixth week of her placement. The exposure initially entailed visits to the high school with her therapist, followed by full days spent in the high school. Lydia initially spent two periods per day in her scheduled classes and worked in a resource classroom the remainder of the day. She slowly added additional classes according to her hierarchy. Her transition into new classes was carefully coordinated with key high school personnel. Lydia was advised that once she committed to reentering a class, she was expected to attend the class daily or receive a set of negative consequences, both at school and at home. All classroom teachers were kept informed about her progress so that consequences could be administered according to the plan if necessary. A set of rewards was also established with Lydia's mother and preferred staff at the high school to provide external incentives for Lydia to progress along her hierarchy.

During the transition, Lydia met twice weekly with her individual therapist, who also consulted with her mother and the treatment team. As each new step on the hierarchy approached, Lydia exhibited increased anxiety. Her anxiety was often expressed in the form of somatic complaints or social stressors, which she would report as obstacles to her progress. Despite her anxiety and resistance, Lydia was able to take each additional step with coaching, and she expressed pride each time she successfully completed a step. Within 5 weeks of returning to the high school, Lydia had reentered all of her academic classes, and therapy sessions were reduced to once weekly. Plans were also made for Lydia to participate in a half-day summer program to reduce the stress of her transition back into school the following fall.

SUMMARY AND FUTURE RESEARCH

As is evident from this review, significant progress has been made in the use of cognitive-behavioral therapy for the treatment of childhood anxiety disorders. During the past decade, several controlled clinical trials have demonstrated the efficacy of behavioral and cognitive-behavioral techniques. In some cases, these results have replicated across independent samples, allowing for increased confidence in reports of efficacy. Following the American Psychological Association's Division 12 Task Force on Promotion and Dissemination of Psychological Procedures (1995) guidelines for identifying and classifying empirically supported treatments, several cognitive-behavioral techniques have been classified as "probably efficacious" or "well-established" treatments for childhood anxiety disorders (Ollendick & King, 1998). Specifically, imaginal and *in vivo* variants of systematic desensitization, live and filmed modeling, and self-instruction training have been designated as "probably efficacious" for treating childhood fears and phobias; participant modeling and reinforced practice are classified as a "well-established" treatment for childhood fears and phobias; and integrated cognitive-behavioral therapy with and without family management procedures has been designated as "probably efficacious" for treating more complex anxiety disorders. Researchers have also published clinical practice parameters for specific anxiety disorders, including PTSD and OCD (Cohen & the Work Group on Quality Issues, 1998; R. A. King et al., 1998).

Although the field has advanced considerably in the past several years, there are still many areas that require further study. First, there is a need for follow-up studies to determine the long-term gains of empirically validated treatments for childhood anxiety disorders (Kendall, 1998). Evidence for the maintenance of treatment gains from integrated cognitive-behavioral programs has been demonstrated in two separate samples during 2- to 5-year follow-up (Kendall & Southam-Gerow, 1996) and 5- to 7-year follow-up (Barrett, Duffy, Dadds, & Rapee, 2001), but there is no current evidence for the effects beyond 7 years. Second, researchers need to begin to dismantle integrated cognitive-behavioral treatments to see which components are most effective for which disorders and to determine the relative potencies of the various treatment components (Kendall, Panichelli-Mindel et al., 1997). Third, researchers need to investigate predictors of treatment outcome. Clinical experience highlights the importance of individual differences as predictors of treatment outcome (Barrett, 2000), and some researchers are beginning to identify specific factors. Early investigations point to the importance of parental psychopathology and level of family dysfunction (Berman, Weems, Silverman, & Kurtines, 2000; Cobham,

Dadds, & Spence, 1998; Crawford & Manassis, 2001; Southam-Gerow, Kendall, & Weersing, 2001), as well as child pretreatment comorbidity, particularly comorbid internalizing symptoms (Berman et al., 2000; Southam-Gerow et al., 2001), although there are some discrepancies (e.g., Kendall, Brady, & Verduin, 2001; Öst et al., 2001). Identification of pretreatment predictors of response could help determine what type of treatment (e.g., individual vs. family) would be most effective for specific children (Kendall, Panichelli-Mindel, et al., 1997). Finally, research needs to move in the direction of studying effectiveness. We need to begin to identify ways to apply programs that have been shown to be efficacious in research trials in outpatient settings. Recognition of the need to balance manualized treatment with individualized care suggests that the research community is beginning to investigate effectiveness. Kendall, Chu, Gifford, Hayes, and Nauta (1998) recently offered suggestions for individualizing a manualized CBT program for anxiety. Analyses of 18 therapists who had treated children with the Coping Cat protocol suggested no relations between therapist flexibility and treatment outcome (Kendall & Chu, 2000), supporting the flexibility of CBT in treating anxiety disorders.

REFERENCES

Albano, A. M. (2000). Treatment of social phobia in adolescents: Cognitive behavioral programs focused on intervention and prevention. *Journal of Cognitive Psychotherapy, 14*, 67–76.

Albano, A. M., Marten, P. A., Holt, C. S., Heimberg, R. G., & Barlow, D. H. (1995). Cognitive-behavioral group treatment for social phobia in adolescence: A preliminary study. *Journal of Nervous and Mental Disease, 183*, 649–656.

American Academy of Child and Adolescent Psychiatry. (1998). Practice parameters for the assessment and treatment of children and adolescents with obsessive–compulsive disorder. *Journal of the American Academy of Child and Adolescent Psychiatry, 37*(Suppl.), 27S–45S.

American Psychological Association Task Force on Promotion and Dissemination of Psychological Procedures. (1995). Training in and dissemination of empirically-validated psychological treatments: Report and recommendations. *Clinical Psychologist, 48*, 3–24.

Bandura, A. (1977). Self-efficacy: Towards a unifying theory of behavioral change. *Psychological Review, 84*, 191–215.

Barlow, D. H., Craske, M. G., Cerny, J. A., & Klosko, J. S. (1989). Behavioral treatment of panic disorder. *Behavior Therapy, 20*, 261–282.

Barrett, P. M. (1998). An evaluation of cognitive-behavioral group treatments for childhood anxiety disorders. *Journal of Clinical Child Psychology, 27*, 459–468.

Barrett, P. M. (2000). Treatment of childhood anxiety: Developmental aspects. *Clinical Psychology Review, 20,* 479–494.

Barrett, P. M., Dadds, M. R., & Rapee, R. M. (1996). Family treatment of childhood anxiety: A controlled trial. *Journal of Consulting and Clinical Psychology, 64,* 333–342.

Barrett, P. M., Duffy, A. L., Dadds, M. R., & Rapee, R. M. (2001). Cognitive-behavioral treatment of anxiety disorders in children: Long-term (6–year) follow-up. *Journal of Consulting and Clinical Psychology, 69,* 135–141.

Barrios, B. A., & O'Dell, S. L. (1998). Fears and anxieties. In E. J. Mash & R. A. Barkley (Eds.), *Treatment of childhood disorders* (2nd ed., pp. 249–337). New York: Guilford Press.

Beidel, D. C., Turner, S. M., & Morris, T. L. (2000). Behavioral treatment of childhood social phobia. *Journal of Consulting and Clinical Psychology, 68,* 1072–1080.

Berman, S. L., Weems, C. F., Silverman, W. K., & Kurtines, W. M. (2000). Predictors of outcome in exposure-based cognitive and behavioral treatments for phobic and anxiety disorders in children. *Behavior Therapy, 31,* 713–731.

Blagg, N. R., & Yule, W. (1984). The behavioral treatment of school refusal: A comparative study. *Behaviour Research and Therapy, 22,* 119–127.

Cobham, V. E., Dadds, M. R., & Spence, S. H. (1998). The role of parental anxiety in the treatment of childhood anxiety. *Journal of Consulting and Clinical Psychology, 66,* 893–905.

Cohen, J. A., & Mannarino, A. P. (1996). A treatment outcome study for sexually abused preschool children: Initial findings. *Journal of the American Academy of Child and Adolescent Psychiatry, 35,* 42–50.

Cohen, J. A., and the Work Group on Quality Issues. (1998). Practice parameters for the assessment and treatment of children and adolescents with posttraumatic stress disorder. *Journal of the American Academy of Child and Adolescent Psychiatry, 37*(Suppl. 10), 4S–26S.

Cornwall, E., Spence, S. H., & Schotte, D. (1996). The effectiveness of emotive imagery in the treatment of darkness phobia in children. *Behaviour Change, 13,* 223–229.

Crawford, A. M., & Manassis, K. (2001). Familial predictors of treatment outcome in childhood anxiety disorders. *Journal of the American Academy of Child and Adolescent Psychiatry, 40,* 1182–1189.

Dadds, M. R., Holland, D. E., Laurens, K. R., Mullins, M., Barrett, P. M., & Spence, S. H. (1999). Early intervention and prevention of anxiety disorders in children: Results at 2–year follow-up. *Journal of Consulting and Clinical Psychology, 67,* 145–150.

Dadds, M. R., Spence, S. H., Holland, D. E., Barrett, P. M., & Laurens, K. R. (1997). Prevention and early intervention for anxiety disorders: A controlled trial. *Journal of Consulting and Clinical Psychology, 65,* 627–635.

Deblinger, E., & Heflin, A. H. (1996). *Treating sexually abused children and their nonoffending parents: A cognitive behavioral approach.* Thousand Oaks, CA: Sage.

Deblinger, E., Lippman, J., & Steer, R. (1996). Sexually abused children suffering posttraumatic stress symptoms: Initial treatment outcome findings. *Child Maltreatment, 1,* 310–322.

Deblinger, E., Steer, R. A., & Lippman, J. (1999). Two-year follow-up study of cognitive behavioral therapy for sexually abused children suffering post-traumatic stress symptoms. *Child Abuse and Neglect, 23,* 1371–1378.

Elliott, J. G. (1999). School refusal: Issues of conceptualization, assessment, and treatment. *Journal of Child Psychology and Psychiatry and Allied Disciplines, 40,* 1001–1012.

Flannery-Schroeder, E., & Kendall, P. C. (1996). *Cognitive-behavioral therapy for anxious children: Therapist manual for group treatment.* Ardmore, PA: Workbook.

Flannery-Schroeder, E., & Kendall, P. C. (2000). Group and individual cognitive-behavioral treatments for youth with anxiety disorders: A randomized clinical trial. *Cognitive Therapy and Research, 24,* 251–278.

Foa, E. B., & Rothbaum, B. O. (1998). *Treating the trauma of rape: Cognitive-behavioral treatment for PTSD.* New York: Guilford Press.

Francis, G., & Gragg, R. A. (1996). *Childhood obsessive–compulsive disorder.* New York: Sage.

Francis, G., & Ollendick, T. (1990). Behavioral treatment of social anxiety. In E. L. Feindler & G. R. Kalfus (Eds.), *Casebook in adolescent behavior therapy* (pp. 127–146). New York: Springer.

Franklin, M. E., Kozak, M. J., Cashman, L. A., Coles, M. E., Rheingold, A. A., & Foa, E. B. (1998). Cognitive-behavioral treatment of pediatric obsessive–compulsive disorder: An open clinical trial. *Journal of the American Academy of Child and Adolescent Psychiatry, 37,* 412–419.

Geffken, G. R., Pincus, D. B., & Zelikovsky, N. (1999). Obsessive–compulsive disorder in children and adolescents: Review of background, assessment, and treatment. *Journal of Psychological Practice, 5,* 15–31.

Goenjian, A. K., Karayan, I., Pynoos, R. S., Minassian, D., Najarian, L. M., Steinberg, A. M., & Fairbanks, L. A. (1997). Outcome of psychotherapy among early adolescents after trauma. *American Journal of Psychiatry, 154,* 536–542.

Hagopian, L. P., & Ollendick, T. H. (1993). Simple phobia in children. *Handbook of Behavior Therapy with Children and Adults, 8,* 123–136.

Harris, C. V., & Goetsch, V. L. (1990). Multi-component flooding treatment of adolescent phobia. In E. L. Feindler & G. R. Kalfus (Eds.), *Adolescent behavior therapy casebook* (pp. 147–164). New York: Springer.

Hayward, C., Varady, S., Albano, A. M., Thienemann, M., Henderson, L., & Schatzberg, A. F. (2000). Cognitive-behavioral group therapy for social phobia in female adolescents: Results of a pilot study. *Journal of the American Academy of Child and Adolescent Psychiatry, 39,* 721–726.

Jones, M. C. (1924). A laboratory study of fear: The case of Peter. *Journal of Genetic Psychology, 31,* 308–315.

Kazdin, A. E., & Weisz, J. R. (1998). Identifying and developing empirically supported child and adolescent treatments. *Journal of Consulting and Clinical Psychology, 66,* 19–36.

Kearney, C. A., Albano, A. M., Eisen, A. R., Allan, W. D., & Barlow, D. H. (1997). The phenomenology of panic disorder in youngsters: An empirical study of a clinical sample. *Journal of Anxiety Disorders, 11,* 49–62.

Kearney, C. A., & Silverman, W. K. (1990). A preliminary analysis of a functional model of assessment and treatment for school refusal behavior. *Behavior Modification, 14,* 340–366.

Kendall, P. C. (1990). *Coping Cat Workbook.* Ardmore, PA: Workbook Publishing.

Kendall, P. C. (1994). Treating anxiety disorders in children: Results of a randomized clinical trial. *Journal of Consulting and Clinical Psychology, 62,* 100–110.

Kendall, P. C. (1998). Empirically supported psychological therapies. *Journal of Consulting and Clinical Psychology, 66,* 3–6.

Kendall, P. C., Brady, E. U., & Verduin, T. L. (2001). Comorbidity in childhood anxiety disorders and treatment outcome. *Journal of the American Academy of Child and Adolescent Psychiatry, 40,* 787–794.

Kendall, P. C., Chansky, T. E., Kane, M. T., Kim, R., Kortlander, E., Ronan, K. R., et al. (1992). *Anxiety disorders in youth: Cognitive-behavioral interventions.* Needham Heights, MA: Allyn & Bacon.

Kendall, P. C., & Chu, B. C. (2000). Retrospective self-reports of therapist flexibility in a manual-based treatment for youths with anxiety disorders. *Journal of Clinical Child Psychology, 29,* 209–220.

Kendall, P. C., Chu, B. C., Gifford, A., Hayes, C., & Nauta, M. (1998). Breathing life into a manual: Flexibility and creativity with manual-based treatments. *Cognitive and Behavioral Practice, 5,* 177–198.

Kendall, P. C., Flannery-Schroeder, E., Panichelli-Mindel, S. M., Southam-Gerow, M., Henin, A., & Warman, M. (1997). Therapy for youths with anxiety disorders: A second randomized clinical trial. *Journal of Consulting and Clinical Psychology, 65,* 366–380.

Kendall, P. C., Panichelli-Mindel, S. M., Sugarman, A., & Callahan, S. A. (1997). Exposure to child anxiety: Theory, research, and practice. *Clinical Psychology: Science and Practice, 4,* 29–39.

Kendall, P. C., & Southam-Gerow, M. A. (1996). Long-term follow-up of a cognitive-behavioral therapy for anxiety-disordered youth. *Journal of Consulting and Clinical Psychology, 64,* 724–730.

King, N. J., Tonge, B. J., Heyne, D., & Ollendick, T. H. (2000). Research on the cognitive-behavioral treatment of school refusal: A review and recommendations. *Clinical Psychology Review, 20,* 495–507.

King, N. J., Tonge, B. J., Heyne, D., Pritchard, M., Rollings, S., Young, D., Myerson, N., & Ollendick, T. H. (1998). Cognitive-behavioral treatment of school-refusing children: A controlled evaluation. *Journal of the American Academy of Child and Adolescent Psychiatry, 37,* 395–403.

King, R. A., Leonard, H., & March, J. (1998). Summary of the practice parameters for the assessment and treatment of children and adolescents with obsessive–compulsive disorder. *Journal of the American Academy of Child and Adolescent Psychiatry, 37,* 1110–1116.

King, R. A., Murphy, G. C., & Heyne, D. (1997). The nature and treatment of social phobia in youth. *Counselling Psychology Quarterly, 10,* 377–387.

Koeppen, A. S. (1974). Relaxation training for children. *Elementary School Guidance and Counseling, 9,* 14–21.

Last, C. G., Hansen, C., & Franco, N. (1998). Cognitive-behavioral treatment of school phobia. *Journal of the American Academy of Child and Adolescent Psychiatry, 37,* 404–411.

March, J. S. (1995). Cognitive-behavioral psychotherapy for children and adolescents with OCD: A review and recommendations for treatment. *Journal of the American Academy of Child and Adolescent Psychiatry, 34*, 7–18.

March, J. S., Amaya-Jackson, L., Murray, M. C., & Schulte, A. (1998). Cognitive-behavioral psychotherapy for children and adolescents with posttraumatic stress disorder after a single-incident stressor. *Journal of the American Academy of Child and Adolescent Psychiatry, 37*, 585–593.

March, J. S., & Mulle, K. (1998). *OCD in children and adolescents: A cognitive-behavioral treatment manual.* New York: Guilford Press.

Meichenbaum, D. H., & Goodman, J. (1971). Training impulsive children to talk to themselves: A means of developing self-control. *Journal of Abnormal Psychology, 77*, 115–126.

Ollendick, T. H. (1995). Cognitive behavioral treatment of panic disorder with agoraphobia in adolescents: A multiple baseline design analysis. *Behavior Therapy, 26*, 517–531.

Ollendick, T. H., & Cerny, J. A. (1981). *Clinical behavior therapy with children.* New York: Plenum Press.

Ollendick, T. H., & King, N. J. (1998). Empirically supported treatments for children with phobic and anxiety disorders: Current status. *Journal of Clinical Child Psychology, 27*, 156–167.

Öst, L. G., Svensson, L., Hellström, K., & Lindwall, R. (2001). One-session treatment of specific phobias in youth: A randomized clinical trial. *Journal of Consulting and Clinical Psychology, 69*, 814–824.

Öst, L. G., Westling, B. E., & Hellström, K. (1993). Applied relaxation, exposure in vivo and cognitive methods in the treatment of panic disorder with agoraphobia. *Behaviour Research and Therapy, 31*, 383–394.

Piacentini, J. (1999). Cognitive behavioral therapy of childhood OCD. *Child and Adolescent Psychiatric Clinics of North America, 8*, 599–616.

Piacentini, J., & Bergman, R. L. (2001). Developmental issues in cognitive therapy for childhood anxiety disorders. *Journal of Cognitive Psychotherapy, 15*, 165–182.

Saigh, P. A. (1986). In vitro flooding in the treatment of a 6–year-old boy's posttraumatic stress disorder. *Behaviour Research and Therapy, 24*, 685–688.

Saigh, P. A. (1987a). In vitro flooding of an adolescent posttraumatic stress disorder. *Journal of Clinical Child Psychology, 16*, 147–150.

Saigh, P. A. (1987b). In vitro flooding of a childhood posttraumatic stress disorder. *School Psychology Review, 16*, 203–211.

Saigh, P. A. (1987c). In vitro flooding of childhood posttraumatic stress disorders: A systematic replication. *Professional School Psychology, 2*, 135–137.

Silverman, W. K., Kurtines, W. M., Ginsburg, G. S., Weems, C. F., Lumpkin, P. W., & Carmichael, D. H. (1999). Treating anxiety disorders in children with group cognitive-behavioral therapy: A randomized clinical trial. *Journal of Consulting and Clinical Psychology, 67*, 995–1003.

Silverman, W. K., Kurtines, W. M., Ginsburg, G. S., Weems, C. F., Rabian, B., & Serafini, L. T. (1999). Contingency management, self-control, and education support in the treatment of childhood phobic disorders: A randomized clinical trial. *Journal of Consulting and Clinical Psychology, 67*, 675–687.

Southam-Gerow, M. A., Kendall, P. C., & Weersing, V. R. (2001). Examining outcome variability: Correlates of treatment response in a child and adolescent anxiety clinic. *Journal of Clinical Child Psychology, 30,* 422–436.

Treadwell, K. R. H., Flannery-Schroeder, E. C., & Kendall, P. C. (1995). Ethnicity and gender in relation to adaptive functioning, diagnostic status, and treatment outcome in children from an anxiety clinic. *Journal of Anxiety Disorders, 9,* 373–384.

Wolpe, J. (1958). *Psychotherapy by reciprocal inhibition.* Stanford, CA: Stanford University Press.

Chapter 15

Pharmacotherapy

MURRAY B. STEIN
SORAYA SEEDAT

Anxiety disorders are the most commonly occurring class of psychiatric disorders in youths, with an estimated prevalence of 5–18% (Costello & Angold, 1995). Recent prospective longitudinal data suggest that, in addition to elevated rates of anxiety and depression in adulthood (Stein et al., 2001), adolescent anxiety is associated with a number of other adverse health outcomes and risky health behaviors, including alcohol and illicit drug dependence, suicidal behavior, educational underachievement (Woodward & Ferguson, 2001), and cigarette smoking (Sonntag, Wittchen, Hofler, Kessler, & Stein, 2000). These data call strongly for early intervention with the hope of preventing these adverse outcomes. Yet it must be acknowledged that the literature on treatment of anxiety disorders in youths is sparse, particularly with regard to controlled studies of pharmacological interventions.

The explanation for the relative dearth of rigorously designed pharmacotherapy trials in youngsters is complex. Despite better insights into the pathophysiology of childhood social phobia, separation anxiety disorder, generalized anxiety disorder, and posttraumatic stress disorder, biological research in the field has been impeded by a plethora of ethical considerations peculiar to this population, for example, developmental immaturity, risks posed by treatment, and problems associated with informed consent procedures. In the absence of definitive efficacy and effectiveness data to inform prescribing practices, clinicians are guided by practice experience and extrapolation of efficacy and safety data from adults. This situation has led to the routine "off-label" application of antianxiety (and other psychotropic [Zito et al., 2000]) drugs with U.S. Food and Drug Administration (FDA) indications in adults to disorders in children and adolescents (Labellarte, Ginsburg, Walkup, & Riddle, 1999). In one report, approximately 72% of pediatricians and family physicians surveyed reported prescribing a selective serotonin reuptake inhibitor (SSRI) for a child or adolescent (Rushton, Clark, & Freed, 2000). In an effort to encourage more direct testing of psychopharmacological agents in children and adolescents (for indications where the medications are already being used or will be used off-label in the future), the FDA has recently offered patent extensions to pharmaceutical companies that conduct additional studies in youths. Several such studies have either recently been completed or are underway at the time of this writing, making it likely that additional high-quality controlled data will soon become available.

INDICATIONS FOR PHARMACOTHERAPY

A general consensus exists among clinicians who treat anxious children that psychosocial interventions should be tried prior to starting medication (e.g., Heyne, King, Tonge, & Cooper, 2001). The rationale for this approach centers on the fact that nonpharmacological interventions are effective for many children, so why expose them needlessly to the potential risks of psychotropic medication? It is hard to argue with this basic premise. We fully agree with the approach to try psychosocial interventions as the first line of treatment for children with anxiety disorders. Ideally, the intervention should be an evidence-based form of psychotherapy, such as cognitive-behavioral therapy (CBT) directed at the primary disorder. In practice, however, given the dearth of clinicians with child CBT expertise, what many children receive falls short of this ideal. Nonetheless, it is reasonable to assume that many children, perhaps those whose anxiety symptoms are less severe (though this has not yet been demonstrated), will respond to nonspecific supportive or more behaviorally oriented interventions, usually administered in conjunction with parental advice and support. What, though, to do about the children who do not respond to this first line of treatment?

Our experience in this situation is that clinicians (and parents) are too slow to move to other treatment modalities when a child is not improving. They will often persist with a psychosocial intervention that is clearly not helping the child, with the well-intentioned hope that it will eventually work. Here, too, we all too often see frustrated counselors begin blaming parents for their child's failure to improve. Though strict guidelines about when to implement pharmacotherapy for anxious youths are lacking, our recommendation is that medication be given serious consideration long before "everything else" has been tried. The potential hazards of using psychotropic medication, particularly with regard to the presently unknown long-term risks, should not be downplayed. But neither should the potential perils of leaving serious anxiety untreated in a young person, perils that include possible deleterious effects on social, emotional, and academic development.

APPROACH TO PHARMACOTHERAPY

Although the treatment of anxiety disorders in youths needs to be multifaceted, pharmacotherapy should be especially considered when dealing with (1) serious and disabling anxiety symptoms and (2) older children and adolescents (Bernstein, Borchardt, & Perwien, 1996). Treatment selection will depend on the presence of comorbidity and the side effect and safety profile of the drug under consideration; however, general consensus is that medication should not be the only intervention but should be used as an adjunct to behavioral or other psychotherapeutic treatments (King & Bernstein, 2001).

When recommending a pharmacotherapeutic intervention, prescribing physicians must provide a rationale for the use of psychotropic medication for anxiety and must be prepared to discuss with the child and parent the various pros and cons of this treatment modality. A detailed discussion of possible side effects—providing information about which effects are common and which are not and which are serious (i.e., those that should prompt an immediate phone call to the physician) and which are unlikely to be serious (i.e., those that should abate in a day or two but that may call for a phone call to the physician if they persist or cause concern)—should help promote compliance. When parent and child opinions about taking medication do not mesh (e.g., parent agrees but child does not), the prescribing physician must be prepared to help the parents negotiate in a productive, nonpunitive fashion with the child. If the child (typically an adolescent) is not highly motivated to take medication for his or her anxiety problem, or if there are other schisms in the family's acceptance of the treatment, compliance will ultimately suffer (Hack & Chow, 2001).

In the case of phobic disorders (including separation anxiety disorder), the prescribing physician must provide (or arrange to have provided by a qualified mental health professional) explicit advice about behavioral interventions that should be employed by the parent. For example, a pediatrician who prescribes an SSRI for a child with "school phobia" should help the parents plan an approach to reintroducing the child to the classroom, including contingencies for how to handle refusals. In many cases, parents catch on quickly to the hierarchical exposure-based model and function effectively as promoters of their child's *in vivo* exposure. In some cases, however, the severity of the child's avoidance or the extent of family dysfunction or both require an intensity of intervention that is usually beyond the expertise of (or, at least, the limited time available to) most family physicians and pediatricians. When this situation arises, it is imperative that an experienced cognitive-behavioral therapist become involved. This aspect of care may be provided by the school psychologist or by another mental health professional. The role of the physician is to coordinate the combined pharmacological and psychological care of the child or adolescent.

PHARMACOKINETIC AND PHARMACODYNAMIC CONSIDERATIONS

As mentioned previously, despite the fact that children and adolescents are being increasingly exposed to psychotropic medications (Zito et al., 2000), little is known about unique pharmacokinetic and pharmacodynamic factors that may be unique to these age groups. Thus it is difficult—indeed, potentially dangerous—to extrapolate dosage determinations from adult studies (Dulcan, Bregman, Weller, & Weller, 1999). Several pharmacokinetic factors are sufficiently well elucidated, however, to make some general comments about dosing possible. On a per-kg body-weight basis, children tend to be more efficient metabolizers of drugs that are primarily metabolized by the liver, leading to the not infrequent need for relatively higher mg per kg doses compared with adults (Jatlow, 1987). This tends to change as children enter puberty, at which time more adult-like levels (on a mg per kg basis) are typically required, necessitating careful monitoring of drug response and adverse effects (and, if available and meaningful, plasma drug levels) during this period of development (Dulcan et al., 1999).

OBSESSIVE–COMPULSIVE DISORDER

Of all the childhood anxiety disorders, OCD is perhaps the one that has most evolved from a pharmacological standpoint. Although both SSRIs and CBT are effective and well-tolerated treatments, CBT should be considered as a first-line treatment for (1) all prepubertal children and (2) adolescents with OCD of mild to moderate severity. Adolescents with severe OCD should preferably be treated with a combination of serotonergic agent and CBT (American Academy of Child and Adolescent Psychiatry, 1998).

Clomipramine

Pharmacological challenge studies and empirical treatment studies with serotonergic agents have provided primary support for the hypothesis that abnormalities in serotonergic activity may, in part, be responsible for OCD (Piacenti & Bergman, 2000). Clomipramine, a tricyclic antidepressant (TCA) with serotonergic reuptake inhibition, has been the most extensively studied serotonergic antidepressant and was the first to gain an FDA indication for pediatric OCD. Double-blind, placebo-controlled, crossover, and parallel studies have found clomipramine to be significantly superior to both placebo (DeVeaugh-Geiss et al., 1992; Flament et al., 1985) and desipramine (Leonard et al., 1989). Flament and colleagues (1985) demonstrated a moderate to marked improvement in nearly 75% of children after 5 weeks of treatment with clomipramine at doses of 100–200 mg per day (approximately 3.0 mg per kg per day). In a 10-week double-blind crossover trial of clomipramine and desipramine, Leonard and colleagues (1989) reported clomipramine to be superior to desipramine, and, in longitudinal follow-up studies, further demonstrated that switching from clomipramine to desipramine after long-term maintenance treatment with clomipramine resulted in relapse in the majority (90%) of patients (Leonard et al., 1991).

Side effects of clomipramine in children and adolescents are typical of TCAs and similar to those reported in adults. They include dry mouth, somnolence, dizziness, headache, constipation, perspiration, and tremor. Clomipramine and other TCAs may also cause increases in heart rate and conduction abnormalities (prolongation of QRS and QTc interval; Leonard et al., 1995). Baseline and periodic electrocardiogram and drug serum level monitoring are recommended.

Dosages of clomipramine of up to 3 mg per kg per day for a minimum 3-month trial period should be considered. Dosages should preferably not exceed 5 mg per kg per day or 250 mg per day owing to the risks of toxicity (i.e. seizures and cardiovascular effects; Thomsen, 2000).

Selective Serotonin Reuptake Inhibitors

In adults, SSRIs have been shown to have powerful and broad-spectrum therapeutic effects in OCD. In children and adolescents with OCD, large multicenter trials of sertraline (March et al., 1998) and fluvoxamine (Riddle, 1998) have led to FDA indications, with fluvoxamine now indicated for use in children ages 8–17 years and sertraline indicated for use in children ages 6–17 years (Labellarte, Walkup, & Riddle, 1998). Fluoxetine has also been observed, in double-blind, acute treatment studies, to be more effective than placebo for OCD in pediatric populations (Geller et al., 2001; Riddle et al., 1992). Although controlled studies are lacking for the other two SSRIs currently available in the United States, citalopram and paroxetine, open studies suggest that they are also likely to show efficacy for treating OCD in youths (Rosenberg et al., 1999; Thomsen, 1997).

Other Pharmacological Agents

In the first reported case of venlafaxine use in a child with attention-deficit/ hyperactivity disorder (ADHD) and comorbid OCD and conduct disorder (Pleak & Gormly, 1995), significant improvements in attention, impulsivity, and obsessive–compulsive symptoms were noted after 6 weeks of venlafaxine treatment (maximum daily dose = 300 mg). In children and adolescents with autism spectrum disorder treated with open-label venlafaxine (maximum daily dose = 50 mg), Hollander, Kaplan, Cartwright, and Reichman (2000) also documented improvements in core autistic behaviors, ADHD, and obsessional symptoms. However, the efficacy and tolerability of venlafaxine in child and adolescent OCD has yet to be demonstrated under double-blind, placebo-controlled conditions.

Pharmacotherapy of OCD-Related Conditions

Several case reports suggest that the SSRIs, primarily fluoxetine, may be effective for other compulsive-like behaviors in children and adolescents, such as trichotillomania (Alexander, 1991; Sheikha, Wagner, & Wagner, 1993), self-injurious behavior (Bass & Beltis, 1991; King, 1991), perseverative and ritualistic behaviors in children with autism (Cook, Rowlett, Jaselskis, & Leventhal, 1992; Ghaziuddin, Tsai, & Ghaziuddin, 1991; McDougle, Price, & Goodman, 1990), and Prader–Willi syndrome (Dech & Budow, 1991). In children with Tourette's disorder and obsessive–compulsive symptoms, SSRIs have been useful in suppressing motor and vocal tics and reducing obsessions (Como & Kurlan, 1991; Kurlan, Como, Deeley, McDermott, & McDermott, 1993; Riddle, Hardin, King, Seahill, & Woolston, 1990).

OCD and PANDAS

The abrupt onset or exacerbation of OCD, tic disorders, or both may be triggered by an infection such as beta-hemolytic streptococcal infection in children or adolescents, resulting in a syndrome known as pediatric autoimmune neuropsychiatric disorders associated with streptococcal infection, or PANDAS (Allen, Leonard, & Swedo, 1995). These children are thought to mount a postinfectious autoimmune reaction to group A beta-hemolytic streptococci (Snider & Swedo, 2000). In children with PANDAS, plasma exchange and intravenous immunoglobulins appear to be more effective than placebo in reducing neuropsychiatric symptoms (Perlmutter et al., 1999), though these are still very much considered to be experimental interventions.

Dose and Duration of Pharmacotherapy for OCD

The favorable side effect profile and therapeutic index of the SSRIs make them a first choice for children and adolescents. With heightened concerns following the sudden deaths of several children who were treated with desipramine at therapeutic doses, TCAs, such as clomipramine, should be considered as second- or third-line options in childhood OCD (Daly & Wilens, 1998).

Although optimal dose–response relationships for the SSRIs have not been established in children and adolescents, a low starting dose (e.g., 10 mg of fluoxetine, citalopram, or paroxetine and 50 mg of sertraline) is recommended to improve tolerability and minimize dose-related side effects. Gradual titration up to 40–60 mg of fluoxetine, citalopram, or paroxetine and 100–200 mg of sertraline is suggested. Treatment should be continued at maximum therapeutic dose for at least 12 weeks before switching or combining treatments. It is worth keeping in mind that as many as 25% may not respond to an initial trial of an SSRI. Although data are limited, it is recommended that a trial of discontinuation only be considered in children who have remained symptom free for at least 1 year. To minimize the risk of relapse, it is further recommended that the dose of the SSRI be reduced by 25% every 2 months, coupled with CBT booster sessions (Piacenti & Bergman, 2000). Some children and adolescents may require longer term maintenance SSRI treatment, although there are indications that CBT may reduce the need for long-term medication treatment (March, 1995).

Long-Term Maintenance

Studies of the long-term effectiveness of SSRIs in children and adolescents with OCD have started to emerge. In a recently published 52-week, open-label extension study of sertraline (50–200 mg per day) in children (N = 72) and adolescents (N = 65) who had completed a 12-week, double-blind, placebo-controlled sertraline study, significant improvements were shown on all outcome measures at the end of treatment (Children's Yale–Brown Obsessive Compulsive Scale, Clinical Global Impression Scale, and National Institute of Mental Health–Global Obsessions and Compulsions Scale; Cook et al., 2001). Improvements were demonstrated regardless of whether participants had received sertraline or placebo in the preceding 12-week study. Adverse events reported at an incidence of ≥10% included headache, insomnia, nausea, diarrhea, somnolence, abdominal pain, hyperkinesia, nervousness, dyspepsia, and vomiting. Sixteen of 37 patients (43%) treated with sertraline in the acute study who were not classified as responders at the 12-week end point became responders with continued sertraline treatment.

Similarly, benefits relating to clinical effectiveness and tolerability have been observed with fluoxetine, citalopram, and clomipramine in children and adolescents followed up for 12 months or more (Thomsen, Ebbesen, & Persson, 2001; Thomsen & Mikkelsen, 1995). Although these studies lacked placebo and comparator arms and did not incorporate quality of life measures, they suggest long-term effectiveness of the SSRIs in pediatric OCD.

Medication versus Cognitive-Behavioral Therapy

Trials that compare SSRI efficacy with CBT are in progress. The only published study comparing a serotonergic agent (clomipramine, mean dose 2.5 mg per kg per day) with exposure-based CBT in children ages 8–18 years with OCD (N = 22) reported significant improvements in OCD symptoms with both treatments; however, CBT was significantly more effective than clomipramine on the Children's Yale–Brown Obsessive Compulsive Scale (CY-BOCS) scores (mean improvement 59.9% vs. 33.4%, respectively; de Haan, Hoogduin, Buitelaar, & Keijsers, 1998).

Augmentation Strategies

Augmentation or combination drug therapy should be considered for children and adolescents who: (1) respond only partially to SSRI treatment, (2) fail at least two trials of an SSRI plus a trial of CBT, or (3) have comorbid disorders not thought to be responsive to the single pharmacotherapeutic agent. Although augmentation strategies have not been systematically evaluated in children, there is some empirical evidence in adults that the addition of risperidone (McDougle et al., 1995; Stein, Bouwer, Hawkridge, & Emsley, 1997), olanzapine (Weiss, Potenza, McDougle, & Epperson, 1999), haloperidol (McDougle et al., 1994), or buspirone (Jenike, Baer, & Buttolph, 1991; Markowitz, Stagno, & Calabrese, 1990) to a serotonergic agent may be a useful strategy. In children and adolescents, case studies have reported benefits from the use of fluoxetine plus clomipramine (Simeon, Thatte, & Wiggins, 1990) and fluoxetine plus bupropion (Alessi & Bos, 1991). In addition, buspirone (5–60 mg per day) added to SSRI treatment has been observed to reduce obsessive–compulsive symptoms in 5 of 6 adolescents treated (Thomsen & Mikkelsen, 1999). Augmentation or combination strategies in children and adolescents should be undertaken judiciously and only after serious consideration of the probable risks and benefits.

GENERALIZED ANXIETY DISORDER

Children and adolescents with generalized anxiety disorder (GAD) have excessive, pervasive, and uncontrollable worries about a number of activities or events (e.g., school performance, family relationships, world events). These worries are associated with symptoms of muscle tension, irritability, fatigue, concentration difficulties, and sleep disturbance. The anxiety and worry persists for at least 6 months and interferes with the child's school, family, and social functioning (American Psychiatric Association, 1994). Formerly subsumed under the category "overanxious disorder" in DSM-III-R (American Psychiatric Association, 1987), GAD frequently co-occurs with other anxiety disorders (e.g., social phobia, panic disorder; Last, Hersen, Kazdin, Finkelstein, & Strauss, 1987; Last, Perrin, Hersen, & Kazdin, 1992). There is also a high rate of comorbidity between GAD and major depression in children and adolescents (Axelson & Birmaher, 2001; Masi, Mucci, Favilla, Romano, & Poli, 1999). Although these facts may argue the need for early intervention for GAD to possibly prevent later major depression, there have been few pharmacological studies in pediatric GAD.

Benzodiazepines

Earlier reports supported a role for high-potency benzodiazepines in GAD. Biederman (1987) reported success with open-label clonazepam (maximum dose = 3 mg per day) in one child with overanxious disorder and two children with separation anxiety disorder and comorbid panic symptoms. Four weeks of open-label alprazolam (maximum dose = 1.5 mg per day) was also effective in reducing anxiety and depressive symptoms in children and adolescents ages 8–16 years (N = 12) with overanxious and/or avoidant disorders (Simeon & Ferguson, 1987).

However, several recent double-blind, placebo-controlled studies have not confirmed efficacy. A 4-week trial of alprazolam (maximum dose = 3.5 mg per day) was not found to be superior to placebo in children and adolescents (N = 30, 8–16 years old) with overanxious or avoidant disorder (Simeon et al., 1992). Similarly, in a double-blind crossover trial of 4 weeks of clonazepam (maximum dose = 2 mg per day) and 4 weeks of placebo, clonazepam was not shown to be superior in 7- to 13-year-old children (N = 15) with primary diagnoses of separation anxiety disorder, six of whom had secondary diagnoses of overanxious disorder (Graae, Milner, Rizzotto, & Klein, 1994). Commonly reported adverse events for clonazepam and alprazolam included daytime drowsiness, fatigue, dry mouth, headaches, agitation, and nausea. Although these trials were of small sample size and brief duration, the use of these agents in youths remains controversial given the potential for abuse, behavioral disinhibition, and dependence. If used at all, short-term treatment (weeks rather than months) is recommended.

Buspirone

In open trials, buspirone, a 5-HT_{1A} receptor agonist, has been beneficial in children and adolescents with GAD, though placebo-controlled data are lacking. In an open-label study of adolescents with overanxious disorder or GAD, buspirone (maximum dose = 30 mg per day) significantly reduced anxiety after 6 weeks of treatment (Kutcher, Reiter, Gardner, & Klein, 1992). A case report of a 13-year-old with overanxious disorder also documented improvement with buspirone (10 mg per day); however, when the dose was increased to 15 mg per day, the boy experienced significant sedation (Kranzler, 1988). Simeon (1993) further reported significant improvements with buspirone (maximum dose = 30 mg per day) in nine children ages 6–14 years with overanxious disorder. Mild and transient side effects included sleep difficulties, nausea, headaches, and stomachaches.

Selective Serotonin Reuptake Inhibitors

There are a few open-label studies of fluoxetine treatment for overanxious disorder. A retrospective report of fluoxetine (mean dose 25.7 mg per day, range 10–60 mg per day) in 21 children and adolescents (ages 11–17) with overanxious disorder showed significant clinical improvements in anxiety in more than 80% of participants (Birmaher et al., 1994). However, many of these children had comorbid separation anxiety, social phobia, or both. Reported side effects, which were mild and short-lived, included nausea, headache, insomnia, stomachaches, and anorexia. Manassis and Bradley (1994) and Fairbanks and colleagues (1997) have also reported success with fluoxetine in mixed pediatric samples (with overanxious disorder plus a variety of other anxiety disorders).

Recently, the efficacy of fluvoxamine was demonstrated in a large ($N = 128$), randomized, placebo-controlled study of girls and boys ages 6–17 years with generalized anxiety disorder, social phobia, and separation anxiety disorder (Research Units of Pediatric Psychopharmacology Anxiety Study Group [RUPP], 2001). These children, nonresponsive to a prior 3-week course of brief psychotherapy, were randomly assigned to receive fluvoxamine (up to a maximum of 300 mg per day) or placebo for 8 weeks.

Children in the fluvoxamine group had significantly greater reductions in symptoms of anxiety and higher rates of clinical response than children in the placebo group. Fluvoxamine was generally well tolerated; adverse events included headache, abdominal discomfort, increased motor activity, drowsiness, and gastrointestinal disturbance.

A second double-blind, placebo-controlled study of an SSRI (sertraline) evaluated children and adolescents ($N = 22$, ages 5–17 years) with generalized anxiety disorder. Children and adolescents treated with sertraline (25 mg per day for the first week and 50 mg per day for weeks 2–9) showed significant improvements over placebo as measured on the Hamilton Anxiety Rating Scale and Clinical Global Severity and Clinical Global Improvement scores (Rynn, Siqueland, & Rickels, 2001). Ten of 11 patients (90%) at treatment end point were "improved" on sertraline compared with only 1 of 11 on placebo (10%). There appeared to be no depression-by-treatment interaction effect and no age effects. Despite significant treatment differences in favor of sertraline from week 4 to study's end, these results will need replication in a larger study group. Given the promising results with SSRIs in pediatric GAD, further controlled studies with these agents are indicated.

A third double-blind, placebo-controlled study of an SSRI (fluoxetine) was conducted in children and adolescents ($N = 74$) with generalized anxiety disorder, separation anxiety disorder, or social phobia (Birmaher et al., 2003). In this study, patients were randomized to receive either fluoxetine 20 mg per day ($N = 37$) or placebo ($N = 37$) for 12 weeks. Fluoxetine was effective in reducing the anxiety symptoms and improving functioning across all measures. Overall, 61% of patients taking fluoxetine and 35% taking a placebo were considered much to very much improved. The authors noted that although many patients improved, many had residual symptoms, pointing to the need for the development of even better treatment approaches for young people with anxiety disorders.

Other Pharmacotherapeutic Agents

No efficacy data exist for TCAs in children and adolescents with GAD. The beta-blocker propranolol has also not been studied as a therapy, but cardiovascular side effects, such as bradycardia and hypotension, limit its use in children (Wagner, 2001). Although earlier studies of antihistamines supported their use in children, subsequent controlled studies in children with mixed psychiatric diagnoses, including "neurotic disorder," were not able to differentiate the anxiolytic effects of antihistamines from the sedative effects (Korein, Fish, Shapiro, Gerner, & Levidow, 1971). Furthermore, the sedative properties of antihistamines do not favor their long-term use in GAD. Venlafaxine and venlafaxine extended release (XR) are currently

FDA-approved for use in adult GAD (Kapczinski, Lima, Souza, & Schmitt, 2003). However, there are no published studies of venlafaxine use for this indication in children and adolescents.

In summary, although preliminary data seem to indicate the usefulness of SSRIs and, to a lesser degree, high-potency benzodiazepines and buspirone in childhood GAD, further studies of SSRIs in this population are needed to establish optimal dose and treatment duration, relapse rates upon discontinuation, and the relative efficacy of SSRIs compared with CBT-based treatments.

SEPARATION ANXIETY DISORDER (AND SCHOOL PHOBIA)

Several published pharmacotherapy trials have apparently included children with separation anxiety disorder, though it is rarely possible from these reports to isolate the effects of treatment on this particular diagnostic group. It should be especially noted that studies of children with "school phobia" almost certainly include an admixture of children whose anxiety-based school refusal is due to separation anxiety disorder or social phobia. Although we have elected to include those studies within this section on separation anxiety disorder, readers should be cognizant of this potential confound. As in all cases of pediatric anxiety disorder, pharmacotherapy for separation anxiety disorder should be administered only in the context of psychoeducation and advice about behavioral management to parents (Heyne et al., 2001).

Tricyclic Antidepressants

Although an early, classic placebo-controlled study of the TCA imipramine for school phobia suggested that it was efficacious (Gittleman-Klein & Klein, 1971), a subsequent study of separation anxiety disorder failed to demonstrate efficacy (Klein, Kopelwicz, & Kanner, 1992). Reasons for this discrepancy are unclear, but they may relate to patient heterogeneity within the "school refusal" rubric.

Bernstein and colleagues (2000) compared 8 weeks of treatment with imipramine versus placebo, *each in conjunction with CBT*, for school-refusing adolescents with comorbid anxiety and major depressive disorders. In this randomized controlled trial, 63 participants entered and 47 completed the study. Outcomes included weekly school attendance rates based on percentage of hours attended. The investigators found that imipramine plus CBT was significantly superior to placebo plus CBT. This study provides the best evidence to date of the utility of imipramine (in conjunction with CBT) for the treatment of school phobia.

Selective Serotonin Reuptake Inhibitors

Several open-label studies with fluoxetine, which had included children with various and "mixed" anxiety disorders (presumably at least some of which included separation anxiety disorder), had hinted at their efficacy for separation anxiety disorder (Birmaher et al., 1994; Fairbanks et al., 1997). The double-blind study by Birmaher and colleagues (2003), referred to earlier in this chapter, included children with separation anxiety disorder and they responded to fluoxetine 20 mg per day. The study conducted by the Research Unit on Pediatric Psychopharmacology (RUPP, 2001), referred to earlier in this chapter, also included children with separation anxiety disorder. This study found that the SSRI fluvoxamine, at doses ranging up to 300 mg per day, was highly effective for pediatric separation anxiety disorder, GAD, and social phobia. Based on these studies, it is reasonable to suggest that doses of SSRIs for separation anxiety disorder be in the range of those used to treat GAD or social phobia (see the next section). Although imipramine apparently continues to be prescribed for treatment of separation anxiety disorder and school phobia, the utility and better margin of safety of SSRIs should render the TCAs nearly obsolete for this indication.

SOCIAL PHOBIA (SOCIAL ANXIETY DISORDER)

As mentioned, it is likely that some of the children included in "school phobia" studies had social phobia as their primary diagnosis. At the time of this writing, we are aware of two published placebo-controlled studies of pediatric social phobia, those being the study by the RUPP group (2001) and Birmaher and colleagues (2003) that included children with separation anxiety disorder, GAD, and/or social anxiety disorder. (These three disorders, it should be noted, are commonly comorbid, making it difficult—and possibly nonrepresentative of the kinds of children encountered in clinical practice—to conduct studies of these disorders in isolation.)

Several open-label studies have demonstrated the efficacy of SSRIs for youths with social phobia. Mancini and colleagues had good success in treating seven children ages 7–18 with social phobia with a variety of SSRIs (Mancini, Van Ameringen, Oakman, & Farvolden, 1999). Compton and colleagues (2001) conducted an open-label study of 14 children and adolescents with sertraline and found that 36% were responders and 29% partial responders after 8 weeks of treatment. Our research group also obtained very promising results from a study combining open-label citalopram with brief psychoeducation for children and adolescents with clinically predominant diagnoses of social phobia (Chavira & Stein, 2002). At the time of this writing, several multicenter randomized clinical trials for child and/or adolescent social phobia are nearing publication. The results of these studies will provide more definitive information about the usefulness of SSRIs (and other antidepressants, which are also being studied) for youths with social phobia. But based on the RUPP (2001) and Birmaher and colleagues (2003) studies, it is to be expected that SSRIs will be highly efficacious for child and adolescent social phobia.

SELECTIVE MUTISM

Most investigators now agree that selective mutism (defined as the inability to speak in the presence of peers, despite normal language skills) is a severe form of social phobia that manifests in childhood (Astendig, 1999; Stein, Chavira, & Jang, 2001), though this is still somewhat controversial (Yeganeh, Beidel, Turner, Pina, & Silverman, 2003). Interestingly, the psychopharmacological treatment literature for selective mutism predates that of social phobia. In fact, Black and Uhde (1994) demonstrated the utility of fluoxetine for selective mutism in a double-blind, placebo-controlled study. More recently, Carlson, Kratochwill, and Johnston (2000) described the utility of sertraline in an open-label case series of 5 children with selective mutism. It is to be expected that, as the literature on the treatment of social phobia in children evolves, this information will be readily applicable to selective mutism.

POSTTRAUMATIC STRESS DISORDER

There are no published placebo-controlled trials of pharmacological agents in children with PTSD. Yet it is clear that medications such as SSRIs are being prescribed for this purpose (Donnelly, 2003). In a recently published survey of current practices of psychiatrists and nonmedical therapists in the treatment of traumatized children and adolescents with PTSD, cognitive-behavioral therapy (CBT) was endorsed as the most preferred first-line treatment among nonmedical therapists and the second most preferred among psychiatrists (Cohen, Mannarino, & Rogal, 2001). Although only 17% of psychiatrists said they preferred psychotropic medications, the majority (95%) prescribed medications for the disorder. Both groups rated SSRIs as the most effective medications for treating overall PTSD symptoms.

Psychotherapy has long been the mainstay of treatment for acute stress reactions and PTSD (Pfefferbaum, 1997). Despite there being compelling evidence that a number of key psychobiological systems are dysregulated in PTSD, very few studies have addressed the benefits of pharmacological treatments in children and adolescents with the disorder (Donnelly, Amaya-Jackson, & March, 1999; March, Amaya-Jackson, & Pynoos, 1996).

Alpha-Adrenergic Agonists

Prior to its investigation as a potential treatment for PTSD, De Bellis, Lefter, Trickett, and Putnam (1994) and Marmar, Foy, Kagan, and Pynoos (1994) suggested that clonidine might be useful in the treatment of sexually abused children diagnosed with ADHD and comorbid PTSD. Harmon and Riggs (1996) subsequently conducted an uncontrolled trial of clonidine in seven preschool children ages 3–6 years with DSM-IV diagnoses of PTSD. The children had not responded to previous individual, family, milieu, or behavioral treatment. Some had concurrent depressive symptoms, attentional problems, and reactive attachment disorders. Oral clonidine was administered to 6 of the 7 children but then replaced by patches (dose of 0.1–0.2 mg per day) to minimize the sedation resulting from the oral formulation. Clonidine was documented to be effective in reducing hyperarousal, insomnia, and aggressive behavior in these children. The patches also appeared to be better tolerated than the oral formulation; however, the authors reiterated the need for close medical monitoring in view of the potential risks of hypotension and tolerance to the therapeutic effects of clonidine with long-term use (Harmon & Riggs, 1996). Guanfacine, another alpha$_2$-agonist that has a longer half-life than clonidine, was reported in a single case study to be beneficial in treating nightmares in a 7-year-old child with PTSD (Horrigan & Barnhill, 1996).

Beta-Blockers

In an open-label study of propranolol (dose of 2.5 mg per kg) in 11 sexually and/or physically abused children, Famularo, Kinscheiff, and Fenton (1988) demonstrated a significant decrease in PTSD symptoms after a 5-week course of treatment, particularly in symptoms of hypervigilance and hyperarousal.

Selective Serotonin Reuptake Inhibitors

There are no controlled studies of SSRIs in child and adolescent PTSD. In a small trial ($N = 8$) of 12 weeks of citalopram treatment in adolescents with moderate to severe PTSD, all seven completers were rated as much improved or very much improved on the Clinical Global Impression (CGI) Scale (Seedat, Lockhat, Kaminer, Zungu-Dirwayu, & Stein, 2001). Core PTSD symptoms (reexperiencing, avoidance, hyperarousal) showed statistically significant improvement at week 12 on the Clinician-Administered PTSD Scale—Child and Adolescent Version (CAPS-CA). Self-reported symptoms of depression failed to improve significantly at end point. Citalopram was well tolerated overall.

Tricyclic Antidepressants and Monoamine Oxidase Inhibitors

No controlled studies of either TCAs or MAOIs in childhood PTSD have been published. In a prospective, double-blind pilot study comparing 7 days of imipramine with chloral hydrate for treatment of acute stress disorder (ASD) in 25 children (ages 2–19 years) who had sustained serious burns, imipramine (1 mg per kg per day, maximum dose =100 mg) was significantly more effective than chloral hydrate (25 mg per kg per day, maximum dose = 500 mg; Robert, Blakeney, Villareal, Rosenberg, & Meyer, 1999).

Anticonvulsants

Loof, Grimley, Kuiler, Martin, and Shunfield (1995) studied the effects of carbamazepine in 28 children with PTSD (dose of 300–1,200 mg per day, serum levels 10.0–11.5 µg per ml). Carbamazepine treatment resulted in remission of symptoms in 22 children, but 6 children continued to experience nightmares related to ongoing abuse experiences despite significant improvements in other PTSD symptoms. Findings of this study should be interpreted cautiously, as several children had comorbid disorders, such as depression, ADHD, polysubstance abuse, or oppositional defiant disorder. Furthermore, many children were on other concomitant treatments, for example, imipramine, fluoxetine, sertraline, clonidine, or methylphenidate.

Other Pharmacotherapeutic Agents

Nefazodone, a 5-HT$_2$ antagonist, was noted to be beneficial in adolescents with PTSD, particularly for addressing symptoms of anger, aggression, restlessness, insomnia, and even concentration (Domon & Andersen, 2000).

Cyproheptadine, an antihistaminic 5-HT antagonist, has been hypothesized to be particularly useful with sleep onset problems and nightmares in children with PTSD, in lights of its sedative properties (Donnelly et al., 1999), but this has yet to be shown.

Morphine has been documented in a recent study of children with burns as a possible preventive agent in PTSD (Saxe et al., 2001). The authors found that the dose of oral morphine (mean equivalency dose = 0.80 mg per kg per day, range 0.01–4.50 mg per kg per day) administered to 24 children, ages 6–16 years, during hospital admission for burn injuries resulted in a significant reduction in PTSD symptoms at 6 months follow-up. Opiates are known to inhibit the noradrenergic system in areas of the brain thought to be responsible for the consolidation of traumatic memory in PTSD, and this was the rationale for using it for prevention. These intriguing results, based on naturalistic observation, await replication under randomized, controlled conditions.

Benzodiazepines are widely used in the treatment of adults with PTSD, though an evidence base for their use in PTSD is, at present, lacking (Braun, Greenberg, Dasberg, & Lerer, 1990; Lowenstein, Hornstein, & Farber, 1988). In children and adolescents, the adverse effects of benzodiazepines make them less than an ideal choice, particularly for chronic use. Their use in children and adolescents on a short-term basis is also not established.

Antipsychotic use in PTSD is not well documented. The first open trial of *risperidone* (average dose = 1.3 mg per day for 16 weeks) conducted in adolescent boys with severe PTSD (N = 18) demonstrated significant improvements in 50% of the sample. However, comorbidity in the sample was high, with 83% meeting criteria for ADHD, 56% for oppositional defiant disorder, 33% for bipolar disorder, 22% for conduct disorder, and 11% for major depression. Only 11% met criteria for psychosis (Horrigan, 1998). Concern about the possible development of tardive dyskinesia (Feeney & Klykylo, 1996), although mitigated in the case of the atypical antipsychotic agents, nonetheless tempers their use for nonpsychotic conditions, particularly in children and adolescents.

Dose and Duration of Treatment

Despite the lack of controlled studies of childhood PTSD, these agents, given their increasingly widespread use and acceptance in adult PTSD, are recommended as a first choice in pharmacological treatment of pediatric PTSD. The starting dose of SSRI should be low, with the dose slowly titrated up into the range used to treat OCD. In children and adolescents, it is recommended that an adequate trial of an SSRI be at least 12 weeks long. After a therapeutic response is observed, treatment should be continued for at least 12 months.

In summary, pharmacological agents are indicated in pediatric PTSD when the disorder is severe or when concurrent symptoms of depression, panic, ADHD, and conduct disorder are present. Although SSRIs are preferred agents in the treatment of pediatric PTSD because of their broad spectrum of effects and favorable side effect profile, the type of comorbidity present should guide the choice of agent. For example, an SSRI may be useful for comorbid depression, whereas psychostimulants or clonidine may be useful for concurrent ADHD symptoms. Much additional research is needed in this area.

OTHER ANXIETY DISORDERS

There is a dearth of literature on the psychopharmacological treatment of panic disorder in children and adolescents; we are aware of only one open-label pilot study in which SSRIs were tried (Renaud, Birmaher, Wassick, & Bridge, 1999). But findings from studies of separation anxiety disorder may be applicable.

The treatment of specific phobias in youth has been similarly ignored, presumably because the mainstay of treatment—in children as well as adults—is exposure therapy, not pharmacotherapy. One area in which we want to mention a potentially efficacious pharmacotherapeutic intervention, however, is for needle phobias. These may be sufficiently severe that the administration of routine vaccines or phlebotomy becomes a highly traumatic experience for the child, parent, and pediatrician alike. Whereas exposure therapy is the ultimate goal, we have found that the use of topical anesthetic cream (see Chen & Cunningham, 2001, for review), in combination with empathic reassurance, can be a remarkably effective interim intervention for needle phobias.

SUMMARY

The psychopharmacological treatment of pediatric anxiety disorders is, pardon the pun, in its infancy. The OCD literature is relatively well developed, with many studies demonstrating the efficacy of clomipramine and SSRIs and several highlighting the importance of conjoint cognitive-behavioral treatment. For most of the other anxiety disorders in youths, there are either few or no randomized controlled trials, though several are in progress thanks in large part to new mandates issued by pharmaceutical regulatory agencies. It is hoped that these studies, once completed, will significantly strengthen the evidence base for these treatments. The next step will then be to determine under what circumstances medication treatments can augment the powerful effects of cognitive and behaviorally oriented interventions and how these can be best provided to children and adolescents in real-world (i.e., outside of academic research) settings.

REFERENCES

Alessi, N., & Bos, T. (1991). Buspirone augmentation of fluoxetine in a depressed child with obsessive–compulsive disorder (Letter). *American Journal of Psychiatry, 148*, 1605–1606.

Alexander, R. C. (1991). Fluoxetine treatment of trichotillomania (Letter). *Journal of Clinical Psychiatry, 52*, 88.

Allen, A. J., Leonard, H. L., & Swedo, S. E. (1995). Case study: A new infection triggered, autoimmune subtype of pediatric OCD and Tourette syndrome. *Journal of the American Academy of Child and Adolescent Psychiatry, 34*, 307–311.

American Academy of Child and Adolescent Psychiatry. (1998). Practice parameters for the assessment and treatment of children and adolescents with obsessive–compulsive disorder. *Journal of the American Academy of Child and Adolescent Psychiatry, 37*, 1110–1116.

American Psychiatric Association. (1987). *Diagnostic and statistical manual of mental disorders* (3rd ed., rev.). Washington, DC: Author.

American Psychiatric Association. (1994). *Diagnostic and statistical manual of mental disorders* (4th ed.). Washington, DC: Author.

Astendig, K. D. (1999). Is selective mutism an anxiety disorder? Rethinking its DSM-IV classification. *Journal of Anxiety Disorders, 13*, 417–434.

Axelson, D. A., & Birmaher, B. (2001). Relation between anxiety and depressive disorders in childhood and adolescence. *Depression and Anxiety, 14*, 67–78.

Bass, J. N., & Beltis, J. (1991). Therapeutic effect of fluoxetine on naltrexone-resistant self-injurious behavior in an adolescent with mental retardation. *Journal of Child and Adolescent Psychopharmacology, 1*, 331–340.

Bernstein, G. A., Borchardt, C. M., & Perwien, A. R. (1996). Anxiety disorders in children and adolescents: A review of the past 10 years. *Journal of the American Academy of Child and Adolescent Psychiatry, 35*(9), 1110–1119.

Bernstein, G. A., Borchardt, C. M., Perwien, A. R., Crosby, R. D., Kushner, M. G., Thuras, P. D., & Last, C. G. (2000). Imipramine plus cognitive-behavioral therapy in the treatment of school refusal. *Journal of the American Academy of Child and Adolescent Psychiatry, 39*, 276–283.

Biederman, J. (1987). Clonazepam in the treatment of prepubertal children with panic-like symptoms. *Journal of Clinical Psychiatry, 48*(Suppl.), 38–42.

Birmaher, B., Axelson, D. A., Monk, K., Kalas, C., Clark, D. B., Ehmann, M., Bridge, J., Heo, J., & Brent, D. A. (2003). Fluoxetine for the treatment of childhood anxiety disorders. *Journal of the American Academy of Child and Adolescent Psychiatry, 42*, 415–423.

Birmaher, B., Waterman, G. S., Ryan, N., Cully, M., Balach, L., Ingram, J., & Brodsky, M. (1994). Fluoxetine for childhood anxiety disorders. *Journal of the American Academy of Child and Adolescent Psychiatry, 33*, 993–999.

Black, B., & Uhde, T. W. (1994). Treatment of elective mutism with fluoxetine: A double-blind, placebo controlled study. *Journal of the American Academy of Child and Adolescent Psychiatry, 33*, 1000–1006.

Braun, P., Greenberg, D., Dasberg, H., & Lerer, B. (1990). Core symptoms of posttraumatic stress disorder unimproved by alprazolam treatment. *Journal of Clinical Psychiatry, 51,* 236–238.

Carlson, J. S., Kratochwill, T. R., & Johnston, H. F. (2000). Sertraline treatment of 5 children diagnosed with selective mutism: A single-case research trial. *Journal of Child and Adolescent Psychopharmacology, 9,* 293–306.

Chavira, D. A., & Stein, M. B. (2002). Combined psychoeducation and treatment with selective serotonin reuptake inhibitors for youth with generalized social anxiety disorder. *Journal of Adolescent and Child Psychopharmacology, 12,* 47–54.

Chen, B. K., & Cunningham, B. B. (2001). Topical anesthetics in children: Agents and techniques that equally comfort patients, parents, and clinicians. *Current Opinion in Pediatrics, 13,* 324–330.

Cohen, J. A., Mannarino, A. P., & Rogal, S. (2001). Treatment practices for childhood posttraumatic stress disorder. *Child Abuse and Neglect, 25,* 123–135.

Como, P. G., & Kurlan, R. (1991). An open-label trial of fluoxetine for obsessive–compulsive disorder in Gilles de la Tourette's syndrome. *Neurology, 41,* 872–874.

Compton, S. N., Grant, P. J., Chrisman, A. K., Gammon, P. J., Brown, V. L., & March, J. S. (2001). Sertraline in children and adolescents with social anxiety disorder: An open trial. *Journal of the American Academy of Child and Adolescent Psychiatry, 40,* 564–571.

Cook, E. H., Jr., Rowlett, R., Jaselskis, C., & Leventhal, B. L. (1992). Fluoxetine treatment of children and adults with autistic disorder and mental retardation. *Journal of the American Academy of Child and Adolescent Psychiatry, 31,* 739–745.

Cook, E. H., Wagner, K. D., March, J. S., Biederman, J., Landau, P., Wolkow, R., & Messig, M. (2001). Long-term treatment of children and adolescents with obsessive–compulsive disorder. *Journal of the American Academy of Child and Adolescent Psychiatry, 40,* 1175–1181.

Costello, E. J., & Angold, A. (1985). Epidemiology. In J. S. March (Ed.), *Anxiety disorders in children and adolescents* (pp. 109–124). New York: Guilford Press.

Daly, J. M., & Wilens, T. M. (1998). The use of tricyclic antidepressants in children and adolescents. *Pediatric Clinics of North America, 45*(5), 1123–1135.

De Bellis, M. D., Lefter, L., Trickett, P. K., & Putnam, F. W., Jr. (1994). Urinary catecholamine excretion in sexually abused girls. *Journal of the American Academy of Child and Adolescent Psychiatry, 33*(3), 320–327.

Dech, B., & Budow, L. (1991). The use of fluoxetine in an adolescent with Prader–Willi syndrome. *Journal of the American Academy of Child and Adolescent Psychiatry, 30,* 298–302.

de Haan, E. D., Hoogduin, K. A., Buitelaar, J. K., & Keijsers, G. P. (1998). Behavior therapy versus clomipramine for the treatment of obsessive–compulsive disorder in children and adolescents. *Journal of the American Academy of Child and Adolescent Psychiatry, 37,* 1022–1029.

DeVeaugh-Geiss, J., Moroz, G., Biederman, J., Cantwell, D., Fontaine, R., Greist, J. H., Reichler, R., Katz, R., & Landau, P. (1992). Clomipramine hydrochloride in childhood and adolescent obsessive–compulsive disorder: A multicenter trial. *Journal of the American Academy of Child and Adolescent Psychiatry, 31,* 45–49.

Domon, S. E., & Andersen, M. S. (2000). Nefazodone for PTSD. *Journal of the American Academy of Child and Adolescent Psychiatry, 39* (8), 942–943.

Donnelly, C. (2003). Pharmacologic treatment approaches for children and adolescents with posttraumatic stress disorder. *Child and Adolescent Psychiatric Clinics of North America, 12,* 251–269.

Donnelly, C. L., Amaya-Jackson, L., & March, J. S. (1999). Psychopharmacology of pediatric posttraumatic stress disorder. *Journal of Child and Adolescent Psychopharmacology, 9*(3), 203–220.

Dulcan, M. K., Bregman, J., Weller, E. B., & Weller, R. (1999). Treatment of childhood and adolescent disorders. In H. I. Kaplan & B. J. Sadock (Eds.), *Comprehensive textbook of psychiatry* (pp. 803–850). Baltimore: Williams & Wilkins.

Fairbanks, J. M., Pine, D. S., Tancer, N. K., Dummitt, E. S., Kentgen, L. M., Martin, J., Asche, B. K., & Klein, R. G. (1997). Open fluoxetine treatment of mixed anxiety disorders in children and adolescents. *Journal of Child and Adolescent Psychopharmacology, 7,* 17–29.

Famularo, R., Kinscheiff, R., & Fenton, T. (1988). Propranolol treatment for childhood posttraumatic stress disorder, acute type: A pilot study. *American Journal of Diseases of Children, 142,* 1244–1247.

Feeney, D. J., & Klykylo, W. (1996). Risperidone and tardive dyskinesia (Letter). *Journal of the American Academy of Child and Adolescent Psychiatry, 36*(7), 867.

Flament, M. F., Rapaport, J. L., Berg, C. J., Sceery, W., Kilts, C., Mellstrom, B., & Linnoila, M. (1985). Clomipramine treatment of childhood obsessive–compulsive disorder: A double-blind controlled study. *Archives of General Psychiatry, 42*(10), 977–983.

Geller, D. A., Hoog, S. L., Heiligenstein, J. H., Ricardi, R. K., Tamura, R., Kluszynski, S., Jacobson, J. G., & Fluoxetine Pediatric OCD Study Team. (2001). Fluoxetine treatment for obsessive–compulsive disorder in children and adolescents: A placebo-controlled clinical trial. *Journal of the American Academy of Child and Adolescent Psychiatry, 40*(7), 773–779.

Ghaziuddin, N., Tsai, L., & Ghaziuddin, N. (1991). Fluoxetine in autism with depression. *Journal of the American Academy of Child and Adolescent Psychiatry, 30,* 508–509.

Good, C., & Petersen, C. (2001). SSRI and mirtazapine in PTSD. *Journal of the American Academy of Child and Adolescent Psychiatry, 40,* 263–264.

Gittleman-Klein, R., & Klein, D. F. (1971). Controlled imipramine treatment of school phobia. *Archives of General Psychiatry, 25,* 204–207.

Graae, F., Milner, J., Rizzotto, L., & Klein, R. G. (1994). Clonazepam in childhood anxiety disorders. *Journal of the American Academy of Child and Adolescent Psychiatry, 33*(3), 372–376.

Hack, S., & Chow, B. (2001). Pediatric psychotropic medication compliance: A literature review and research-based suggestions for improving treatment compliance. *Journal of Child and Adolescent Psychopharmacology, 11,* 59–67.

Harmon, R. J., & Riggs, P. D. (1996). Clonidine for posttraumatic stress disorder in preschool children. *Journal of the American Academy of Child and Adolescent Psychiatry, 35,* 1247–1249.

Heyne, D., King, N. J., Tonge, B. J., & Cooper, H. (2001). School refusal: Epidemiology and management. *Paediatric Drugs, 3,* 719–732.

Hollander, E., Kaplan, A., Cartwright, C., & Reichman, D. (2000). Venlafaxine in children, adolescents and young adults with autism spectrum disorders: An open retrospective clinical report. *Journal of Child Neurology, 15,* 132–135.

Horrigan, J. P. (1998). *Risperidone appears effective for children, adolescents with severe PTSD.* Paper presented at the annual meeting of the American Academy of Child and Adolescent Psychiatry, Anaheim, CA.

Horrigan, J. P., & Barnhill, L. J. (1996). The suppression of nightmares with guanfacine. *Journal of Clinical Psychiatry, 57,* 371.

Jatlow, P. I. (1987). Psychotropic drug disposition during development. In C. Popper (Ed.), *Psychiatric pharmacosciences of children and adolescents* (pp. 27–44). Washington, DC: American Psychiatric Press.

Jenike, M. A., Baer, L., & Buttolph, L. (1991). Buspirone augmentation of fluoxetine in patients with obsessive compulsive disorder. *Journal of Clinical Psychiatry, 52,* 13–14.

Kapczinski, F., Lima, M. S., Souza, J. S., & Schmitt, R. (2003). Antidepressants for generalized anxiety disorder. *Cochrane Database System Review,* CD003592.

King, B. H. (1991). Fluoxetine-induced self-injurious behavior in an adolescent with mental retardation. *Journal of Child and Adolescent Psychopharmacology, 1,* 321–329.

King, N. J., & Bernstein, G. A. (2001). School refusal in children and adolescents: A review of the past 10 years. *Journal of the American Academy of Child and Adolescent Psychiatry, 40,* 197–205.

Klein, R. G., Kopelwicz, H. S., & Kanner, A. (1992). Imipramine treatment in children with separation anxiety disorder. *Journal of the American Academy of Child and Adolescent Psychiatry, 31,* 21–28.

Korein, J., Fish, B., Shapiro, T., Gerner, E. W., & Levidow, T. (1971). EEG and behavioral effects of drug therapy in children: Chlorpromazine and diphenhydramine. *Archives of General Psychiatry, 24,* 552–563.

Kranzler, H. (1988). Use of buspirone in an adolescent with overanxious disorder. *Journal of the American Academy of Child and Adolescent Psychiatry, 27,* 789–790.

Kurlan, R., Como, P. G., Deeley, C., McDermott, M., & McDermott, M. P. (1993). A pilot controlled study of fluoxetine for obsessive–compulsive symptoms in children with Tourette's syndrome. *Clinical Neuropharmacology, 16,* 167–172.

Kutcher, S. P., Reiter, S., Gardner, D. M., & Klein, R. G. (1992). The pharmacotherapy of anxiety disorders in children and adolescents. *Psychiatric Clinics of North America, 15,* 41–67.

Labellarte, M. J., Ginsburg, G. S., Walkup, J. T., & Riddle, M. A. (1999). The treatment of anxiety disorders in children and adolescents. *Biological Psychiatry, 46,* 1567–1578.

Labellarte, M. J., Walkup, J. T., & Riddle, M. A. (1998). The new antidepressants: Selective serotonin reuptake inhibitors. *Pediatric Clinics of North America, 45*(5), 1137–1155.

Last, C. G., Hersen, M. L., Kazdin, A. E., Finkelstein, R., & Strauss, C. C. (1987). Comparison of DSM-II separation anxiety and overanxious disorders: Demographic characteristics and patterns of comorbidity. *Journal of the American Academy of Child and Adolescent Psychiatry, 26,* 527–531.

Last, C. G., Perrin, S., Hersen, M., & Kazdin, A. E. (1992). DSM-III-R anxiety disorders in children: Sociodemographic and clinical characteristics. *Journal of the American Academy of Child and Adolescent Psychiatry, 31,* 1070–1076.

Leonard, H. L., Meyer, M. C., Swedo, S. E., Richter, D., Hamburger, S. D., Allen, A. J., Rapoport, J. L., & Tucker, E. (1995). Electrocardiographic changes during desipramine and clomipramine treatment in children and adolescents. *Journal of the American Academy of Child and Adolescent Psychiatry, 34,* 1460–1468.

Leonard, H. L., Swedo, S. E., Lenane, M. C., Rettew, D. C., Cheslow, D. L., Hamburger, S. D., & Rapoport, J. L. (1991). A double-blind desipramine substitution during long-term clomipramine treatment in children and adolescents with obsessive–compulsive disorders. *Archives of General Psychiatry, 48,* 922–927.

Leonard, H. L., Swedo, S. E., Rapoport, J. L., Koby, E. V., Lenane, M. C., Cheslow, D. L., & Hamburger, S. D. (1989). Treatment of childhood obsessive–compulsive disorder with clomipramine and desipramine in children and adolescents: A double-blind crossover comparison. *Archives of General Psychiatry, 46,* 1088–1092.

Looff, D., Grimley, P., Kuiler, F., Martin, A., & Shunfield, L. (1995). Carbamazepine for posttraumatic stress disorder [Letter]. *Journal of the American Academy of Child and Adolescent Psychiatry, 34,* 703–704.

Lowenstein, R. J., Hornstein, N., & Farber, B. (1988). Open trial of clonazepam in the treatment of post-traumatic stress symptoms in multiple personality disorder. *Dissociation, 1,* 3–12.

Manassis, K., & Bradley, S. (1994). Fluoxetine in anxiety disorders [Letter]. *Journal of the American Academy of Child and Adolescent Psychiatry, 33,* 761.

Mancini, C., Van Ameringen, M., Oakman, J. M., & Farvolden, P. (1999). Serotonergic agents in the treatment of social phobia in children and adolescents: A case series. *Depression and Anxiety, 10,* 33–39.

March, J. S. (1995). Cognitive-behavioral psychotherapy for children and adolescents with OCD: A review and recommendations for treatment. *Journal of the American Academy of Child and Adolescent Psychiatry, 34,* 7–18.

March, J. S., Amaya-Jackson, L., & Pynoos, R. S. (1996). Pediatric posttraumatic stress disorder. In J. M. Weiner (Ed.), *Textbook of child and adolescent psychiatry* (2nd ed.). Washington, DC: American Psychiatric Press.

March, J. S, Biederman, J., Wolkow, R., Safferman, A., Mardekian, J., Cook, E. H., Cutler, N. R., Dominguez, R., Ferguson, J., Muller, B., Riesenberg, R., Rosenthal, M., Sallee, F. R., Wagner, K. D., & Steiner, H. (1998). Sertraline in children and adolescents with obsessive–compulsive disorder: A multicenter randomized controlled trial. *Journal of the American Medical Association, 280*(20), 1752–1756.

Markowitz, P. J., Stagno, S. L., & Calabrese, J. R. (1990). Buspirone augmentation of fluoxetine in obsessive–compulsive disorder. *American Journal of Psychiatry, 147,* 798–800.

Marmar, C. K., Foy, D., Kagan, B., & Pynoos, R. S. (1993). An integrated approach for treating posttraumatic stress. In R. S. Pynoos (Ed.), *Posttraumatic stress disorder: A clinical review* (pp. 99–132). Lutherville, MD: Sidran Press.

Masi, G., Mucci, M., Favilla, L., Romano, R., & Poli, P. (1999). Symptomatology and comorbidity of generalized anxiety disorder in children and adolescents. *Comprehensive Psychiatry, 40*, 210–215.

McDougle, C. J., Fleischmann, R. L., Epperson, C. N., Wasylink, S., Leckman, J. F., & Price, L. H. (1995). Risperidone addition in fluvoxamine-refractory obsessive–compulsive disorder: Three cases. *Journal of Clinical Psychiatry, 56*, 526–528.

McDougle, C. J., Goodman, W. K., Leckman, F. J., Lee, N. C., Heninger, G. R., & Price, L. H. (1994). Haloperidol addition in fluvoxamine-refractory obsessive–compulsive disorder: A double-blind, placebo-controlled study in patients with and without tics. *Archives of General Psychiatry, 51*, 302–308.

Perlmutter, S. J., Leitman, S. F., Garvey, M. A., Hamburger, S., Feldman, E., Leonard, H. L., & Swedo, S. E. (1999). Therapeutic plasma exchange and intravenous immunoglobulin for obsessive–compulsive disorder and tic disorders in childhood. *Lancet, 354*, 1153–1158.

Pfefferbaum, B. (1997). Posttraumatic stress disorder in children: A review of the past 10 years. *Journal of the American Academy of Child and Adolescent Psychiatry, 36*(11), 1503–1511.

Piacentini, J., & Bergman, R. L. (2000). Obsessive–compulsive disorder in children. *Psychiatric Clinics of North America, 23*(3), 519–533.

Pleak, R. R., & Gormly, L. J. (1995). Effects of venlafaxine treatment for ADHD in a child. *American Journal of Psychiatry, 152*, 1099.

Renaud, J., Birmaher, B., Wassick, S. C., & Bridge, J. (1999). Use of selective serotonin reuptake inhibitors for the treatment of childhood panic disorder: A pilot study. *Journal of Child and Adolescent Psychopharmacology, 9*, 73–83.

Research Units of Pediatric Psychopharmacology Anxiety Study Group. (2001). Fluvoxamine for the treatment of anxiety disorders in children and adolescents. *New England Journal of Medicine, 344*, 1279–1285.

Riddle, M. (1998). Obsessive–compulsive disorder in children and adolescents. *British Journal of Psychiatry, 35*(Suppl.), 91–96.

Riddle, M. A., Hardin, M. T., King, R., Scahill, L., & Woolston, J. L. (1990). Fluoxetine treatment of children and adolescents with Tourette's and obsessive–compulsive disorders: Preliminary clinical experience. *Journal of the American Academy of Child and Adolescent Psychiatry, 29*, 45–48.

Riddle, M. A., Scahill, L., King, R. A., Hardin, M. T., Anderson, G. M., Ort, S. I., Smith, J. C., Leckman, J. F., & Cohen, D. J. (1992). Double-blind, crossover trial of fluoxetine and placebo in children and adolescents with obsessive–compulsive disorder. *Journal of the American Academy of Child and Adolescent Psychiatry, 31*, 1062–1069.

Robert, R., Blakeney, P. E., Villareal, C., Rosenberg, L., & Meyer, W. K., III. (1999). Imipramine treatment in pediatric burn patients with symptoms of acute stress disorder: A pilot study. *Journal of the American Academy of Child and Adolescent Psychiatry, 38*(7), 873–882.

Rosenberg, D. R., Stewart, C. M., Fitzgerald, K. D., Tawile, V., & Carroll, E. (1999). Paroxetine open-label treatment of pediatric outpatients with obsessive–compulsive disorder. *Journal of the American Academy of Child and Adolescent Psychiatry, 38*, 1180–1185.

Rushton, J. L., Clark, S. J., & Freed, G. L. (2000). Pediatrician and family physician prescription of selective serotonin reuptake inhibitors. *Pediatrics, 105,* E82.

Rynn, M. A., Siqueland, L., & Rickels, K. (2001). Placebo-controlled trial of sertraline in the treatment of children with generalized anxiety disorder. *American Journal of Psychiatry, 158,* 2008–2014.

Saxe, G., Stoddard, F. J., Courtney, D., Cunningham, K., Chawla, N., Sheridan, R., King, D. W., & King, L. A. (2001). Relationship between acute morphine and the course of PTSD in children with burns. *Journal of the American Academy of Child and Adolescent Psychiatry, 40,* 915–921.

Seedat, S., Lockhat, R., Kaminer, D., Zungu-Dirwayi, N., & Stein, D. J. (2001). An open trial of citalopram in adolescents with posttraumatic stress disorder. *International Clinical Psychopharmacology, 16,* 21–25.

Sheikha, S. H., Wagner, K. D., & Wagner, R. J., Jr. (1993). Fluoxetine treatment of trichotillomania and depression in prepubertal children. *Cutis, 51,* 50–52.

Simeon, J. G. (1993). Use of anxiolytics in children. *Encephale, 19,* 71–74.

Simeon, J. G., & Ferguson, H. B. (1987). Alprazolam effects in children with anxiety disorders. *Canadian Journal of Psychiatry, 32*(7), 570–574.

Simeon, J. G., Thatte, S., & Wiggins, D. (1990). Treatment of adolescent obsessive–compulsive disorder with a clomipramine–fluoxetine combination. *Psychopharmacology Bulletin, 26,* 285–290.

Simeon, J. G., Ferguson, H. B., Knott, V., Roberts, N., Gauthier, B., Dubois, C., & Wiggins, D. (1992). Clinical, cognitive, and neurophysiological effects of alprazolam in children and adolescents with overanxious and avoidant disorders. *Journal of the American Academy of Child and Adolescent Psychiatry, 31*(1), 29–33.

Snider, L. A., & Swedo, S. E. (2000). Pediatric obsessive–compulsive disorder. *Journal of the American Medical Association, 284,* 3104–3106.

Sonntag, H., Wittchen, H.-U., Hofler, M., Kessler, R. C., & Stein, M. B. (2000). Are social fears and DSM-IV social anxiety disorder associated with smoking and nicotine dependence in adolescents and young adults? *European Psychiatry, 15,* 67–74.

Stein, D. J., Bouwer, C., Hawkridge, S., & Emsley, R. A. (1997). Risperidone augmentation of serotonin reuptake inhibitors in obsessive–compulsive and related disorders. *Journal of Clinical Psychiatry, 58,* 119–122.

Stein, M. B., Chavira, D. A., & Jang, K. L. (2001). Bringing up bashful baby: Developmental pathways to social phobia. *Psychiatric Clinics of North America, 24,* 661–675.

Stein, M. B., Fuetsch, M., Muller, N., Höfler, M., Lieb, R., & Wittchen, H.-U. (2001). Social anxiety disorder and the risk of depression: A prospective community study of adolescents and young adults. *Archives of General Psychiatry, 58,* 251–256.

Thomsen, P. H. (1997). Child and adolescent obsessive–compulsive disorder treated with citalopram: Findings from an open trial of 23 cases. *Journal of Child and Adolescent Psychopharmacology, 7,* 157–166.

Thomsen, P. H. (2000). Obsessive–compulsive disorder: Pharmacological treatment. *European Child and Adolescent Psychiatry, 9,* I/76–I/84.

Thomsen, P. H., Ebbesen, C., & Persson, C. (2001). Long-term experience with citalopram in the treatment of adolescents with OCD. *Journal of the American Academy of Child and Adolescent Psychiatry, 40*(8), 895–902.

Thomsen, P. H., & Mikkelsen, H. U. (1995). Course of obsessive–compulsive disorder in children and adolescents: A prospective follow-up study of 23 Danish cases. *Journal of the American Academy of Child and Adolescent Psychiatry, 34*, 1432–1440.

Thomsen, P. H., & Mikkelsen, H. U. (1999). The addition of buspirone to SSRI in the treatment of adolescent obsessive–compulsive disorder: A study of six cases. *European Child and Adolescent Psychiatry, 8*, 143–148.

Wagner, K. D. (2001). Generalized anxiety disorder. *Psychiatric Clinics of North America, 24*, 139–153.

Weiss, E. L., Potenza, M. N., McDougle, C. J., & Epperson, C. N. (1999). Olanzapine addition in obsessive–compulsive disorder refractory to selective serotonin reuptake inhibitors: An open-label case series. *Journal of Clinical Psychiatry, 60*, 524–527.

Woodward, L. J., & Ferguson, D. M. (2001). Life course outcomes of young people with anxiety disorders in adolescence. *Journal of the American Academy of Child and Adolescent Psychiatry, 40*(9), 1086–1093.

Yeganeh, R., Beidel, D. C., Turner, S. M., Pina, A. A., & Silverman, W. K. (2003). Clinical distinctions between selective mutism and social phobia: An investigation of childhood psychopathology. *Journal of the American Academy of Child and Adolescent Psychiatry, 42*, 1069–1075.

Zito, J. M., Safer, D. J., dosReis, S., Gardner, J. F., Boles, M., & Lynch, F. (2000). Trends in the prescribing of psychotropic medication to preschoolers. *Journal of the American Medical Association, 283*(8), 1025–1030.

Chapter 16

Combining Medication and Psychosocial Treatments

An Evidence-Based Medicine Approach

SCOTT N. COMPTON
CATHERINE D. MCKNIGHT
JOHN S. MARCH

Over the past 40 years the field of childhood and adolescent clinical psychology and psychiatry has witnessed the development of diverse, sophisticated, and empirically supported cognitive-behavioral and psychopharmacological interventions for the treatment of a wide range of childhood-onset anxiety disorders (March, 1999; Turner & Heiser, 1999). However, in the complex world of clinical practice, selecting an appropriate treatment for the anxious child from among the many possible treatment options is rarely a straightforward task. Many clinicians and researchers now believe that the combination of disorder-specific cognitive-behavioral therapy and medication, administered within the conceptual framework of evidence-based medicine (EBM), is the initial treatment of choice for many if not most children and adolescents with a diagnosable anxiety disorder (for example, see March, Frances, Kahn, & Carpenter, 1997). Within the framework of EBM, this chapter provides guidelines for how best to combine psychosocial and drug treatments for the individual patient.

THE BIOPSYCHOSOCIAL MODEL

Although there is no universally accepted model regarding the etiology and maintenance of anxiety disorders in children, the biopsychosocial disease management model is as effective a change strategy in psychiatry and psychology as it is in other areas of medicine. Within the biopsychosocial approach, combined treatment is the rule rather than the exception, as it is across most areas of medicine (cf. the treatment of hypertension with antihypertensives and weight reduction or the treatment of juvenile rheumatoid arthritis with ibuprofen and physical therapy). From within the biopsychosocial approach, the treatment of the anxious child can be thought of as partially analogous to the treatment of juvenile-onset diabetes, with the caveat that the treatment of the disorder requires psychosocial interventions of much greater complexity. The treatment of diabetes and anxiety disorder both involve medications—insulin in diabetes and, typically, a selective serotonin reuptake inhibitor (SSRI) in anxiety. Each also involves an evidence-based psychosocial intervention. In diabetes, the psychosocial treatment of choice is diet and exercise, and in anxiety it is exposure-based cognitive-behavior therapy (CBT).

WHY COMBINE PSYCHOSOCIAL AND DRUG TREATMENTS?

Psychosocial treatments are often combined with medications for the following reasons. First, two treatments provide a greater "dose" and thus may provide a more rapid and efficient response. For this reason, many patients with obsessive–compulsive disorder (OCD) opt for combined treatment, even though CBT alone may offer equal benefit (March & Leonard, 1998). Second, the presence of comorbidity often requires two treatments. For example, treating an 8-year-old child who has attention-deficit/ hyperactivity disorder (ADHD) and mild separation anxiety disorder with a psychostimulant and CBT is a reasonable treatment strategy (March et al., 2000). Third, in the case of partial response to one therapy, adding another treatment may result in greater symptom reduction in the domain targeted by the initial treatment. For example, CBT can be added to an SSRI for the treatment of OCD to improve OCD-specific outcomes. Likewise, a second treatment may be added to an initial treatment in order to positively affect one or more additional outcome domains (e.g., an SSRI can be added to CBT for OCD to treat comorbid symptoms of depression or panic disorder).

COGNITIVE-BEHAVIORAL THERAPY
IN A MEDICAL CONTEXT

Rather than focusing primarily on historical events, CBT targets problem behaviors and symptoms that are negatively affecting the patient's current level of functioning. Thus, unlike most other psychotherapeutic approaches, CBT fits beautifully into an evidence-based-medicine framework in which the current symptoms of the illness and associated functional impairments are specifically targeted for treatment. The cornerstone of CBT is a collaborative therapeutic relationship and a careful functional analysis of problem behaviors that is governed by several important assumptions. First, repertoires of behavior (including both maladaptive and adaptive behaviors) are shaped and maintained by contingencies of reinforcement (e.g., all consequences that increase or decrease the strength of behavior). Second, the antecedents and consequences of target behaviors, as well as target behaviors themselves, must be operationally defined and accurately measured. Third, as behavior may differ across settings, multi-informant, multimodal, multi-domain assessment is critical. Fourth, treatment planning depends on careful assessment, including periodic reassessment of how behaviors have changed, and subsequent revision of the treatment as necessary. Although these assumptions and procedures are not necessarily incompatible with pharmacological treatment, the level of specificity involved in conducting a functional analysis is generally greater with CBT than with medication management. On the other hand, the level of monitoring for change should be similar for both psychosocial and pharmacological interventions, as it is symptomatic change and improvement in functional outcomes that govern patient and clinician assessment of degree of improvement. Put experimentally, CBT lends itself to viewing the treatment of each patient through the lens of one of several possible single-case designs (Hayes, 1981), which in turn makes combining pharmacological and cognitive-behavioral interventions relatively straightforward.

EVIDENCE-BASED MEDICINE

One of the more common criticisms of an evidence-based approach to clinical practice is that clinical trials are only weakly related to what the average clinician does in the "real world." The external validity of many efficacy studies—defined as the extent to which the results of the research are generalizable to clinical populations—is limited by filters imposed by the methods for sample selection, assessment, and treatment. Thus the results from many internally valid experiments are not fully relevant to clinical practice because the treatments used or the nature of the patients studied is dissimilar to those in practice settings. This is one of the reasons that the National Institute of Mental Heath (NIMH) has moved away from funding efficacy trials conducted in "relatively pure" patients toward effectiveness trials, such as the Multimodal Treatment Study of ADHD (MTA), conducted with "messy" clinical samples and "messy" clinical settings (Norquist & Magruder, 1998).

From the point of view of an individual practitioner hoping to conform to best-practice standards in caring for anxious children, it is critical to ascertain how the results of a particular study are relevant to clinical practice. EBM provides a simple, straightforward framework for accomplishing this task. It can be thought of as a set of tools that allow clinicians to systematically integrate current best evidence in making decisions about the care of the individual (Guyatt, Sackett, & Cook, 1993, 1994; Guyatt, Sinclair, Cook, & Glasziou, 1999).

Whether approaching diagnosis, prognosis, or treatment, EBM begins with (1) selecting a clinically relevant question presented by the care of a specific patient, (2) searching the literature for evidence relevant to that question, and (3) evaluating the strength of the evidence using a standardized set of decision rules (Sackett, Richardson, Rosenberg, & Haynes, 2000).

The first step in evaluating a relevant question in EBM is to frame the question in terms of P-E-C-O: What is the Population, the Exposure to active treatment, the Control (or Comparison) condition, and the desired Outcome? A simple PECO might be: In children with OCD, what is the evidence that a serotonin reuptake inhibitor is better than placebo in reducing symptoms of OCD? Having framed the question as a PECO, the clinician can then turn for an answer to the increasingly EBM-optimized resources available on the Internet (Guyatt, Haynes, et al., 2000). More specifically, EBM provides a clear hierarchy of search strategies that move from EBM reviews (which have summarized all the relevant literature on a given topic) to critically appraised topics (CATS, which summarize one or two relevant articles) to searching and critiquing the literature oneself. Full text articles for many journals can be retrieved from OVID, which is available either as a subscription service or free from most academic libraries. Assuming that the designs and outcomes are similar, the most recent or the most powerful study likely is sufficient to construct a CAT. Conversely, where the literature is rich with randomized trials, the most recent EBM review might be the most important source of information (Guyatt, Meade, Jaeschke, Cook, & Haynes, 2000; see Sackett et al., 2000, for a more detailed discussion of search strategies, systematic reviews, and CATS).

After one identifies an article that is directly relevant to the question of interest, the next step is to evaluate the article for its validity and applicability to the patient. The EBM approach to reviewing an article requires a close reading of (1) the abstract, to get an overall summary of the question addressed, the research methods used, and the main findings; (2) the methods section, to assess validity and to identify the population studied; and (3) the results section, to understand the direction and clinical importance of the outcome. The introduction and discussion sections can often be skipped as an inefficient use of time (although such information might be extremely useful for other purposes).

Four relatively easy and commonsensical steps then provide an answer to the question of clinical relevance to the patient:

• *Step 1. Is the study valid?* Did the investigators use a randomized, controlled, double-blind design? Did the study include a follow-up period of sufficient length so that the durability of the treatment can be assessed? Apart from intrinsic differences in the treatments themselves, were all patients treated the same way? Without affirming these relatively straightforward parameters, it is impossible to know whether differences in the outcome reflect true differences in the impact of the treatments or some other characteristic of the study.

• *Step 2. What were the results?* Ideally, the results should be presented both dimensionally, using rating scales with normative data so that the reader can judge improvement toward or into the normal range, and categorically, to allow easy calculation of magnitude of clinical improvement. If the results are presented as a change score (the mean at posttreatment minus the mean at pretreatment for each treatment group), the actual mean scores and standard deviations for each treatment group at baseline should also be included so that the clinician can judge whether the amount of change moved the average patient into the normal range. If comorbidity is a factor, initial levels of comorbid symptomatology and changes in comorbidity over time should also be presented. Finally, the same questions that are asked about treatment effectiveness can be asked about harm to answer the critical question: Is a treatment safe? (Levine et al., 1994).

• *Step 3. Are the results clinically meaningful?* This is an important variable for clinicians who want to determine whether the results of a given clinical trial can be applied to their clinical patients. Traditionally in psychiatry and psychology, the magnitude of the effect has been portrayed in terms of small (0.2), medium (0.5), or large (> 0.8) effect sizes in standard deviation units (Cohen, 1969). EBM uses a much simpler rubric, the "number needed to treat," or NNT. In practice, NNT represents the number of patients that need to be treated with the active treatment to produce one additional positive outcome beyond that obtainable with the control or comparison condition. For example, an NNT of 10 describes the number of patients you would need to treat with the active treatment rather than the control treatment to see one additional positive outcome.[1] A very small NNT (i.e., an NNT that approaches 1) means that a favorable outcome occurs in nearly every patient who receives the treatment and in relatively few patients in the comparison group. An NNT of 2 or 3 indicates that a treatment is quite effective. In contrast, NNTs above 30 or 40 fall in the realm of public health effects, although they may still be considered clinically relevant. Used in this fashion, the NNT can be useful for interpreting results of clinical trials and for making therapeutic decisions for a given patient.

Results from studies that use a dimensional response metric can be recast into an intuitive statistic similar to the NNT, called the "binomial effect size display" (BESD; Rosenthal, Rosnow, & Rubin, 2000; Rosenthal & Rubin, 1982). Like the NNT, the BESD uses the difference between two proportions (e.g., difference in success rates between the treatment and control group) as a way of describing the practical importance of an experimental effect. The BESD, however, can be calculated directly from more traditional effect size statistics (e.g., Cohen's d or the correlation r), as well as from results of statistical tests (e.g., t test, and F test; for details on how to calculate BESD, see Rosenthal et al., 2000; Rosenthal & Rubin, 1982).

- *Step 4. Is the result applicable to my patient?* Before applying the results of a study to the care of an individual patient, it is important to understand the similarities between the patients who participated in the research study and the patients treated by a practitioner in his or her office. This can be accomplished quickly by asking the following questions: Is my patient represented in the research sample, or were patients like mine excluded from the trial? Were the clinically important outcomes both functional

---

[1]Starting with a dimensional response metric, ES is a measure of the average response in standard deviation units calculated as $MC - ME/SD_{pooled}$, where ME represents the mean of the experimental treatment, MC represents the mean of the control treatment, and SD_{pooled} represents pooling of the standard deviations from within both groups at the end of treatment. Starting with a categorical response metric, NNT is a measure of the average response presented as the probability of response in single patient units. Arithmetically, the NNT is the inverse of the absolute risk reduction (1/ARR), defined as the percent response in the experimental group – the percent response in the control condition. When benefit (a positive response) rather than risk (e.g., mortality) is the outcome, the ARR is often rephrased as the absolute benefit increase, or ABI. For example, if 80% of patients respond to treatment X and 30% to a PBO control condition, the ABI is 50% and the NNT is 2, a very robust response. Confidence intervals can be calculated around the NNT to estimate the precision of the treatment effect. Confidence intervals (CI) are a useful measure of the certainty that you, the clinician, can provide when informing your patient about the expected outcome of treatment. The wider the confidence interval, the less confident you can be about predicting correctly.

(e.g., return to school) and disorder specific (e.g., less anxiety)? How were the outcomes measured, are they clinically meaningful, and can I apply these measures in my practice? To the extent that my patient offers a better or worse prognosis than the average patient in the study, would an adjusted NNT[2] bias my choice of treatments, for example, toward combined drug and psychosocial treatment in a very ill multiply comorbid patient? Are the treatments worth the potential benefits, harms, and costs? Can colleagues work together to provide the treatment in our clinical setting(s)? Will the patient accept the treatment? The answers to these questions bring the research study to the level of direct patient care.

COMBINED TREATMENT FOR ANXIETY, DEPRESSION, AND SCHOOL REFUSAL

One of the most challenging clinical problems in pediatric psychiatry and psychology is teenagers with severe anxiety, depression, and associated school refusal. These patients present with multiple behavioral and family problems and are often, if inappropriately, thought of as treatment refractory even before treatment begins (Bernstein, Borchardt, & Perwien, 1996; Bernstein, Warren, Massie, & Thuras, 1999). The treatment of these teenagers provides an excellent example of how EBM can be used to guide the combining of medication and psychosocial treatments in clinical practice.

In a recently published study (Bernstein et al., 2000), Bernstein and colleagues asked the following question (framed as a PECO): In school-refusing teenagers with combined anxiety and depressive disorders (the population), is imipramine plus CBT (the exposure) more effective than CBT plus pill placebo (the control) in returning patients to school (the outcome) after 8 weeks of treatment? They used a balanced randomized parallel-group design, complete follow-up, an intent-to treat analysis, blind assessment, pill placebo to balance the CBT-alone condition, and equal treatment characteristics in each group apart from the intervention. Over 8 weeks, they found a statistically significant difference favoring

---

[2]Modifications to the NNT can be introduced depending on the extent to which the individual patient resembles the patients assembled in the treatment study. Specifically, the NNT can be adjusted for a specific patient by estimating the patient's likelihood of change relative to the average control patient in the trial report, expressing the likelihood as a decimal fraction, F, and then dividing the reported NNT by F. For example, if your patient is judged to have half the probability of a positive response as the average control patient, then F = 0.5 and the NNT/F = twice the unadjusted NNT.

combined treatment over CBT alone for depression outcomes and in returning patients to school. The magnitude and precision of the NNT (NNT = 3, CI 1–4) for this notoriously difficult-to-treat population was quite impressive, suggesting that combined CBT and medication is better than CBT alone.

The study by Bernstein and colleagues (2000) was initiated before SSRIs came into wide use with children and adolescents. A large number of studies have shown that the tricyclic antidepressants (TCAs) are not effective on average for children and adolescents with major depression (the results of a different EBM search) and are riskier and more complicated to use than SSRIs (Birmaher, 1998; Leonard, March, Rickler, & Allen, 1997). Thus we might want to ask, "Can we substitute an SSRI for the TCA imipramine in combination with CBT in this patient population?" A recently published study from the Research Units on Pediatric Psychopharmacology Anxiety Study Group (RUPP) that compared fluvoxamine to pill placebo in children and adolescents with generalized, social, and separation anxiety disorders provides an unambiguous affirmative answer (RUPP, 2001). With an NNT of 2 (CI 1–3) in this study, we could reasonably assume that the Bernstein findings would have been as good or even better had they used fluvoxamine, though of course there is as yet no randomized evidence pointing in that direction. Given this new evidence and substantial expert opinion favoring the SSRIs over the TCAs in this patient population (Bernstein & Shaw, 1997; March, 1999), the substitution of an SSRI for imipramine is a clinically reasonable treatment strategy to take.

COMBINED TREATMENT FOR CHILDREN WITH ADHD COMORBID WITH ANXIETY

A large body of literature suggests that treatment with a psychostimulant is effective for externalizing symptoms in children with ADHD (Swanson, 1993). However, it has long been speculated that comorbid anxiety may adversely influence the outcome of drug treatment for ADHD (Pliszka, 1998). Whether this is true or whether it would confer an advantage for behavioral or combined treatment was, until recently, unknown (Jensen, Martin, & Cantwell, 1997). Thus, given a patient with ADHD and anxiety, we might wish to know (framed as a PECO) whether, in the treatment of young children with ADHD comorbid with an anxiety disorder (the population), combined treatment (the exposure) has an advantage over treatment with medication or parent training alone (the comparison condition). A search of PubMed using the "clinical queries" option and the search terms "ADHD," "anxiety," "child," and "combined treatment" would identify the primary outcome papers from the NIMH collaborative Multimodal Treatment Study of Children with ADHD (MTA Cooperative Group, 1999a, 1999b) and a subsequent secondary analysis from the MTA Cooperative Group specifically addressing the impact of anxiety on treatment outcome (March et al., 2000).

The MTA study was designed to address a priori questions about the individual and combined effects of pharmacological and psychosocial (behavioral) treatment for children between the ages of 7 and 9 with ADHD (Arnold et al., 1997). The rationale and design of the MTA, which serves as a heuristically valuable example of how CBT and medication can and should be combined, have been reported elsewhere (Arnold et al., 1997). Briefly, 579 children meeting dimensional criteria for hyperactivity and DSM-IV criteria for ADHD, combined subtype, were randomly assigned to an intensive behavior therapy program (BT), a titration-adjusted optimized medication management strategy (MM), an interactive combination of BT and MM (COMB) in which dose and timing of interventions were adjusted for one treatment depending on response to the other, and a comparison group that was assessed and then referred to local community care resources (CC). Children and parents received comprehensive assessments at baseline and at 3, 9, and 14 months (treatment end point; Hinshaw et al., 1997). The BT consisted of 14 months of parent training that was provided in individual and group format, 4 months of classroom behavioral management training provided by a paraprofessional working with the teacher, and an intensive 8-week summer treatment program (Wells et al., 2000). Optimal medication dosage was attained by acutely titrating medication (starting with methylphenidate and switching to other drugs as needed) and subsequently adjusting the dose and timing of drug administration based on teacher and parent symptom ratings over the course of the study (Greenhill et al., 1996).

As recently summarized by Jensen and colleagues (Jensen et al., 2001), COMB and MM interventions proved superior to BT and CC interventions for ADHD symptoms (MTA Cooperative Group, 1999a). Despite the fact that CC children were frequently medicated, these effects were clinically meaningful, with an NNT for COMB or MM relative to CC of 2, indicating that well-delivered treatment that includes medication is superior to less intensive community care. For other functional domains (social skills, academics, parent–child relations, oppositional behavior, anxiety/depression), results suggested modest incremental benefits of the COMB intervention over the single-component (MM, BT) treatments and community care (MTA Cooperative Group, 1999b).

Initial moderator analyses of the MTA findings suggested that childhood anxiety, ascertained by parent report on the Diagnostic Interview

Schedule for Children Version 2.3 (DISC Anxiety), differentially moderated the outcome of treatment (MTA Cooperative Group, 1999b). However, questions regarding the nature of DISC Anxiety, the impact of comorbid conduct problems on the moderating effect of DISC Anxiety, and the clinical significance of DISC Anxiety as a moderator of treatment outcome were left unanswered. Exploratory analyses by March and colleagues (March et al., 2000) suggested that DISC Anxiety reflected parental attributions regarding child negative affectivity and associated behavior problems, particularly in the area of social interactions, rather than fearfulness, another core component of anxiety that is more typically associated with phobic symptoms. Analyses using hierarchical linear modeling (HLM) indicated that the moderating effect of DISC Anxiety continued to favor the inclusion of psychosocial treatment for anxious children with ADHD, irrespective of the presence or absence of comorbid conduct problems. This effect, although clinically meaningful, was confined primarily to parent-reported outcomes involving disruptive behavior, internalizing symptoms, and inattention and was generally stronger for combined than for unimodal treatment. Contradicting earlier studies, no adverse effect of anxiety on medication response for core ADHD or other outcomes in anxious or nonanxious children with ADHD was demonstrated (March et al., 2000). In particular, the effect sizes for the comorbid group were often double those for the nonanxious group (large versus small), irrespective of treatment modality, with COMB often showing a large treatment effect and BT and MM medium treatment effects. Thus granting defensible (Jensen, 1999) limitations in generalizability (Boyle & Jadad, 1999), the results of the MTA study would suggest that the clinician, when confronted with a child comorbid with ADHD and anxiety, would be wise to recommend a combination of intensive MM and parent training, whereas for the youngster without such complications, MM alone will likely suffice as the initial treatment of choice.

DOSE–RESPONSE AND TIME–RESPONSE ISSUES

When initiating any type of treatment, the ability to construct a dose–response curve and to analyze time–action effects is critical. The former refers to the relationship between dose of drug and the presence of benefits and adverse effects. Establishing these relationships depends on understanding time–action parameters, namely the relationship between the timing of administration and onset of response, maximum responsiveness, and loss or offset of drug effect. Departures from a linear dose–response pattern are common, with some children showing a threshold effect (no response below a threshold level) and others a quadratic response (linear at lower doses and degradation at higher doses). Thus each child requires an individually constructed dose–response curve, taking into consideration the time–action effects of drug or psychosocial treatment at each dose before making dosage adjustments. With a single-drug treatment, many clinicians start with the lowest possible dose, titrating upward toward the end of the expected time–response window until benefits are maximized or the patient shows prohibitive side effects. With psychosocial treatment, dose is usually conceptualized as "number of sessions," with a minimum number of sessions (typically 10–20 over as many weeks) serving as the definition of an acceptable course of treatment.

When combining drug and psychosocial treatments, it is often possible to capitalize on between-treatment differences in dose–response and time–response parameters. With respect to dose–response, there is some evidence that treatments can be additive (e.g., the impact of the dose of both treatments is the same as the impact of each treatment separately, added together) or multiplicative (two treatments act synergistically such that the benefit of combined treatment is greater than the additive combination). This may be the case for OCD, in which partial response to medication is the rule rather than the exception (March et al., 1997, 1998). Similarly, when combining treatments, a lower dose of one or both treatments may be necessary, with a resultant decrease in expense, inconvenience, or adverse events. For example, the MTA study implemented a very high-dose behavioral therapy—a 14-month combination of parent training, a summer treatment program, and a classroom intervention (Wells et al., 2000)—that resulted in an slightly lower methylphenidate dose in the combined group (28 mg per day in divided doses) as compared with the medication-alone group (36 mg per day in divided doses). Even when dose does not differ, capitalizing on differences in time–response parameters can lead to reduced patient suffering. For example, by blocking full panic episodes and quelling anticipatory anxiety, the combination of clonazepam with an SSRI in the acutely separation-anxious youngster allows more rapid reintroduction to school than either CBT or SSRI alone might permit (Birmaher, Yelovich, & Renaud, 1998; March, 1999). Finally, time–response parameters can be matched to the patient's benefit, as when the patient receiving CBT for OCD experiences maximum benefit from an SSRI just at the time he or she reaches the top of the stimulus hierarchy (March, 1998).

FUTURE OF RESEARCH

As child and adolescent psychiatry has matured, large multisite comparative treatment trials, such as the Multimodal Treatment of Children with

ADHD study (MTA), play a more prominent role in treatment outcome research. Such trials typically are performed when three conditions are fulfilled. First, the treatment literature for the respective monotherapies must indicate that the monotherapy treatment (either medication or psychosocial treatment) is efficacious for a given disorder when compared with suitable control conditions. At the same time, reasons for inclusion of a combined-treatment group and the rationale for testing the treatments in the same patient population must be compelling. Second, the disorder to be treated must be of significant public health importance, as indicated by high prevalence and substantial suffering and functional impairment. Third, the outcome of the trial must have the potential for a positive impact on the clinical outcomes of children and, depending on the results, the cost of care for the specified disorder. In addition to the MTA, four such trials are currently underway: (1) the Pediatric OCD Treatment Study (POTS; Franklin, Foa, & March, 2003), (2) the Treatment of Adolescent Depression Study (TADS, 2003), (3) the Child Anxiety Management Study (CAMS), and (4) the Treatment of Adolescent Suicide Attempters (TASA). With the exception of TASA, each clinical trial uses a balanced 1 × 4 experimental design to contrast treatment with an SSRI, cognitive-behavior therapy, and their combination against a pill-placebo control condition. Taken together, these studies, and others about to be undertaken on anxiety, eating, and conduct disorders, begin to approach the question of which treatment—drug, psychosocial, or combination—is best for which child with what set of predictive characteristics (Jensen, 1999; March & Curry, 1998).

CONCLUSION

Empirically supported unimodal treatments are now available for most disorders seen in clinical practice, including the various anxiety disorders, ADHD, OCD, Tourette's disorder, major depression, schizophrenia, and autism. Despite limitations in the research literature with regard to the long-term outcome of combined treatment, effectiveness of drugs and psychosocial interventions across divergent outcome domains and ages is increasing. As our understanding of the pathogenesis of mental illness in youth increases, dramatic treatment innovations inevitably will accrue, including knowledge about when and how to combine treatments. Hence, the clinician facing the daunting task of keeping up with the rapid advances in evidence regarding the diagnosis and treatment of mental illness in children and adolescents would be well advised to acquire at least a basic understanding of the tools of evidence-based medicine (Sackett et al., 2000).

ACKNOWLEDGMENTS

This work was supported by NIMH Grant No. 1 K24 MHO1557 to John S. March and by contributions from the Robert and Sarah Gorrell family. Adapted from March (2002).

REFERENCES

Arnold, L. E., Abikoff, H. B., Cantwell, D. P., Conners, C. K., Elliott, G., Greenhill, L. L., et al. (1997). NIMH Collaborative Multimodal Treatment Study of Children with ADHD (the MTA): Design, methodology and protocol evolution. *Journal of Attention Disorders, 2*(3), 141–158.

Bernstein, G. A., Borchardt, C. M., & Perwien, A. R. (1996). Anxiety disorders in children and adolescents: A review of the past 10 years. *Journal of the American Academy of Child and Adolescent Psychiatry, 35*(9), 1110–1119.

Bernstein, G. A., Borchardt, C. M., Perwien, A. R., Crosby, R. D., Kushner, M. G., Thuras, P. D., & Last, C. G. (2000). Imipramine plus cognitive-behavioral therapy in the treatment of school refusal. *Journal of the American Academy of Child and Adolescent Psychiatry, 39*(3), 276–283.

Bernstein, G. A., & Shaw, K. (1997). Practice parameters for the assessment and treatment of children and adolescents with anxiety disorders. *Journal of the American Academy of Child and Adolescent Psychiatry, 36*(10, Suppl.), 69S–84S.

Bernstein, G. A., Warren, S. L., Massie, E. D., & Thuras, P. D. (1999). Family dimensions in anxious-depressed school refusers. *Journal of Anxiety Disorders, 13*(5), 513–528.

Birmaher, B. (1998). Should we use antidepressant medications for children and adolescents with depressive disorders? *Psychopharmacology Bulletin, 34*(1), 35–39.

Birmaher, B., Yelovich, A. K., & Renaud, J. (1998). Pharmacologic treatment for children and adolescents with anxiety disorders. *Pediatric Clinics of North America, 45*(5), 1187–1204.

Boyle, M. H., & Jadad, A. R. (1999). Lessons from large trials: The MTA study as a model for evaluating the treatment of childhood psychiatric disorder. *Canadian Journal of Psychiatry, 44*(10), 991–998.

Cohen, J. (1969). *Statistical power analysis for the behavioral sciences.* Hillsdale, NJ: Erlbaum.

Franklin, M., Foa, E., & March, J. S. (2003). The Pediatric Obsessive–Compulsive Disorder Treatment Study (POTS): Rationale, design and methods. *Journal of Child and Adolescent Psychopharmacology, 13*(Suppl. 1), S39–S51.

Greenhill, L. L., Abikoff, H. B., Arnold, L. E., Cantwell, D. P., Conners, C. K., Elliott, G., Hechtman, L., Hinshaw, S. P., Hoza, B., Jensen, P. S., March, J. S., Newcorn, J., Pelham, W. E., Severe, J. B., Swanson, J. M., Vitiello, B., & Wells, K. (1996). Medication treatment strategies in the MTA Study: Relevance to clinicians and researchers. *Journal of the American Academy of Child and Adolescent Psychiatry, 35*(10), 1304–1313.

Guyatt, G. H., Haynes, R. B., Jaeschke, R. Z., Cook, D. J., Green, L., Naylor, C. D., Wilson, M. C., & Richardson, W. S. (2000). Users' guides to the medical literature: Vol. 25. Evidence-based medicine: Principles for applying the Users' Guides to patient care. *Journal of the American Medical Association, 284*(10), 1290–1296.

Guyatt, G. H., Meade, M. O., Jaeschke, R. Z., Cook, D. J., & Haynes, R. B. (2000). Practitioners of evidence-based care: Not all clinicians need to appraise evidence from scratch but all need some skills [Editorial]. *British Medical Journal, 320*(7240), 954–955.

Guyatt, G. H., Sackett, D. L., & Cook, D. J. (1993). Users' guides to the medical literature: 2. How to use an article about therapy or prevention. A. Are the results of the study valid? *Journal of the American Medical Association, 270*(21), 2598–2601.

Guyatt, G. H., Sackett, D. L., & Cook, D. J. (1994). Users' guides to the medical literature: 2. How to use an article about therapy or prevention. B. What were the results and will they help me in caring for my patients? *Journal of the American Medical Association, 271*(1), 59–63.

Guyatt, G. H., Sinclair, J., Cook, D. J., & Glasziou, P. (1999). Users' guides to the medical literature: Vol. 16. How to use a treatment recommendation. *Journal of the American Medical Association, 281*(19), 1836–1843.

Hayes, S. (1981). Single case experimental design and empirical clinical practice. *Journal of Consulting and Clinical Psychology, 49*, 193–211.

Hinshaw, S., March, J., Abikoff, H., Arnold, L., Cantwell, D., Conners, C., et al. (1997). Comprehensive assessment of childhood attention-deficit/hyperactivity disorder in the context of a multisite, multimodal clinical trial. *Journal of Attention Disorders, 1*(4), 217–234.

Jensen, P. S., Hinshaw, S. P., Kraemer, H. C., Lenora, N., Newcorn, J. H., Abikoff, H. B., March, J. S., Arnold, L. E., Cantwell, D. P., Conners, C. K., Elliott, G. R., Greenhill, L. L., Hechtman, L., Hoza, B., Pelham, W. E., Severe, J. B., Swanson, J. M., Wells, K. C., Wigal, T., & Vitiello, B. (2001). ADHD comorbidity findings from the MTA study: Comparing comorbid subgroups. *Journal of the American Academy of Child and Adolescent Psychiatry, 40*(2), 147–158.

Jensen, P. S. (1999). Fact versus fancy concerning the multimodal treatment study for attention-deficit/hyperactivity disorder. *Canadian Journal of Psychiatry, 44*(10), 975–980.

Jensen, P. S., Martin, D., & Cantwell, D. P. (1997). Comorbidity in ADHD: Implications for research, practice, and DSM-V. *Journal of the American Academy of Child and Adolescent Psychiatry, 36*(8), 1065–1079.

Leonard, H. L., March, J., Rickler, K. C., & Allen, A. J. (1997). Pharmacology of the selective serotonin reuptake inhibitors in children and adolescents. *Journal of the American Academy of Child and Adolescent Psychiatry, 36*(6), 725–736.

Levine, M., Walter, S., Lee, H., Haines, T., Holbrook, A., & Moyer, V. (1994). Users' guides to the medical literature: 4. How to use an article about harm. *Journal of the American Medical Association, 271*(20), 1615–1619.

March, J. S. (1998). Cognitive behavioral psychotherapy for pediatric OCD. In M. Jenike, L. Baer, & W. Minichello (Eds.), *Obsessive–compulsive disorders* (3rd ed., pp. 400–420). Philadelphia: Mosby.

March, J. S. (1999). Current status of pharmacotherapy for pediatric anxiety disorders. In D. Beidel (Ed.), *Treating anxiety disorders in youth: Current problems and future solutions* (pp. 42–62). Washington, DC: Anxiety Disorders Association of America.

March, J. S. (2002). Combining medication and psychosocial treatments: An evidence-based medicine approach. *International Review of Psychiatry, 14*(2), 155–163.

March, J. S., Biederman, J., Wolkow, R., Safferman, A., Mardekian, J., Cook, E. H., Cutler, N. R., Dominguez, R., Ferguson, J., Muller, B., Riesenberg, R., Rosenthal, M., Sallee, F. R., Wagner, K. D., & Steiner, H. (1998). Sertraline in children and adolescents with obsessive-compulsive disorder: A multicenter randomized controlled trial. *Journal of the American Medical Association, 280*(20), 1752–1756.

March, J. S., & Curry, J. F. (1998). Predicting the outcome of treatment. *Journal of Abnormal Child Psychology, 26*(1), 39–51.

March, J., Frances, A., Kahn, D., & Carpenter, D. (1997). Expert consensus guidelines: Treatment of obsessive–compulsive disorder. *Journal of Clinical Psychiatry, 58*(Suppl. 4), 1–72.

March, J. S., & Leonard, H. L. (1998). OCD in children: Research and treatment. In M. Richter (Ed.), *Obsessive–compulsive disorder: Theory, research, and treatment* (pp. 367–394). New York: Guilford Press.

March, J. S., Swanson, J. M., Arnold, L. E., Hoza, B., Conners, C. K., Hinshaw, S. P., et al. (2000). Anxiety as a predictor and outcome variable in the Multimodal Treatment Study of Children with ADHD (MTA). *Journal of Abnormal Child Psychology, 28*(6), 527–541.

MTA Cooperative Group. (1999a). A 14–month randomized clinical trial of treatment strategies for attention-deficit/hyperactivity disorder: Multimodal Treatment Study of Children with ADHD. *Archives of General Psychiatry, 56*(12), 1073–1086.

MTA Cooperative Group. (1999b). Moderators and mediators of treatment response for children with attention-deficit/hyperactivity disorder: The Multimodal Treatment Study of Children with Attention-Deficit/Hyperactivity Disorder. *Archives of General Psychiatry, 56*(12), 1088–1096.

Norquist, G. S., & Magruder, K. M. (1998). Views from funding agencies. National Institute of Mental Health. *Medical Care, 36*(9), 1306–1308.

Pliszka, S. (1998). Comorbidity of attention-deficit/hyperactivity disorder with psychiatric disorder: An overview. *Journal of Clinical Psychiatry, 59*(Suppl. 7), 50–58.

Research Units of Pediatric Psychopharmacology Anxiety Study Group. (2001). Fluvoxamine for the treatment of anxiety disorders in children and adolescents. *New England Journal of Medicine, 344*(17), 1279–1285.

Rosenthal, R., Rosnow, R. L., & Rubin, D. B. (2000). *Contrasts and effect sizes in behavioral research: A correlational approach*. Cambridge, UK: Cambridge University Press.

Rosenthal, R., & Rubin, D. B. (1982). A simple general purpose display of magnitude of experimental effect. *Journal of Educational Psychology, 74*, 166–169.

Sackett, D., Richardson, W., Rosenberg, W., & Haynes, B. (2000). *Evidence-based medicine* (2nd ed.). London: Churchill Livingston.

Swanson, J. (1993). Effect of stimulant medication on hyperactive children: A review of reviews. *Exceptional Child, 60,* 154–162.

TADS. (2003). Treatment for Adolescents with Depression Study (TADS): Rationale, design, and methods. *Journal of the American Academy of Child and Adolescent Psychiatry, 42*(5), 531–542.

Turner, S., & Heiser, N. (1999). Current status of psychological interventions for childhood anxiety disorders. In D. Beidel (Ed.), *Treating anxiety disorders in youth: Current problems and future solutions* (pp. 63–76). Washington, DC: Anxiety Disorders Association of America.

Wells, K. C., Pelham, W. E., Jr., Kotkin, R. A., Hoza, B., Abikoff, H. B., Abramowitz, A., et al. (2000). Psychosocial treatment strategies in the MTA study: Rationale, methods, and critical issues in design and implementation. *Journal of Abnormal Child Psychology, 28*(6), 483–505.

Chapter 17

Prevention Strategies

PAULA M. BARRETT
CYNTHIA M. TURNER

In the past decade, prevention of mental health problems has become a priority for governments, both in terms of funding research initiatives and in practice. As a result, the literature pertaining to preventative interventions has increased considerably over the past 3–4 years (e.g., see Greenberg, Domitrovich, & Bumbarger, 2001, for a recent review of prevention programs for school-age children and adolescents). However, as a science, the field of prevention is still in its infancy, and to date there has been a limited focus on preventative interventions for childhood anxiety disorders.

Nonetheless, the rationale for pursuing the prevention of childhood anxiety remains strong. Earlier chapters in this volume have highlighted the fact that anxiety disorders in children represent one of the most common and debilitating forms of psychopathology, and although significant progress has been made in the development of effective treatment approaches (e.g., Barrett, 1998; Barrett, Dadds, & Rapee, 1996; Kendall, 1994; Silverman & Kurtines, 1999), the majority of children with anxiety disorders do not attend any agency for treatment (Tuma, 1989; Zubrick et al., 1997). For those who do seek professional help, treatment remains ineffective for a significant proportion, with between 12 and 40% still meeting diagnostic criteria for an anxiety disorder at the end of treatment (e.g., Barrett et al., 1996; Kendall, 1994). Thus treating children who are already experiencing significant anxiety problems may not be the most effective or efficient means of reducing the incidence of childhood anxiety in the general population or of reducing the suffering of children and families. The potential of prevention programs, which intervene prior to the development of significant anxiety problems, therefore deserves to be investigated.

This chapter aims to (1) examine current intervention technologies that are or could be employed in this area, (2) review existing prevention and early intervention programs that are described in the literature, (3) highlight the role of risk and protective factors in preventative research, (4) examine some practical issues relevant to implementing prevention programs, and (5) discuss important methodological issues for conducting preventative interventions. Accordingly, we aim to motivate clinicians and researchers to build on the foundation research that is beginning to emerge in the area of childhood anxiety prevention.

APPROACHES TO PREVENTION

Before we proceed, we believe that it is important to discuss the current approaches to prevention and the terminology used to describe these methods. Traditionally, three levels of prevention have been described: primary, secondary, and tertiary (Caplan, 1964). Primary prevention referred to interventions that sought to reduce the incidence of psychopathology by intervening prior to the onset of a disorder. Secondary prevention sought to reduce the prevalence of pathology by intervening once problems had been identified but before they became severe. Tertiary prevention involved treatment of existing disorders and prevention of relapse. The disadvantages of this classification system were that the secondary and tertiary levels related more to treatment than to prevention and that the classifications assumed that a clear distinction existed between the presence or absence of a disorder (Spence, 1996).

In reality, most forms of psychopathology lie on a continuum, from few or mild symptoms to more severe and/or numerous symptoms. The prevention literature has therefore adopted an alternative approach to classifying interventions, based on the presence and extent of risk factors related to the development of a disorder (Gordon, 1987). These approaches, labeled "universal," "selective," and "indicated," have been adopted by the Institute of Medicine (Mrazek & Haggerty, 1994) and are truly prevention focused in that they are reserved for only those interventions that occur before the initial onset of a disorder.

Universal interventions are those applied to whole populations, regardless of their risk status. In some instances, universal preventative interventions are designed to enhance general mental health or to build resiliency, whereas others are targeted at one specific disorder. Selective preventative efforts are applied to those individuals or subgroups of the population whose imminent or lifetime risk of developing a mental health disorder is significantly higher than average. Indicated prevention approaches are those applied to individuals or groups who are found to manifest mild symptomatology, identifying them as being at extremely high risk for the future development of full-blown mental health disorders. This chapter discusses programs in terms of universal, selective, and indicated interventions, as this model is currently the most widely accepted.

REVIEW OF PREVENTATIVE INTERVENTIONS

Although there has been an encouraging increase in the number of psychological academic journal articles related to prevention of childhood anxiety, the majority of papers have been theoretical in nature (e.g., Donovan & Spence, 2000; Spence, 1996, 2001; Spence & Dadds, 1996) rather than empirical evaluations of preventative interventions. Studies reviewed for inclusion in this chapter were restricted to published preventative interventions that targeted improvements in anxious symptomatology or a reduction in risk for the later development of an anxiety disorder. Programs were excluded if their target was generic mental health risk factors (e.g., parental separation/divorce, transition to high school) or if they sought to prevent anxiety associated with medical or dental procedures. Only four published studies that have addressed the question of anxiety prevention in children met these review criteria.

LaFreniere and Capuano (1997) reported on an indicated preventative intervention for preschool children who exhibited anxious–withdrawn behavior. Forty-three anxious–withdrawn children (20 boys, 23 girls) and their mothers participated. Children ranged in age from 2½ years to 5½ years (mean age = 4.45 years) and were identified as anxious–withdrawn on the basis of a teacher-report questionnaire examining social competence and behavior. Of the 137 children identified, 43 of their mothers (31.4%) consented to participate, and families were randomly assigned to either an intervention or a monitoring control condition. A pre–post test design evaluated children's social-emotional behavior (as reported by teachers), and measures of parental stress, maternal warmth, and discipline were also taken.

Through an intensive 20-session home-based intervention, the researchers sought to provide mothers with education about children's developmental needs, to promote parenting competence through parent-skills-training techniques, and to alleviate maternal stress through the provision of social support. It was expected that the intervention would have a positive impact on parenting stress, parent–child interactions, and child anxious–withdrawn behavior in the preschool context.

Results suggested a number of encouraging findings. As predicted, levels of maternal stress were reduced, and parent–child interactions showed an increase in maternal warmth and support and a decrease in levels of intrusive, overcontrolling behavior. Teachers rated children as more socially competent, but although positive changes in anxious–withdrawn behavior were also noted, these changes fell short of reaching significance (LaFreniere & Capuano, 1997).

Unfortunately, this study did not include a follow-up assessment to ascertain whether positive changes in childhood anxious–withdrawn behavior would continue. Krohne and Hock (1991) suggest that parental overcontrol is a specific risk factor for childhood anxiety disorder because it tends to interfere with children's acquisition of effective problem solving, resulting in a failure to learn to deal successfully with stressful life situations and undermining children's belief in their ability to succeed. Reducing levels of parental overcontrol should therefore have a positive impact on child anxiety; however, a follow-up period is essential to examine this possibility. Long-term follow-up is crucial in prevention research, as it may take time for preventative effects to emerge (Greenberg et al., 2001); several studies with long-term follow-up have found increases in preventative effects over time (Gillham, Shatte, & Reivich, 2001).

A second indicated preventative intervention relating to childhood anxiety has become known as the Queensland Early Intervention and Prevention of Anxiety Project (QEIP-AP; Dadds, Spence, Holland, Barrett, & Laurens, 1997). This study represented a combination of indicated prevention and early intervention, because it targeted children who were free of disorders but who exhibited anxious symptomatology (prevention indicated), as well as children who met criteria for an anxiety disorder but were in the less severe range (early intervention indicated).

Children were selected for participation in this school-based program following a four-stage screening process that incorporated children's, teachers', and parents' reports. Screening on an initial cohort of 1,786 children reduced the final sample to 128 children ages 7–14 years, who were invited to participate in the program. Students were assigned to either the intervention or the monitoring condition on the basis of the school they attended, and all participating schools were matched for size and sociodemographics.

The intervention offered was the *Coping Koala* program, a 10-session cognitive-behavioral program with demonstrated effectiveness as both an individual and a group-based intervention for the treatment of childhood anxiety disorders (Barrett, 1998; Barrett et al., 1996). The intervention, conducted by a trained clinical psychologist and cofacilitated by graduate students, assisted participants in developing and implementing their own plans for graduated exposure to fear stimuli using physiological, cognitive, and behavioral coping strategies. Three parent sessions were offered, and parents were introduced to parent management skills and were helped to apply these skills to the management of their child's anxiety.

This study is one of the few preventative interventions to examine diagnostic status as an outcome measure, and results were favorable. Immediately postintervention, the percentage of children meeting diagnostic criteria decreased for both intervention and monitoring groups, and there was no significant difference between them. However, by 6-month follow-up, 57% of monitoring participants received an anxiety disorder diagnosis, compared with 27% of intervention participants. The intervention effect remained evident in a 2-year follow-up (Dadds, Spence, Laurens, Mullins, & Barrett, 1999). However, these results collapse across pretreatment diagnostic status, and it was of interest to us to specifically examine the preventative effects.

A clear preventative effect was demonstrated when results were examined only for those participants who were diagnosis free at pretreatment. At postintervention, approximately 10% of children in both groups had developed an anxiety disorder, but a difference emerged by the 6-month follow-up, at which 54% of children in the monitoring group, compared with 16% of children in the intervention group, received an anxiety diagnosis. Unfortunately, 2-year follow-up analyses combined data across pretreatment diagnostic status, and it was not possible to examine the longer term preventative effects.

Nonetheless, these results provide encouraging support for the potential of school-based preventative interventions, and the success of this study inspired our research team to examine the utility of a universal preventative strategy. We have recently published two pilot studies examining the effectiveness of a universal school-based prevention strategy (Barrett & Turner, 2001; Lowry-Webster, Barrett, & Dadds, 2001). The aims of the first study, reported by Barrett and Turner (2001), were threefold: (1) to examine the effectiveness of a universal anxiety preventative intervention in comparison with a monitoring condition, (2) to compare the effectiveness of teachers versus clinically trained psychologists as group leaders, and (3) to examine the effectiveness of a universal preventative strategy for those children who exhibit risk for future anxiety disorders.

Participants were 489 grade 6 children ages 10–12 years. Schools, rather than individuals, were selected as the unit for random assignment, and schools were randomly assigned to one of three intervention conditions: a psychologist-led intervention, a teacher-led intervention, or a standard curriculum with monitoring. The intervention offered was the *Friends for Children* program (Barrett, Lowry-Webster, & Turner, 2000a, 2000b), a

10-session cognitive-behavioral program designed to address limitations that existed within the *Coping Koala* program. *Friends for Children*, described in detail by Barrett (1999), assists children in learning skills that help them cope with and manage anxiety. Skills taught include relaxation, cognitive restructuring, attention training, graduated exposure, and family and peer support.

The results were consistent with predictions and offered preliminary support for the effectiveness of a universal strategy. Intervention participants reported fewer symptoms of anxiety at postintervention, compared with monitoring participants. These intervention effects were demonstrated equally across both the psychologist-led and the teacher-led interventions. Most encouraging, however, were the positive effects shown for children who displayed high levels of anxious symptomatology at preintervention. In comparison with the monitoring condition, the intervention conditions resulted in a significant reduction in the number of children who reported clinical levels of anxious symptomatology at postintervention.

The second universal prevention trial conducted by our team was reported by Lowry-Webster and colleagues (2001). They report on a series of studies designed to examine the effectiveness of a teacher-training package and the subsequent effectiveness of a universal preventative intervention when implemented solely by schoolteachers. Study 1 sought to train teachers in the skills and techniques associated with the prevention of childhood anxiety and to assess whether the training was associated with increases in teachers' knowledge of and confidence about implementing a prevention program. Study 2 sought to evaluate whether teachers could successfully implement the intervention and whether the intervention was associated with a positive outcome for children.

They found that training was beneficial for teachers and that teachers who completed the training workshops reported a level of knowledge equivalent to that of psychologists who worked with children and youths. Their preliminary results for the effectiveness of the intervention mirror those from the Barrett and Turner (2001) study. That is, teachers were able to effectively implement the *Friends for Children* intervention, and the intervention had a positive impact upon children's anxious symptomatology when compared with a monitoring control condition.

Although encouraging, both of these studies are preliminary and must be interpreted cautiously. The breadth of the intervention effect is unlikely to be known until follow-up assessments are completed. Indeed, Sandler (1999) suggests that the effects of prevention programs should be judged by how well they change targeted outcomes over time, rather than in terms of immediate effects. Consequently, although the preliminary results of the reviewed studies are encouraging, the most important questions about the public health benefit of preventative interventions have yet to be answered.

THE ROLE OF RISK AND PROTECTIVE FACTORS IN PREVENTATIVE RESEARCH

One thing becomes apparent from reviewing existing anxiety prevention programs. Each of the studies identified a particular risk or protective factor (or set of factors) that the researchers sought to modify via the intervention that was offered. For example, LaFreniere and Capuano (1997) sought to modify parental behavior, because poor parent–child relationships and overcontrolling parental behavior have been documented as risk factors for childhood anxiety. Dadds and colleagues (1997), Barrett and Turner (2001), and Lowry-Webster and colleagues (2001) all sought to modify intrinsic child characteristics known to be associated with childhood anxiety. Risk factors targeted were avoidant coping and a pessimistic thinking style, whereas protective factors targeted were problem-focused coping skills and positive self-talk.

Space constraints prevent us from extensively reviewing the literature associated with the known risk factors for childhood anxiety, but let it suffice to say that there is now a considerable body of knowledge pertaining to the biological, psychological, and environmental risk factors for childhood anxiety disorders. These risk factors include anxious–resistant attachment (e.g., Warren, Huston, Egeland, & Sroufe, 1997), behavioral inhibition (e.g., Kagan & Snidman, 1991), parental anxiety (Last, Hersen, Kazdin, Francis, & Grubb, 1987; Thapar & McGuffin, 1995), parenting characteristics (e.g., Barrett, Dadds, Rapee, & Ryan, 1996; Krohne & Hock, 1991), and negative or stressful life events (e.g., Goodyer & Altham, 1991; Yule & Williams, 1990).

In comparison with risk-factor research, the search for protective factors has not been as intensive, and investigation of protective factors for childhood anxiety has been largely restricted to the areas of social support (e.g., Compas, 1987) and children's coping skills (e.g., Folkman & Lazarus, 1985). Clearly more work is needed regarding identification of protective factors. Nonetheless, if we are to effect prevention of childhood anxiety, it is essential that we use the existing knowledge base regarding risk and protective factors as the basis for designing and evaluating preventative interventions.

It is relatively easy to identify children who have experienced a trauma or an event that might place them at risk of later developing an anxiety disorder (e.g., being witness to a natural disaster). However, proactive prevention of anxiety disorders will require researchers and clinicians to accurately and reliably detect risk factors such as behavioral inhibition and anxious–resistant attachment and parenting characteristics such as overcontrol (Spence, 2001). Once these factors are identified, effective methods must be made available to bring about lasting change within them.

SOME PRACTICAL CONSIDERATIONS

Whether we are designing a new program or planning the implementation of an existing preventative intervention, we need to consider some of the practicalities and the potential advantages or disadvantages associated with the different prevention approaches. Because universal strategies, by definition, target an entire population, there are a number of potential difficulties. First are the large sample sizes and the long-term follow-up that is required to discern differences between groups. These necessarily require substantial funding and resources, which are typically difficult to obtain and highly competitive. A second potential difficulty is gaining access to entire populations of children and youths. Schools have been identified as one potential access point; however, utilizing school systems is often a complex process that requires ongoing support from educational authorities, school principals, teaching and administrative staff, and parents and students. The benefits of a school-based intervention must be highly valued by these consumers if long-term follow-up is involved and if one identified goal is the ongoing implementation of a universal intervention (e.g., an anxiety prevention program included in the classroom curriculum).

A third potential disadvantage is the relatively low dose effect that a universal strategy may offer and whether this would be sufficient exposure (in duration or intensity) to alter the developmental pathways of children already at risk for anxiety. And a final and related point that could be argued is that much of the effort in implementing a universal strategy would be spent on children who would not develop an anxiety disorder anyway.

Universal strategies do, however, offer a number of significant advantages. Evidence to date suggests that children do receive sufficient exposure to a universal intervention, at least enough exposure to provide a short-term positive impact (e.g., Barrett & Turner, 2001; Lowry-Webster et al., 2001). Second, arguing that considerable resources may be spent on children who are at low risk of developing a disorder is an argument more applicable to types of psychopathology with a very low prevalence in the general population (e.g., schizophrenia). However, universal strategies have the potential to be of enormous benefit in terms of reducing the prevalence of childhood anxiety, as anxiety disorders are one of the most prevalent forms of psychopathology in children and youths. Furthermore, given that all children are targeted, those who do need assistance to overcome anxiety problems but who might never come to the attention of a mental health professional are nonetheless engaged in a program of change.

A universal strategy avoids the need for screening and "identifying" children who are at risk and, therefore, avoids any potentially negative effects of labeling or falsely identifying children who in reality do not exhibit any risk signs. As comorbidity between childhood mental health disorders is high and risk and protective factors can be common to many disorders, a single universal preventative intervention has the potential to affect multiple problems (Greenberg et al., 2001). And finally, the value of promoting competence and positive mental health cannot be overlooked. The acquisition of resilience skills is useful even for children and parents who are not at risk, as they may be successfully employed in a number of everyday occurrences (Greenberg et al., 2001; Shure, 2001).

To date, there have been no published accounts of selective interventions for the prevention of childhood anxiety disorders. A number of studies have documented changes in anxious symptomatology as one of several outcome measures resulting from programs designed to counter general psychosocial risk factors. For example, selective preventative interventions have been offered to children experiencing parental divorce (e.g., Pedro-Carroll & Cowen, 1985) and children making the transition from primary to secondary school (e.g., Felner & Adan, 1988). Although a review of these programs is beyond the scope of this chapter, they do highlight some of the costs and benefits involved in employing selective prevention strategies, and many of the costs and benefits associated with selective strategies can be equally applied to indicated strategies.

When compared with universal strategies, selective or indicated prevention strategies are likely to be more attractive to funding bodies because they are able to demonstrate and calculate cost, time, and labor efficiency (Donovan & Spence, 2000). There are, however, issues related to the identification or selection of children that must be addressed. As selective strategies target children at risk of disorder, the identification of risk and protective factors must first be addressed. Valid, reliable, and cheap methods of screening for risk factors (e.g., parental overcontrol, behavioral inhibition) must be found.

Indicated prevention screens children on the basis of symptoms rather than risk factors. A number of valid and reliable questionnaires and interview schedules with sound psychometric properties allow for the accurate assessment of anxious symptomatology in children and youths (e.g., Spence Children's Anxiety Scale, Spence, 1997; Anxiety Disorders Interview Schedule for Children (ADIS-IV-C), Silverman & Albano, 1997). However, when and how often children should be assessed for anxiety symptoms becomes critical. If subclinical symptomatology is indicative of the development of later disorder, timing the assessment and the indicated program to ensure that it is implemented prior to the onset of a clinical disorder is likely to require some skill. Furthermore, implementation of selective and indicated programs requires the consent and motivation of schools, parents and caregivers, and children themselves to withdraw from other activities and become involved in a preventative intervention.

METHODOLOGICAL ISSUES

The science of prevention is clearly in its infancy. Much of the published research relating to the effectiveness of preventative interventions is limited by methodological problems. Methodological issues include the use of small, nonrepresentative samples, the lack of appropriate comparison groups, inadequate measures of central constructs, a limited breadth of measurement, reliance on self-report measures to provide data on multiple variables, low recruitment rates, high attrition rates, and relatively short follow-up periods. Within the area of childhood anxiety prevention, the work of Dadds and colleagues (1997; Dadds et al., 1999) is a notable exception, and this study provides evidence that preventative interventions can be based on sound conceptual and empirical foundations, with rigorous design and evaluation strategies.

Rather than dwell on the limitations of the published research, we review the Institute of Medicine's Committee on Prevention of Mental Disorders criteria for designing and reporting methodologically sound interventions (Mrazek & Haggerty, 1994, pp. 217–222). The first criterion pertains to the risk and protective factors that are purported to be addressed by the research. These factors are required to be well documented and specifically related to the developmental tasks of the target population. The second criterion is a clear description of the targeted or experimental group, the control group, the recruitment and consent process, and the prevention technology that is employed. The third criterion is a description of the intervention itself. All too often, treatment and preventative interventions lack adequate description, sometimes due to restrictions imposed by journal publication formats; in other cases, it is simply missing information that impedes appropriate evaluation and replication. (See Mrazek & Haggerty, 1994, for the elements that each program description should include.)

The fourth criterion addressed is a description of the research methodology. Mrazek and Haggerty (1994) suggest that the ideal research design in a prevention trial is a randomized, controlled trial of adequate sample size embedded in a longitudinal design. However, they concede that a variety of other designs, such as pre- and posttest comparisons, are often employed and may be necessary for large-scale community interventions. Details of the research design should include an appropriate description and use of statistical methods. The researchers caution that it is frequently necessary to confirm that randomized assignment has had its intended effects by comparing experimental and control groups on sociodemographic characteristics and on other relevant characteristics in addition to outcome. Furthermore, they add that designs that employ baseline measures are highly desirable because variables that frequently appear extraneous have the potential to be significant.

The fifth criterion comprises details concerning the implementation of the project. For example, how well were the intended objectives and processes of the intervention actually implemented? Finally, there ought to be a description of the outcomes. Most fundamentally, evidence should be provided that risk and protective factors have been changed and that the intervention was successful. Other obvious sources of evidence for a preventative intervention would be an actual reduction in the observed rate of new cases of a disorder or the delayed onset of a disorder in the experimental group.

Methodological issues in clinical research are so important that the American Psychological Society established a task force, led by Richard Price, to develop a set of criteria to guide the development and evaluation of effective preventative programs (Price, Cowen, Lorion, & Ramos-McKay, 1989). Many of the criteria correspond to those listed previously, however, additional inclusions are (1) a statement of the rationale for the intervention, (2) a description of how the program relates to community groups, (3) the transferability of the intervention to other settings, and (4) the roles of professionals and paraprofessionals in providing caregiver resources.

The final comment we make concerning methodology is that the quality of measures is of utmost importance in evaluating programs and being able to compare evaluations with existing data. It is beneficial when researchers use similar, well-established measures to facilitate comparison of findings.

FUTURE DIRECTIONS

Our research team has recently initiated a large-scale universal preventative intervention for child and youth anxiety within Queensland, Australia. In doing so, we have tried to design a study that will stand up to the rigorous methodological requirements of scientific research, yet at the same time provide the local community with a valuable and sustainable program that will provide children and youths with life skills that will promote resilience and prevent the onset of anxiety disorders, both now and in the longer term. We outline this study here as an example of how the Institute of Medicine's (Mrazek & Haggerty, 1994) methodological recommendations can be operationalized in community-based preventative research.

As a result of the successful pilot studies we conducted utilizing a universal strategy within schools (Barrett & Turner, 2001; Lowry-Webster et al., 2001), we expanded this design to include secondary, as well as primary, schools and to examine the question of which developmental stage (late childhood or early adolescence) offers the best window of opportunity for anxiety prevention. The intervention offered was the *Friends* program (Barrett et al., 2000a, 2000b), as this intervention is based on sound theoretical principles relating to the treatment and prevention of childhood anxiety. The program, reviewed previously, seeks to address many of the intrinsic child characteristics that are known to be risk factors for anxiety disorders (e.g., lack of personal problem-solving and coping skills, lack of social support systems, and negative interpretations of everyday situations).

Participants were grade 6 or grade 9 students within one of seven coeducational schools extending from preschool through grade 12. Schools, rather than participants, were randomly assigned to either an intervention or a monitoring control condition, and consent was sought from the local educational authorities, the school principals and teachers, and from parents and students themselves. Measures of school environment were completed by teachers at all participating schools in an effort to ensure that the school systems were not vastly different from one another. Students, parents, and teachers were asked to complete questionnaire assessments, in a pre- and posttest design, with follow-up periods scheduled to fall at 12, 24, and 36 months following the intervention. Analyses of initial results are currently underway and will be reported in the literature once complete.

We present this project outline specifically to highlight the difficulties associated with utilizing methodological recommendations in applied scientific research. Some compromises were required. For example, it was considered desirable to complete diagnostic interviews for all participants, so that we could accurately determine whether we could prevent the onset of new cases of anxiety disorder. However, a compromise had to be made between methodological rigor and available resources, and diagnostic interviews were therefore completed only for those participants who scored above a predetermined cutoff score on a self-report anxiety measure. The use of teacher report forms is another example of compromise. Ideally, a multi-informant strategy is used in childhood research. However, because a universal approach was adopted and a large sample was recruited, teachers were being asked to complete large numbers of questionnaires. Many felt that they did not have the time or the knowledge of individual students to complete the forms accurately and carefully. Therefore, in an effort to maintain the cooperation and motivation of teachers, we made a decision not to include teacher report forms.

These compromises clearly deviate from an ideal and rigorous methodological design. However, the sacrifices were made because of the perceived value of the research to the community and to the scientific literature. Although we attempted to operationalize all of the methodological guidelines that have been established for prevention research, we found this an impossible goal. Decisions to lower our methodological standards were made along the way. Nonetheless, it is anticipated that our study will significantly contribute to the field of anxiety prevention, and perhaps by highlighting some of the difficulties that we have encountered, others will be able to plan ahead and develop strategies that will overcome these difficulties and substantially build on our research. Other prevention researchers are similarly encouraged to report programs that have been shown not to work and methodologies that were too difficult to achieve.

SUMMARY AND CONCLUDING REMARKS

The significant advances that have been made in the field of mental health prevention have resulted in governments around the world prioritizing prevention initiatives. To date, however, there has been limited research in the area of childhood anxiety prevention. We are hopeful that this will change, given the increase in the number of psychological academic journal articles related to anxiety prevention and to the inclusion of chapters such as this one in childhood anxiety texts.

This chapter has presented a clear rationale for pursuing the prevention of childhood anxiety disorders and has reviewed four published studies that have addressed the question of anxiety prevention in children. Of these studies, one indicated preventative intervention sought to address parental factors involved in the etiology of anxiety disorder (Lafreniere & Capuano, 1997), whereas the other three sought to modify intrinsic child characteristics. All demonstrated some success, although only one of the studies to date has included a long-term follow-up period and has demonstrated a positive impact on the later development of anxiety disorder (Dadds et al., 1997, 1999). Nonetheless, all studies have clearly acknowledged the important role of risk and protective factors in preventative research, and all have clearly articulated the factors that were targeted in their programs.

The field of prevention science has developed significantly in the past 10 years, and there are now established approaches to prevention, with a common dialogue among prevention researchers. This has allowed researchers to share some of the difficulties they have found with implementing preventative interventions, as well as some of the significant advantages to each of the prevention approaches. Prevention programs are now truly focused on intervening prior to the onset of disorder, and researchers are beginning to move beyond the question, Does prevention work? to address questions such as, What preventative approaches will work best and for whom?

The area of childhood anxiety prevention is in its infancy. However, the small amount of evidence available paints an optimistic picture regarding the effectiveness of preventative interventions for child anxiety disorders. We are now beginning to build a substantial knowledge base regarding risk and protective factors and the complex interplay between biological, psychological, and environmental factors. Furthermore, models exist for designing preventative interventions, based on the target population, the available resources, and the methodological designs. Large-scale studies, which assess the long-term impact of preventative interventions, in comparison with no intervention and placebo approaches, are now needed. Reliable and valid outcome measures of maladaptive fears and anxiety problems should be included, in addition to a broader range of outcomes, which involve information from a variety of sources (e.g., child, parent, and clinician) across a range of settings (e.g., home and school). Furthermore, follow-ups should be of adequate duration to permit evaluation of the long-term impact of any preventative intervention.

We can draw on the experiences and recommendations of prevention scientists to assist in establishing sustainable, cost-effective anxiety prevention programs. Recommendations (summarized by Greenberg et al., 2001) include recognizing the need for multiyear programs integrated into existing networks, communities, and systems of treatment that focus on changing institutions and environments, as well as individuals.

REFERENCES

Barrett, P. M. (1998). Evaluation of cognitive-behavioral group treatments for childhood anxiety disorders. *Journal of Clinical Child Psychology, 27,* 459–468.

Barrett, P. M. (1999). Interventions for child and youth anxiety disorders: Involving parents, teachers, and peers. *Australian Educational and Developmental Psychologist, 16,* 5–24.

Barrett, P. M., Dadds, M. R., & Rapee, R. (1996). Family treatment of childhood anxiety: A controlled trial. *Journal of Consulting and Clinical Psychology, 64,* 333–342.

Barrett, P. M., Dadds, M. R., Rapee, R., & Ryan, S. (1996). Family enhancement of cognitive style in anxious and aggressive children. *Journal of Abnormal Child Psychology, 24,* 187–203.

Barrett, P. M., Lowry-Webster, H., & Turner, C. M. (2000a). *Friends for Children group leader manual.* Brisbane, Australia: Australian Academic Press.

Barrett, P. M., Lowry-Webster, H., & Turner, C. M. (2000b). *Friends for Children participant workbook.* Brisbane, Australia: Australian Academic Press.

Barrett, P. M., & Turner, C. M. (2001). Prevention of anxiety symptoms in primary school children: Preliminary results from a universal school-based trial. *British Journal of Clinical Psychology, 40,* 399–410.

Caplan, G. (1964). *Principles of preventive psychiatry.* New York: Basic Books.

Compas, B. (1987). Coping with stress during childhood and adolescence. *Psychological Bulletin, 101,* 393–410.

Dadds, M. R., Spence, S. H., Holland, D., Barrett, P. M., & Laurens, K. . (1997). Prevention and early intervention for anxiety disorders: A controlled trial. *Journal of Consulting and Clinical Psychology, 65,* 627–635.

Dadds, M. R., Spence, S. H., Laurens, K., Mullins, M., & Barrett, P. M. (1999). Early intervention and prevention of anxiety disorders in children: Results at a 2-year follow-up. *Journal of Consulting and Clinical Psychology, 67,* 145–150.

Donovan, C. L., & Spence, S. H. (2000). Prevention of childhood anxiety disorders. *Clinical Psychology Review, 20,* 509–531.

Felner, R. D., & Adan, A. M. (1988). The School Transition Environment Project: An ecological intervention and evaluation. In R. H. Price, E. L. Cowen, R. P. Lorion, & J. Ramos-McKay (Eds.), *Fourteen ounces of prevention: A casebook for practitioners* (pp. 111–122). Washington, DC: American Psychological Association.

Folkman, S., & Lazarus, R. S. (1985). If it changes it must be a process: Study of emotion and coping during three stages of a college examination. *Journal of Personality and Social Psychology, 48,* 150–170.

Gillham, J. E., Shatte, A. J., & Reivich, K. (2001). Needed for prevention research: Long-term follow-up and the evaluation of mediators, moderators, and lay providers. *Prevention and Treatment, 4.*

Goodyer, I. M., & Altham, P. M. (1991). Lifetime exit events and recent social and family adversities in anxious and depressed school-aged children. *Journal of Affective Disorders, 21,* 219–228.

Gordon, R. (1987). An operational classification of disease prevention. In J. A. Steinberg & M. M. Silverman (Eds.), *Preventing mental disorders* (pp. 20–26). Rockville, MD: Department of Health and Human Services.

Greenberg, M. A., Domitrovich, C., & Bumbarger, B. (2001). The prevention of mental disorders in school-aged children: Current state of the field. *Prevention and Treatment, 4.*

Kagan, J., & Snidman, N. (1991). Infant predictors of inhibited and uninhibited profiles. *Psychological Science, 2,* 40–43.

Kendall, P. C. (1994). Treatment of anxiety disorders in children: A randomized clinical trial. *Journal of Consulting and Clinical Psychology, 62,* 100–110.

Krohne, H. W., & Hock, M. (1991). Relationships between restrictive mother–child interactions and anxiety of the child. *Anxiety Research, 4,* 109–124.

LaFreniere, P. J., & Capuano, F. (1997). Preventive intervention as a means of clarifying direction of effects in socialization: Anxious–withdrawn preschoolers case. *Development and Psychopathology, 9,* 551–564.

Last, C. G., Hersen, M., Kazdin, A. E., Francis, G., & Grubb, H. J. (1987). Psychiatric illness in the mothers of anxious children. *American Journal of Psychiatry, 144,* 1580–1583.

Lowry-Webster, H., Barrett, P. M., & Dadds, M. R. (2001). A universal prevention trial of anxiety and depressive symptomatology in childhood: Preliminary data from an Australian study. *Behaviour Change, 18,* 36–50.

Mrazek, P. J., & Haggerty, R. J. (1994). *Reducing risks for mental disorders: Frontiers for preventive intervention research.* Washington, DC: National Academy Press.

Pedro-Carroll, J. L., & Cowen, E. L. (1985). The Children of Divorce Intervention Project: An investigation of the efficacy of a school-based prevention program. *Journal of Consulting and Clinical Psychology, 53,* 603–611.

Price, R. H., Cowen, H. L., Lorion, R. P., & Ramos-McKay, J. (1989). The search for effective prevention programs: What we learned along the way. *American Journal of Orthopsychiatry, 59,* 49–58.

Sandler, I. (1999). Progress in developing strategies and theory for the prevention and treatment of anxiety and depression. *Prevention and Treatment, 2.*

Silverman, W. K., & Albano, A. M. (1997). *Anxiety Disorders Interview Schedule for DSM-IV: Child Version.* San Antonio, TX: Graywing.

Silverman, W. K., & Kurtines, W. M. (1999). Short-term treatment for children with phobic and anxiety problems: A pragmatic view. *Crisis Intervention and Time Limited Treatment, 5,* 119–131.

Shure, M. B. (2001). What's right with prevention? Commentary on "Prevention of mental disorders in school-aged children: Current state of the field." *Prevention and Treatment, 4.*

Spence, S. H. (1996). A case for prevention. In P. Cotton & H. Jackson (Eds.), *Early intervention and prevention in mental health* (pp. 87–107). Melbourne, Australia: Australian Psychological Society.

Spence, S. H. (1997). Structure of anxiety symptoms in children: A confirmatory factor-analytic study. *Journal of Abnormal Psychology, 106,* 280–297

Spence, S. H. (2001). Prevention strategies. In M. W. Vasey & M. R. Dadds (Eds.), The developmental psychopathology of anxiety (pp. 325–351). New York: Oxford University Press.

Spence, S. H., & Dadds, M. R. (1996). Preventing childhood anxiety disorders. *Behaviour Change, 13,* 241–249.

Thapar, A., & McGuffin, P. (1995). Are anxiety symptoms in childhood heritable? *Journal of Child Psychology and Psychiatry, 36,* 439–447.

Tuma, J. M. (1989). Mental health services for children: The state of the art. *American Psychologist, 44,* 188–199.

Warren, S. L., Huston, L., Egeland, B., & Sroufe, L. A. (1997). Child and adolescent anxiety disorders and early attachment. *Journal of the American Academy of Child and Adolescent Psychiatry, 36,* 637–644.

Yule, W., & Williams, R. (1990). Post-traumatic stress reactions in children. *Journal of Traumatic Stress, 3,* 279–295.

Zubrick, S. R., Silburn, S. R., Teoh, H. J., Carlton, J., Shepherd, C., & Lawrence, D. (1997). *Western Australian child health survey: Education, health and competency.* Perth, Australia: Australian Bureau of Statistics.

Index